Dying
in the
Human
Life
Cycle

Dying in the Human Life Cycle

Psychological, Biomedical, and Social Perspectives

Walter J. Smith, S. J.

Fairfield University

Holt, Rinehart and Winston

New York ■ Chicago ■ San Francisco ■ Philadelphia ■ Montreal ■ Toronto

London ■ Sydney ■ Tokyo ■ Mexico City ■ Rio de Janeiro ■ Madrid

Publisher: Robert L. Woodbury
Acquisitions Editor: Susan Meyers
Project Editor: Maruta Mitchell
Production Manager: Robin B. Besofsky
Text Design: Gloria Gentile
Cover Design: Gloria Gentile

Library of Congress Cataloging in Publication Data

Smith, Walter J.
    Dying in the human life cycle.

    Bibliography: p.
    Includes index.   1. Death—Psychological aspects. 2. Bereavement—
Psychological aspects. 3. Terminal care. 4. Hospice care. 5. Death. I. Title.
BF789.D4S65   1985   155.9′37   85-5459

ISBN 0-03-071742-6

CBS COLLEGE PUBLISHING
Holt, Rinehart and Winston
The Dryden Press
Saunders College Publishing

For my parents, Walter and Mary Smith,
who first helped me to appreciate life.

To the Society of Jesus, which has nurtured, encouraged,
and supported me as I have tried to understand and
help those who are dying.

Preface

Without any strategic plan, my own education and professional growth provided me with a rich exposure to the human life cycle and led over many years to the writing of this book. My career as a psychologist evolved naturally from earlier academic preparation in philosophy, theology, language, and literature. As a high school foreign language teacher, I sought to understand the developmental crises of my adolescent students. Working with these students brought me into closer contact with their parents and the struggles they were facing in their marriages and careers.

The desire to provide better counsel to my students and their parents led me to enroll in a number of summer graduate courses in psychology. However, these courses and the psychologists who taught them whetted my appetite for the discipline and opened the doors to many new experiences. A predoctoral internship in a child guidance clinic in Cambridge, Massachusetts, introduced me to a broad range of developmental issues, including childhood grief and bereavement, adolescent depression, and suicide. Reaching to the other end of the age spectrum, my dissertation research investigated aging effects among widows. In the course of this research I intensively interviewed more than 100 widows, ranging from 30 to 90 years of age. As a staff psychologist in a community mental health center and a community hospital, I continued to encounter a broad range of developmental issues faced by adults.

The past ten years, which I have spent in teaching undergraduate courses in human development and the psychology of death and dying, have provided a unique opportunity to reflect upon and integrate many of these previous experiences. This book is the product of those reflections.

Dying in the Human Life Cycle: Psychological, Biomedical, and Social Perspectives places death in its proper context. Death is a *life-cycle* concern, not something relegated to the eighth and ninth decades of a human life. This book presents death and dying as essentially rooted in the dynamics of the human life cycle. In organizing the text, I have endeavored to choose topics that provide important information about and insight into specific developmental periods of the life cycle.

I hope that as an educational tool, this book will prove *formative* as well as *informative* for readers at various stages of their own personal growth and development. Undergraduate students in nursing, premedical curricula, psychology, and sociology will find the material indispensable to their professional growth. The book can serve medical schools in their desire to integrate a comprehensive study of death and dying into their curricula. Finally, this book may help those health care professionals who desire to deepen their understanding and appreciation of death, the dying, and the bereaved throughout the course of life.

The use of the word *dying* in the title of this text emphasizes process: I have consistently focused on how research and theory translates into effective care of dying persons and those family members who survive them. In doing so, I have relied heavily upon case study material. Most of the cases reported in the various chapters are gleaned from my own clinical and pastoral experiences. The rest have been taken from published reports. In many of these, details have been altered to preserve the privacy of the individuals and families involved. Each of the cases is intended to exemplify, clarify, and reinforce important developmental issues. Actual cases help us to see how psychological, biomedical, and social research can influence practice in significant ways. They provide a springboard for considering strategies of intervention with persons in similar circumstances. They vividly remind us that caring for dying and bereaved persons is a profoundly human engagement.

The presentation of the book follows a chronological as well as topical plan. Beginning with a discussion of prenatal, perinatal, and neonatal issues, we then consider a topic receiving much popular attention, Sudden Infant Death Syndrome. Because many people assume that young children cannot understand death, they easily dismiss the notion that children grieve. Childhood bereavement is a fascinating topic and an important clinical issue. The final chapter in the childhood section considers how children and adolescents face life-threatening and possibly terminal illnesses. The specific focus of this chapter is leukemia, its diagnosis and treatment.

Suicide is a national problem. Particularly disturbing are the increasing numbers of teenagers and young adults who take their own lives. The high incidence of fatal heart attacks among middle-aged and older adults poses another concern of national scope which implicates the stressful lifestyle of many Americans. Major burns and multiple-trauma accidents likewise threaten many people and throw victims and families into crisis situations. Each of these major issues receives close attention in this book.

The word *cancer* for many people means death. Although significant advances have been made in the diagnosis and treatment of neoplasms, many people die each year of cancer. The psychological aspects of the disease are interesting and important. Hospice care makes use of current data and new insights in attempting to provide effective holistic assistance to terminally ill persons and their families. The concept of palliative care exemplified by the hospices is finding many creative applications today in American medicine and nursing.

The text concludes with a focus on older persons in the final stage of the life cycle. In addition to a treatment of some psychological issues related to death and the elderly, a brief introduction to the ethical issues involved in the euthanasia debate is provided.

As a scientist, I value methodology and research. As a clinician, I have a keen investment and natural attraction for application and practice. I have attempted throughout the book to strike a balance between these competing objectives. Each of the chapters presents the relevant dimensions of psychological, biomedical, and social theory and research. To complement this, some clinical applications are suggested. However, though I have tried to maintain balance in the theory-and-research versus application equation, my own clinical bias will be evident. Further, I have consistently stressed a humanistic approach to death, dying persons, and bereaved families, believing strongly that it is on the basis of what comprises optimal holistic care for dying persons that contemporary medical and psychiatric practice must ultimately be judged.

I am deeply indebted to the many colleagues in the international community of scholars, whose works are cited in the extensive bibliography which follows the text of the book. In particular, I wish to thank a number of distinguished professionals who enabled me to gain valuable first-hand experience in their institutions, who read earlier drafts of the manuscript, and offered useful suggestions for revision, or who provided counsel and guidance in research. Among these people I would like to recognize: Dr. Alan L. Berman, Professor of Psychology, American University, Washington, D.C., and President of the American Association of Suicidology; Dr. Stanley J. Berman, Staff Clinical Psychologist, Dana-Farber Cancer Institute, Boston, Massachusetts; Dr. Norman R. Bernstein, Professor of Psychiatry, University of Illinois Medical Center; Dr. Robert Blauner, Department of Sociology, University of California, Berkeley, California; Dr. T. L. Brink, Department of Psychology, College of Notre Dame, Belmont, California; Sue S. Cahners, Chief, Department of Social Work, Shriners Hospital for Crippled Children, Burns Institute, Boston, Massachusetts; Dr. Paula J. Clayton, Professor and Chair, Department of Psychiatry, University Hospitals, University of Minnesota, Minneapolis, Minnesota; Dr. John D. DeFrain, Professor, Department of Human Development and Family, University of Nebraska, Lincoln, Nebraska; Dr. Holcombe Grier, Pediatric Oncologist, Children's Hospital, Boston, Massachusetts; Dr. Elaine E. Holder, Department of Psychology and Human Development, California Polytechnic State University, San Luis Obispo, California; Dr. Charles W. Johnson, Department of Psychology, University of Evansville, Indiana; Dr. Emanuel Lewis, Consultant Psychiatrist, Tavistock Clinic, London; Dr. Robert MacAleese, Chair, Department of Psychology, Spring Hill College, Mobile, Alabama; Dr. Matilda S. McIntire, Professor of Pediatrics and Director of Ambulatory Pediatrics, Department of Pediatrics, Creighton University School of Medicine, Omaha, Nebraska; Dr. Richard L. Naeye, Professor and Chairman, Department of Pathology, Milton S. Hershey Medical Center, Pennsylvania State University, Hershey, Pennsylvania; Dr. Carol Nowak, University of Buffalo, Center for the Study of Aging, Buffalo, New York; Dr. Colin Murray Parkes, Professor of Psychiatry, London Hospital Medical College, University of London; Dorothy Patton, Head, Pediatric Oncology Nursing, Children's Hospital, Boston, Massachusetts; Dr. David J. C.

Read, Associate Professor of Physiology, Department of Physiology, University of Sydney, Sydney, Australia; Dame Cicely Saunders, Medical Director, Saint Christopher's Hospice, Sydenham, England; Dr. Sara Taubin, Department of Human Behavior and Development, Drexel University, Philadelphia, Pennsylvania; Dr. James M. Toolan, Psychiatrist (private practice), Old Bennington, Vermont; Dr. R. G. Twycross, Consultant Physician, Sir Michael Sobell House, Churchill Hospital, Oxford, England; and Dr. Sylvia Zaki, Director of Nursing, Medical Center–General Hospital, Cranston, Rhode Island.

I would also like to express my appreciation to Fairfield University and the Fairfield University Jesuit Community for the support they provided me during the preparation of this book. I would be remiss if I did not single out the special assistance I received from Joan Overfield, Nancy Haag, and so many other members of the Nyselius Library staff. Without their patient and friendly support, it is unlikely that this project could have been completed. My work-study student assistant, Maryellyn Haffner, was an invaluable aide. Her organizational and secretarial skills greatly facilitated my work. My colleagues in the Psychology Department assumed additional burdens so that I could benefit from a sabbatical leave to visit a number of clinical training centers in the United States and Europe and pursue the research and writing of this text. Finally, I wish to thank the undergraduate students enrolled in my Psychology of Death and Dying course in the spring term of 1984 who studied the manuscript edition of this book. Their many constructive suggestions have helped to guide its revision.

The editors at Holt, Rinehart and Winston have been a constant source of support and guidance through the various stages of production. The book has been the responsibility of two acquisition editors, Nedah Abbott and Susan Meyers. Maruta Mitchell, project editor, has coordinated each of the tasks of editing, design, and production with gentleness, understanding, and extraordinary patience. Her burdens were lightened by the able assistance of Robin Besofsky, production manager. The author is particularly indebted to Laurie Root, copy editor, whose careful work on the manuscript has improved it significantly.

There is as much diversity in the philosophies and theories of death as there is in the ways we actually attempt to care for the dying. In surveying some of the important moments in the life cycle when death intrudes upon human beings, we come to appreciate the significance and value of these varied theoretical and clinical approaches. However, their greatest value is apparent when they allow deeper insight and help provide more effective assistance to those who face life-threatening or terminal situations. My deepest gratitude is therefore expressed to the many individuals and families who have allowed me to be part of their living and part of their dying. More than anyone else, these people have contributed to this book.

Walter J. Smith, S. J.
Fairfield University
Department of Psychology

Contents

Preface   vii

1   **Stillbirth and Perinatal Death**   1

Introductory Remarks   2
Experiencing Stillbirth and Perinatal Death   2
- Inadequate recognition of actual loss   5
- Doctor-patient relationship in fetal death encounters   7

Effective Management of Grieving Parents   9
- Establishing the personal identity of the infant   9
  - Naming the child   10
  - Seeing the baby   11
- Photographing the deceased infant   13
  - Funeral arrangements   13

Psychiatric Sequelae to Stillbirth and Perinatal Death   14
- Parental grief   15
- Replacement pregnancy   16
- Reactions of other children   17
- Stress in marital relationship   18

Related Issues of Special Concern   19
- Prenatal preparation for possibility of child loss   20
- Newborns with major congenital malformations   21
  - Loss by adoption   22

Summary   22

2   **Sudden Infant Death Syndrome**   25

Clinical Description of the Syndrome   27
- General descriptive features   27
  - Gross examination   28
- Microscopic examination   28

Epidemiology of Sudden Infant Death Syndrome   29
- Age distribution   29
- Medical, familial, socioeconomic, and climatic variables   29

xi

Theoretical Approaches to Sudden Infant Death Syndrome   31
              ■ Apnea theory   31
         ■ Psychophysiological theories   33

Psychological Issues for Families of SIDS Victims   35
         ■ Initial impact of discovery of a dead infant   36
         ■ Concern for other children in the family   40
              ■ Impact on marital relationship   41
                   ■ Replacement child   43
         ■ Population at special risk: the single parent   45

                   Summary   45

         ③   **Childhood Bereavement   50**

         Children and the Experience of Death   51
         Children's Understanding of Death   52
              ■ Piagetian developmental phases   52
    ■ Maria Nagy and the child's conceptual awareness of death   53
              ■ Recent research and theories   54

                   Children's Fear of Death   56
                   Grief and Mourning   58
         Adjustment to Parental Death in Childhood   61
              ■ Analytic theories of childhood mourning   61
    ■ Surviving parental efforts to protect child from reality of death   62
              ■ Children's guilt reactions   64

         Traumatic Aspects of Parental Death   66
              ■ Variability and extent of trauma   66
         ■ Psychological outcome of childhood trauma   69
    ■ Normal responses of children to trauma of parental death   70

              Therapeutic Considerations   71
                   Summary   73

         ④   **Childhood and Adolescent Cancer   76**

              Overview   77
    Acute Lymphocytic Leukemia: The Disease and its Treatment   78
              ■ Description of the disease   78
         ■ The diagnosis of leukemia: first-stage treatment   79
         ■ Neurological complications of chemotherapy   81
    ■ Central nervous system irradiation: second-stage treatment   82
         ■ Maintenance modalities: third-stage treatment   82

Psychological Issues in the Care and Management of Pediatric Cancer Patients 83

- Loss of control 83
- Separation 85
- Therapeutic aspects of play activities 86
- Normalization of hospital life 88
- Primary nursing care 89
- Hypnosis and relaxation techniques 89
- Children as mutual resources 90
- Reentry to home and school 91

**Relapse and the Problem of Terminal Diagnosis 92
Anticipatory Grief and Death 96
Summary 98**

5 **Suicide in Adolescence and Young Adulthood 101**

**Some Demographic and Statistical Data 102
Etiology of Adolescent Suicide 104**

- Genetic predispositions 104
- Biochemical factors 104
- Emotional disorders 105
- Familial and sociocultural determinants 110

Suicidal Behaviors 112

- Intentional suicidal behaviors 113
- Marginally intentional suicidal behaviors 115
- Accidents raising the suspicion of suicidal intent 116

Diagnostic and Treatment Issues 116

- Recognition and identification of symptoms 117
- Hospitalization 117
- Psychotherapy 119
- Psychopharmacological treatment 120

Prevention of suicide 121

- Primary prevention 121
- Secondary prevention 123
- Tertiary prevention 123

Summary 124

6 **Catastrophic Life-threatening Events in Adulthood 129**

**Myocardial Infarction and Sudden Death, Burns and Lethal Thermal Injuries, Multiple-trauma Accidents 130
Coronary Heart Disease 131**

■ Psychological prodromata of myocardial infarction   131
■ Physical activity and coronary heart mortality   132
■ Richter's paradigmatic research on hopelessness and sudden death   134
■ Human physiology and sudden death   135
■ The psychological problems of hospitalization and convalescence   138
■ The coital coronary   139
■ Intervention with the family survivors of cardiac death   140

Life-threatening Thermal Injuries   143
■ Life-death choices   143
■ Prediction of burn mortality   144
■ Postburn adjustment and adaptation   145
■ Disfigurement and "social death"   147
■ Effective coping strategies   148
■ Special needs of burned children, adolescents, and their parents   149
■ Geriatric thermal injury   151
■ Burn death   152

Multiple-trauma Injuries   153
■ The nature of "critical care"   153
■ Anxieties concerning survival and recovery   155
■ Psychological dynamics of coping   156

Summary   160

7   **Conjugal Bereavement   165**

Introduction   166
Psychodynamics of Grief and Mourning   166
■ Pathological grief   167
■ Early analytic formulations   167

Contemporary Approaches to the Process of Normal Grieving   170
Anticipatory Grief   175
■ Freudian thought on anticipatory grief   175
■ Neoanalytic formulations of anticipatory grief   176
■ Sociopsychological and sociocultural aspects of anticipatory grieving   177
■ Assessment of the preventive value of anticipatory grief   178

Sequelae of Conjugal Bereavement   181
■ Physical and psychological morbidity during bereavement   181
■ Psychiatric morbidity during bereavement   183
■ Vulnerability to suicide   185
■ Mortality patterns among the bereaved   185
■ Epidemiological conclusions   186

Clinical Management of the Bereaved   187

- Age as a factor of adjustment   187
- Health care management of the bereaved   191

Summary   192

⑧   **Psychological Aspects of Cancer   196**

Brief Historical Overview and Introduction   197
Psychological Factors in Cancer Etiology   198
- Personality traits   200
- Some specific psychosocial predictors of cancer   201
- Psychophysiological mechanisms   202

Communication   203
- The patient's desire to know and the physician's willingness to tell   205
- Informed consent and communication patterns   207
- Special problems encountered in communicating with cancer patients   209

Iatrogenic Stresses   210
Defense Mechanisms and Coping Behavior   212
- The crisis of diagnosis   213
- The crisis of treatment   216
- Sexuality, sexual functioning, and self-esteem   221

Summary   225

⑨   **Hospice Terminal Care   229**

Introduction: the Hospice Concept   230
The Management of Terminal Disease   232
- Palliative vs. curative care   232
- The polypharmacology of hospice care   233
- Related physical, psychological and spiritual concerns of the terminally ill   238

Flexible Approaches to the Terminally Ill   243
- The psychosocial needs of the dying person   243
- Family members: primary hospice workers in a home care setting   245
- Continuity of care: the inpatient hospice   246

Hospice Bereavement Services   248
- Initial viewing of the body after death   248
- Funeral rites   249
- Contacts with surviving family members   250

Closure to Hospice Care   251
Summary   252

10   The Elderly and Death   255

Introduction   256

Some Dimensions of Death in the Later Years   257
- The context of the dying process   257
  - Expectation of death   258
- Environmental events predicting death   260

Terminal Drop Theory   263
- Cross-sectional analysis of longitudinal data   264
- Longitudinal analysis of longitudinal data   264

Disengagement Theory   265

Psychology of the Dying Older Person   267
- Preoccupation with death   268
- Role of regression in the dying process   269
- Life review as developmental process   271
- Physical illness, depression, and death   272
  - Care of the dying older person   273

The Process of Dying and Ethical Considerations   274
- The "Right-to-die" question   274
- Voluntary and involuntary euthanasia   275
  - Active and passive euthanasia   276
  - Direct and indirect euthanasia   276
- The American Medical Association's policy on euthanasia   276
  - The elderly and euthanasia   277

Summary   279

Epilogue: The Health Care Professional, Death, and Dying   282

Chapter Bibliographies   293

Chapter 1	293	Chapter 6	315
Chapter 2	297	Chapter 7	321
Chapter 3	301	Chapter 8	325
Chapter 4	305	Chapter 9	330
Chapter 5	311	Chapter 10	335
		Epilogue	339

Name Index   345
Subject Index   355

Dying in the Human Life Cycle

1
Stillbirth and Perinatal Death

Introductory Remarks

Experiencing Stillbirth and Perinatal Death

- Inadequate Recognition of Actual Loss
- Doctor-patient Relationship in Fetal Death Encounters

Effective Management of Grieving Parents

- Establishing the Personal Identity of the Infant
  - Naming the Child
  - Seeing the Baby
- Photographing the Deceased Infant
  - Funeral Arrangements

Psychiatric Sequelae to Stillbirth and Perinatal Death

- Parental Grief
- Replacement Pregnancy
- Reactions of Other Children
- Stress in Marital Relationship

Related Issues of Special Concern

- Prenatal Preparation for Possibility of Child Loss
- Newborns with Major Congenital Malformations
  - Loss by Adoption

Summary

Introductory Remarks

Pregnancy and the birth of a child are normally joyful experiences for parents and families. The decision to have a child often represents a significant developmental progression in a couple's relationship. Many conscious and unconscious expectations are linked to this choice for parenthood, and the months of pregnancy provide the time during which these dreams are elaborated. The interruption of this process by miscarriage, fetal death, or the death of the newborn due to congenital abnormalities or birthing complications is a devastating event for the parents.

A decline in the number of fetal and perinatal deaths in the United States is attributable in part to improved diagnostic techniques, competent prenatal obstetrical care, and sophisticated neonatal intensive care. However, it is estimated that 1 to 2 percent of all pregnancies that continue beyond 26 weeks of gestational age end with the death of the fetus or newborn. Translated into more concrete terms, any major obstetrical unit that delivers a weekly average of 100 babies will have one or two stillbirths or perinatal deaths each week. Hospital centers with neonatal intensive care units (NICUs) have a proportionately increased number of neonatal deaths despite the best efforts of specialized staff and rescue procedures. About one in seven neonates admitted to an NICU dies in the hospital.

Parents are often not prepared for this crisis, and many of those involved in neonatal care are similarly unprepared. This chapter will explore a number of important issues related to stillbirth and perinatal death and to the care of bereaved parents. Special attention will be focused on the role of health care professionals in their relationships with families experiencing fetal or perinatal death.

Experiencing Stillbirth and Perinatal Death

The conspiracy of silence that has characterized the medical community's response to fetal and perinatal death has been broken in recent years. Many personal accounts of stillbirth experiences have been published, particularly in nursing journals. Not infrequently, these are the stories of individual nurses who themselves have had stillbirths and whose reflections are insightful and useful to others in the health care field. Teresa Kochmar Crout is coordinator of nursing education at the Christ Hospital School of Nursing in Cincinnati, Ohio. She published her own personal story (Crout, 1980), part of which follows in edited form.

For 9 years, my husband Jack and I had been trying to have a child. After several diagnostic workups, two surgical interventions, and what seemed like an endless regimen of pharmacotherapy, we were finally looking forward to the joyous day of "Little Kid's" arrival. I couldn't have ordered an easier pregnancy—not a single bout of morning sickness. . . . Being a 33-year-old primigravida, I was grateful that I didn't have to cope with any complications. . . .

Two days after a surprise baby shower, I noticed that our previously active baby seemed unusually quiet. He was due in less than 5 weeks, and I told myself that by now "Little Kid" had probably grown to the point where confined uterine space was limiting his movement. I went to work as usual without any real concern. Toward the end of the next day, however, I began to worry that the baby seemed a little *too* quiet. Hesitantly, I called my obstetrician. He suggested that Jack and I put our minds at ease by going to the hospital for an assessment of fetal heart tones. I was so sure that I had nothing to worry about that I didn't even pack a bag.

By 11 P.M., I found myself in an examining room in the labor and delivery area. As the next hour passed, my confidence dwindled, and all my suppressed fears were magnified. Examiners came and went, one by one, each face as masklike and unreadable as the last. I lay rigidly on the bed, silently begging them to tell me *something*—anything that would answer the question I was too frightened to ask.

Finally, a staff physician whom I knew only slightly conducted the last examination and delivered the verdict.

"Mrs. Crout, I'm sorry, but your baby is dead."

"Oh my God," I groaned. It couldn't be. Not our long-awaited "Little Kid." As I cried for my husband, a nurse took my hand and said gently, "Go ahead, let it out."

Jack was with me in a moment, and we clung to each other like two shipwrecked survivors. It was well after midnight before either of us could think about anything but our pain. Then I realized that I was surrounded by laboring women giving birth to live, healthy babies. I asked for a private room on another floor. I felt instinctively that I needed a secluded place where Jack and I could grieve openly without containing our emotions for the sake of others. As I was wheeled down the hall with my chart, I could read my diagnosis: "undetermined intrauterine death."

. . . Later that day, I was reexamined, X-rayed, and transferred to the labor suite for induction. My labor was mercifully brief. Under minimal anesthesia, administered at the last possible moment, I delivered a 4-pound 15-ounce (2.2-kg.) baby girl. Jack and I had decided not to see her. I'm told she was perfect in every way but one. Her umbilical cord, though short, had wrapped itself around her tiny neck and shoulders, cutting off her life support. It was a cruel turn of fate that no one could have anticipated or prevented. Still, I was haunted by doubts.

Should I have called my doctor when I first noticed the baby's diminished activity? Would it have made any difference? I'd always followed the obstetrician's instructions to the letter, but that didn't stop me from going back over every month, week and day of my pregnancy, searching for something I might have done wrong. Intellectually, I knew I was innocent. Emotionally, I still felt guilty.

I also felt incredibly angry. Why did this have to happen to us? So many babies were unwanted, abused or aborted, while ours would have been so cherished.

Perhaps stronger than any emotion was my overwhelming sense of loss and emptiness. I'd become so accustomed to "Little Kid" inside me, that I missed her without even knowing her. I felt cheated.

And so did Jack. He seemed to be coping unrealistically well. Actually, he was throwing all his energy into creating a strong front and denying his own emotions. He needed as much release and support as I did, and I wanted to help him, but I just didn't know how.

Finally, I wished we knew how soon our grief would become tolerable. Would it ever? I think it will—not right away, but someday.

Teresa and Jack Crout's experiences with the stillbirth of their daughter highlight some feelings shared in common with other parents. This articulate account of the final days of her pregnancy and the delivery of her stillborn child provides a suitable background for the discussion of fetal and perinatal death.

Unless a woman has had a previous miscarriage or still-birth, she does not ordinarily consider the possibility of a neonatal death. Pregnancy today is generally a conscious choice. It represents for many couples both planning and preparation. For some couples, like the Crouts, it may have involved special efforts. In such circumstances, the verification of the fact of pregnancy is frequently greeted with enthusiasm and excitement.

As the pregnancy advances, the degree of anticipation is heightened. If all routine obstetrical examinations fail to note any complications, most couples enter the final trimester with the full expectation that their child will be healthy and normal. When some dramatic antepartum change occurs, as Mrs. Crout described, or when an intrapartum complication develops, the whole process of preparing for the baby is violently interrupted. Not only does the couple have to face a situational crisis of death, but they simultaneously must negotiate the maturational crisis of failure at parenthood (Quirk, 1979).

In any crisis situation, an individual has limited personal resources on which to call. Much of one's available psychic energy is exhausted in trying to maintain basic equilibrium in the face of critical events. People in such situations are vulnerable and dependent. Because of their heightened sensitivity, they can be hurt by well-intentioned, but inappropriate, comments. They need understanding and skillful assistance to regroup their energies in order to make the necessary decisions that will influence the course of their recovery.

In dealing with the parents of stillborns and perinatal deaths, medical and nursing personnel have not always been responsive. The most reasonable explanation for this fact is that many health care professionals, like the parents themselves, are not emotionally prepared for a stillbirth or the death of a neonate. They are preparing for birth, not death. It has been suggested that some individuals opt for specializations in obstetrics and gynecology precisely because the encounter with death in this specialty may be significantly less than in some other medical areas. Whether this assumption could be demonstrated or not, it is generally acknowledged that many nurses and physicians find it difficult to deal with the parents of a stillborn or deceased neonate. Parents report feeling abandoned by hospital personnel; some say that their doctors appear to have avoided them. The anecdotal literature about parents' recollections of this avoidance behavior is voluminous, and provides a rich source of material for reflection and learning.

Inadequate Recognition of Actual Loss

The language medicine uses to describe a stillborn is revealing. A *stillbirth* or late fetal death (after the 28th week of gestation) may be defined as "the failure of the product of conception to show evidence of respiration, heart beat, or definite movement of voluntary muscle after expulsion from the uterus, with no possibility of resuscitation" (Dorland's Medical Dictionary, 26th edition, p. 348). In practice, some physicians find it difficult to say that a baby is dead. Parents report physicians' use of a term like "gestationally nonviable infant" to avoid acknowledging simply that the child died. But whether the death occurs *in utero* or during the process of labor and delivery, the parents experience the loss as significant, having already formed a personal relationship with the deceased child.

The grief resulting from a fetal death increases in proportion to the length of the pregnancy. Parents clearly form attachments to the fetus; this is particularly evident in the woman. In the case reported above, the Crouts, who referred to the developing fetus as "Little Kid," demonstrate this early bonding. Too often this loss is minimized. In an effort to console the parents, nurses, physicians, friends, and family members attempt to put aside the loss. They assume, especially in the case of a stillborn, that the parents had no time to establish a personal relationship to the deceased fetus. Therefore, based on this assumption, their words and behaviors may ignore its existence. Hospital procedures may speak of "disposal" of the body rather than of "burial." Mothers may be encouraged by some to "forget" what has happened. "You're young; you can have another child," a nurse or a family friend may casually remark.

When a neonate with birth complications dies in an NICU, doctors and nurses may be prone to offer the comment, "It's merciful that he died; he would have had serious brain damage had he survived." Comments such as these, while intended to be helpful to parents, are often a source of additional distress, and not infrequently they are recalled many years later. These kinds of words and behaviors further isolate the parents in their grief at a time when they need someone with whom to share their inner and outer loss. Comments that signal some "magical repair" or facile solution are neither helpful nor constructive.

In retrospect, many parents say that they would have appreciated someone just to listen to them, to share their confusing and ambivalent feelings, and to acknowledge with them their sense of profound loss. The lack of understanding of their feelings and the reality of the situation creates additional psychological burdens for them at a time when they most need support and compassion.

A number of studies have bolstered the thesis that attending medical personnel, especially physicians, are resistent to acknowledging the degree of loss experienced as a result of a stillbirth or perinatal death. In one of the earliest and seminal studies of the impact of stillbirth on the family, Bourne (1968) noted certain disturbing features of the physician-patient relationship. He identified this disturbance as being caused by physicians' reluctance "to know, notice or remember anything about the patient who has had a stillbirth" (p. 103). His research design included surveying 100 family-practice physicians who delivered stillbirths and a control group of 100 physicians whose patients delivered healthy, normal babies. Apart from a significant difference in the responses received from the questionnaires mailed to the two groups of physicians, the quality of the responses was notable. The physicians who had delivered stillborns returned fewer completed surveys and tended to provide less information than those who had not and checked "don't recall," or "don't remember," or "don't know" answers. This seems to support the position that stillbirth does affect an attending physician, who may seek some relief from anxiety in defensive blocking or denial. Such denial may behaviorally translate into minimizing the impact of the loss or its importance to the parents.

Wolff, Neilson, and Schiller (1969) surveyed 50 women who had lost a baby at birth or shortly thereafter. They followed 40 of these women over a 3-year period and monitored not only their emotional reactions to the loss but also behavioral patterns that determined the resolution of the loss. More than half of the women surveyed were unwilling to discuss their attitudes about their doctors, nurses, or attendants. Those who did respond were quite articulate. More than half of them found their physicians cold and reported attending nurses as having similar characteristics. Although the reason for these judgments is not fully explained, there is enough evidence from other sources to conclude that stillbirth or perinatal death can effectively isolate medical staff from the bereaved parents.

Some health care professionals would like to believe that reported hostility or anger of parents experiencing stillbirth toward attending nurses and physicians is simply a normal manifestation of grief. Though some initial affect of this sort may be grief-related, follow-up interviews with parents are uncovering more serious faults in the way in which parents are treated in the immediate crisis situation. These disturbed interventions may affect not only the early course of parents' reactions to the stillbirth or perinatal death but may determine the course of recovery. The following discussion details how more competent assistance can be provided to parents in similar circumstances.

Doctor-patient Relationship in Fetal Death Encounters

Knapp and Peppers (1979) surveyed 100 middle-class mothers and fathers who had lost infants. These parents seemed to agree that the lack of community recognition of the loss compounded their grief. They turned to their physicians for counsel and support, assuming that their doctors would be understanding and empathic. The research sociologists note that many physicians seem unable to meet such parents' needs and expectations because they either find it difficult to deal with death on a personal level or because they struggle with the required role shift from healer to counselor.

The authors cite one case that clearly is not typical but which dramatizes the lack of sensitivity of some hospital personnel. A 24-year-old woman was taken to the emergency room, with severe vaginal bleeding.

> I had no idea what was going on, only that I was bleeding very badly. Then all of a sudden the doctor held up for me to see a mass of flesh about four or five inches long and an inch or two wide, all bloody and dripping, and said rather dryly, "Well, there's your baby, lady; you lost it." I still can't talk to anyone about this and it happened over two years ago." (Knapp & Peppers, 1979, p. 776)

For the emergency room physician this may have been a routine procedure, like any vacuum curettage, but the woman certainly did not consider the event to be "routine." The failure to anticipate and understand the feelings of any person in these or similar circumstances precludes effective care and may actually be more damaging to her ability to cope with the loss.

One explanation the authors offer to explain the less than adequate level of human responsiveness in some physicians to parents who have lost a baby is the following. The physicians may themselves be involved in a mourning-separation process similar, though distinct, from that of the parents. The doctor may be confronted with feelings of inadequacy, failure, helplessness, and some lingering doubts about his or her own responsibility for the death. Obstetricians will often withdraw from involvement with the parents after the delivery and desire to pass responsibility for care to the pediatrician. Some pediatricians refuse to assume this responsibility since there is no child to care for in the case of a stillborn. In another study Peppers and Knapp (1980) report an interview that underscores this point.

> I knew something was wrong when I was hurriedly sedated and whisked out of the delivery room. My husband told me later that the OB and pediatrician were actually arguing outside in the hall. Neither of them would take the responsibility of telling me. As it worked out, one of the nurses told my husband and he relayed the news to me. I felt totally helpless. Neither of them saw me for two days. (p. 158)

Obviously distorted relations can exist between doctors and patients in these and similar circumstances. Fortunately, education and experience can offer productive solutions (Lake, *et al.*, 1983). Health care personnel are in privileged positions to respond to and help grieving parents. There are a number of practical measures that can be taken to reduce the traumatic impact a stillborn or perinatal death will have on the survivors.

Physicians should communicate directly and immediately with the parents. Some physicians delay in informing parents about verified information of the fetal death. In retrospect, most parents say that they would have preferred knowing the facts as soon as they were diagnosed to having to interpret the nonverbal behaviors of physicians and attendants.

In the case of ***antepartum stillbirth***, when the death of the fetus is diagnosed *in utero* and before delivery, communication of this information is essential. The communication skill of the physician and his or her sensitivity to timing and place are important variables. Ideally, both parents should be informed together, and the doctor needs to be comfortable in expressing his or her own feelings of loss and disappointment to the parents. The details about delivery will have to be reviewed with the parents, and they will need time to assimilate this as well as the news of the death.

An ***intrapartum stillbirth***, involving death during some phase of the birthing process, requires similar procedures. Doctors need to inform the parents as soon as possible of the outcome of the delivery. Because death is always a tragic event, the survivors instinctively turn to others for support. Parents need each other and they need the comfort and consolation a nurse or physician can supply. They remember the language used in communicating the news of the death, so this is not the time to use circumlocution or jargon. The more simple and compassionate the expression of the facts, the more receptive the parents will be in receiving them. After the basic facts have been communicated, there is no need to offer more detail unless this is immediately requested. Parents are stunned by the unwelcome news and require time to digest the reality. There will be ample opportunity later to review other important topics, but for the present, it is more important that the physician be a physical presence and a sympathetic ear to the grief-stricken parents.

In live births with serious complications, medical decision making is necessarily rapid and transfer of the baby to specialized care units may be required. It is understandable in these emergency situations that early consultation with parents may be postponed. As soon as possible, a complete and simple review of the perinatal emergency should be made to the parents. If the neonatologist is available, he or she should be included in the discussion along with the primary care physician to describe the intervention strategy for care of the newborn. It is important to keep hope alive for parents, but not at the sacrifice of honesty. If the degree of the abnormality offers little hope of survival, this needs to be told to parents. It is not useful to protect parents from the facts; they deal better with truthful information than with deception, no matter how noble may be the motivation that attempts to shield them from the truth.

The underlying common denominator in all three of these distinct but related scenarios is immediacy of communication, comprehensiveness of information in clear and understandable terminology, and a warm, supportive, and comforting presence in the face of a highly emotional state of the parents. Every report on parents' recollections of their losses emphasizes the importance of how and when the information was received, and the way in which the information was transmitted.

Effective Management of Grieving Parents

Professionals are becoming more aware of the degree of trauma that parents experience when faced with stillbirth or the early death of a newborn. With greater sensitivity to the psychological impact of hospital management of the crisis, a number of important issues concerning hospital care have been identified. Some of these have stirred controversy among health care professionals and have provoked extensive discussion in the fields of pediatrics, psychiatry, and social work. We shall review the principal issues of the debate with particular attention to how these can ease the grief of parents.

Establishing the Personal Identity of the Infant

In describing stillbirth Bourne (1968) called it a "non- event" in which there is guilt and shame, but no tangible person to mourn. Other researchers have supported this theme. Lewis (1976, 1979) observes that a stillborn is someone who did not exist, a nonperson, often nameless. As such, stillbirth is an "empty tragedy." In reality, this concept is diametrically opposed to the parental experience of the developing fetus.

Another study reports that the course of pregnancy initiates the bonding process and engages a narcissistic preoccupation with the baby, not only in the mother but in the father as well (Winnicott, 1958). This "primary maternal preoccupation" prepares a parent to provide the required physical and psychological care for the expected child. This fact is corroborated by Mrs. Crout's account of the stillbirth of her daughter. "Little Kid" already participated in a personal relationship with her parents, and their expectations were that she would be a perfectly healthy child.

The most difficult paradox which parents like the Crouts must resolve is that what had promised fulfillment has produced a painful void. It is into this emptied world that the health care professional and other family members must enter to encounter the grieving parents. If we allow the family to remain alone and unattended in this experience of loss, we must contend with the possibility that the mental health of the parents and family can be negatively affected by such inattention.

The term "conspiracy of silence" has frequently been used to describe the ways in which some people attempt to manage a stillbirth or death of a newborn. Lewis (1978) maintains that this avoidance of discussion of the events of the neonate's death gives parents the message that what has happened is too tragic, too horrible for words and that the best approach to dealing with it is to try to forget that it ever happened. But this avoidance only further isolates the parents in their grief. In fact, the last thing they need to do is to deny the existence of their baby who has died.

In some hospitals, mothers who have delivered a stillborn child are routinely transferred from the obstetrical unit to either a gynecological unit or general medical service. This is intended to ease the psychological burden of being with other women who have successfully delivered a healthy child and who are engaged in the ordinary feeding and nursing care of their newborns. While the transfer may in fact be desirable for some women and may actually be requested, the mere fact of the shift may be the first step in the process of institutional denial. If a woman elects to return to her assigned room or ward, the other women will need to be informed of the outcome of her delivery and assisted in their efforts to be supportive. Although it may be difficult for a bereaved mother to encounter other live babies, it can be a therapeutic experience. Some have actually been able to participate in the care of their roommates' infants and have formed friendships with these women that have continued after discharge.

Sedation and overmedication is another way in which hospitals may inadvertently conspire to avoid the grief of stillbirth. If a woman has been anesthetized for delivery, she may be unaware of the outcome of the procedure. If she has been awake, she may be quickly sedated. To continually repeat orders for such medication may be a convenient way to avoid dealing with the facts.

One of the most important aids to the establishment of the deceased infant's identity is the naming of the child and the viewing of the body. Both of these acts can be enormously helpful to parents and can have significant importance in the resolution of grief.

Naming the Child

According to Furman (1978), the mourning process is contingent upon two somewhat different mechanisms. The first is *detachment*, which involves the recollection of memories about the deceased that link that individual to the family—these ties have been severed by death and must be surrendered. The second mechanism is *identification*, by which survivors incorporate certain aspects of the deceased into themselves, thus easing the pain of loss. Since it is virtually impossible to identify with a being as undeveloped as a newborn. the parents of a stillborn are deprived of the relief this part of the mourning process would bring. They are left to suffer the pain of detachment. What is done in the first days of mourning can significantly affect its entire course.

For this reason it is important to facilitate those experiences of the deceased infant that can be cherished by the bereft parents. Because there is no legal requirement for a forename in the case of stillbirth, it has not been judged important up to now that the parents provide one. However, since naming helps to establish a personal identity, the parents should be encouraged to name their baby and staff should use this name in talking about the child, not "him", "her," or "it." Often parents have already considered names for the baby, and these names have a personal importance to them. Choosing a name helps them to relate to their child and to share with others the meaning and importance that may be attached to the name they have chosen.

Some parents may wish to ritualize this naming in a religious context. Nurses frequently report that parents requested baptism for the deceased fetus or asked hospital chaplains to christen a neonate in the NICU. Whatever the parents' choice in this matter, they should be encouraged to provide a name for their baby, and this name should become the vehicle for further discussion of the deceased child with the parents.

Seeing the Baby

Of all of the issues concerning the care of the parents of a stillborn child, none has stirred more controversy than that of whether parents should be encouraged and permitted to view and hold the body of the deceased. Kennell, Slyter, and Klaus (1970) in what is becoming a classic discussion of the mourning responses of parents to stillbirth, see viewing as part of the full expression of grief. One strong argument for not encouraging or permitting parents to see the deceased baby is that such an encounter can precipitate a reaction that would only further intensify the pain already being experienced. While this may be true in some cases, it is not possible to generalize such a position.

The overwhelming consensus among those who have worked with the parents of stillborns is that viewing is one of the most important variables affecting the course of bereavement. In the case of Mrs. Crout above, she herself opted not to view the body of her stillborn daughter. Now she wishes that she had consented to see her for she appreciates the importance of such an encounter. Almost all of the research supports this position, although the decision of parents in this matter must be respected. Presented with the option, many parents will initially be opposed to viewing the dead baby. In a study of parents assisted in a perinatal bereavement clinic at Downstate-Kings County Hospital Medical Center in New York, researchers report the parents favor a hospital policy that permits viewing and holding the body of the deceased baby (Cohen et al., 1978). Although little useful data are available concerning the impact of "nonviewing" on psychological adjustment, the early impression of the Downstate team is that more of the mothers referred to their bereavement center's psychiatric service for additional assistance were nonviewers.

Hospitals traditionally have been opposed to such a policy. Changes in it have resulted from adamant requests expressed by some parents to see the child or from the intuitive interventions of staff who were willing to risk the possible negative outcome of such viewing. Today, the wisdom of this action is more widely appreciated.

Staff ordinarily must take the initiative in exploring the option of viewing with parents. Occasionally parents will need some help in understanding why it is beneficial. The thought of seeing the body of their dead child is distressing, particularly if there is serious distortion in the infant's body. With sensitive explanation and without any coercion, the majority of parents will consent to seeing the baby. Nurses and physicians should take care to prepare the parents for what they will see. The physical characteristics of the baby should be described in careful detail before the body is presented to the parents. Discoloration, bruises, deformities, and maceration need to be explained. With this kind of careful preparation, parents are able to see the baby and are less likely to be distressed by these factors.

The common experience of most parents is that their mental pictures of the child do not correspond to reality. When a group of mothers who had not seen their stillborn children were later asked to draw pictures of how they had first envisioned their babies, their sketches revealed greater distortion and deformity than the actual fact (Shokeir, 1979).

Some nurses have demonstrated great sensitivity in presenting the bodies of deceased infants to their parents. They have carefully wrapped the cold and rigid bodies in warm blankets and have carried the body in natural positions, close to their own bodies. This nonverbal gesture of acceptance disposes the mother and father to a similar openness. Nurses take their cues from the parents and present the body when they are ready. Some parents spontaneously reach out to hold the body; others may be content to have the nurse hold the body while they view it from a distance.

In an article on the issues of viewing a stillborn, Parrish (1980) describes a mother who was experiencing her second stillbirth. She had not viewed the first child but was insistent that she be permitted to see this one. At 38 weeks of gestational age, intrauterine death had been confirmed and the delivery had been induced by the saline method.

Rose had repeatedly informed the nursing staff that regardless of how the baby looked, she wanted to see her child. She had been denied seeing her first stillborn at another hospital, two years previously. Following the delivery of a macerated stillborn female infant, Rose received the routine post delivery care and was transferred to the recovery room to await the arrival of her husband whom she felt would also want to see the baby. She did not wait however. About 15 minutes later she called me, said she was ready to see the baby and was it possible to have her mother present. Rose was prepared for what she was to see as we had talked about this on several occasions during the days before delivery.

When I brought the baby to her, Rose sat upright in bed but kept her arms and hands close to her body. I unwrapped the blanket to expose the body which was moderately macerated and misshapen. Although the skin was peeling and some fluid escaping, I had deliberately left my gloves off not wanting to convey anything to Rose that might suggest I found the baby undesirable. I lifted the baby's hands and feet and we counted the toes and fingers together. Rose asked to see the baby's back.

Since the fetal skull had collapsed, the baby had very little resemblance to the baby once fantasized. Rose wistfully remarked that she had hoped to see some family resemblance. I gently encased the baby's head in my hands, molding as much as possible to create some facial symmetry. Rose suddenly responded with a cry of delight, "Yes, there is a resemblance. She looks like John! Oh yes, I can tell that this is our baby!" Then she held her hands out and asked if she could touch the baby in the same way. Gently she explored the baby with her fingertips. Finally she wrapped the baby in the blanket, held her close for a moment and then with a peaceful look said, "Thank you nurse, this has meant so much to me. You see, I never saw my first baby." (Parrish, 1980, p. 36)

Photographing the Deceased Infant

It is contraindicated to force parents to view the body of their dead baby. A decision to waive the option must be respected, and nothing must be done to make parents feel guilty for this decision. It is understandable that some parents feel such an encounter with the lifeless body of their infant would be macabre and too upsetting. They may judge that they are not psychologically disposed for what they perceive to be traumatic.

It may be weeks or months later that parents may regret their decision not to view the infant, particularly as the process of mourning advances. In these instances it is helpful if there is a photograph of the infant that can be given to the parents. Some hospitals routinely make some file photographs of still-borns and neonates who die in their intensive care units. Later, if in follow-up interviews parents express regret for not seeing the child, photographs are available.

Photographs can be the only tangible evidence that the child existed and can be important assets in grief resolution. Some hospital staff still oppose photographing the body of a dead infant, but more and more reports of the advisability of doing so are appearing in the literature (Lewis, 1976; Hilderbrand & Schreiner, 1980; Chase, 1980; Clyman *et al.*, 1980; Harrington, 1982). These photographs, presented and described by those staff members who had actual contact with the deceased infant, have incalculable therapeutic benefit to parents. This issue will be discussed later as it relates to follow-up work with bereaved families.

Funeral Arrangements

In many places, the hospital is prepared to arrange for the burial of the infant's body, providing cremation or inhumation in an unmarked grave in a municipal potter's field. Though generally considered helpful, this may not serve the interests of the surviving parents, who may first hear the service referred to as "disposal." Jolly (1976) recalls the case of a mother who had delivered a stillborn child. On the day after the delivery, when she had recovered enough to plan in her own mind the funeral arrangements she desired, she discovered that the hospital had already cremated her baby.

There is enough evidence already available from grief work with parents to conclude that involvement in funeral arrangements is important. Some husbands, in order to spare their wives additional stress, have privately arranged for the burial of the baby's body. Jolly (1976) describes a letter he received from a woman who wrote: "It is only now after 34 years that I have been able to ask my husband where our son was buried." Other women, deprived of involvement in the infant's burial arrangements, have experienced painful fantasies. Not knowing where the baby's grave is or not being able to identify the precise grave can be unnecessarily stressful for a grieving parent.

Parents should be encouraged to assume whatever control they desire in making funeral plans for their infant. Some wish to have a religious service or some memorial service. Funeral directors can be helpful in providing whatever assistance may be necessary to executing parents' wishes. The hospital staff can be instrumental in providing parents whatever referrals they may require in making appropriate arrangements. In any case, the burial should not take place until the mother is physically able to be present.

Parents who have been receptive to viewing the body of the infant may be favorably inclined to assist in the preparation of the body for burial. The active participation of parents in this preparation facilitates the grieving process. They may select certain clothing and dress the body for burial. Parents who participated in the preparation and burial of their infant children stress the importance to them of these recollections and memories. The value of these involvements should not be underestimated by hospital staff in making disposal arrangements.

Psychiatric Sequelae to Stillbirth and Perinatal Death

The medical responsibility for parents of a stillborn does not terminate upon discharge of the mother from the hospital, but continues during the weeks and months of the normal period of bereavement. Clyman and his associates (1979; 1980) reported that 76 percent of the 108 families in their survey group who had experienced a neonatal death chose to have physician follow-up in the weeks after the death.

These researchers concluded that at a time when so many parents feel isolated and abandoned by other family members and friends, contact with doctors and other health professionals who shared their loss can be very beneficial. Physician-initiated contact with the family signals the importance the doctor places on the stillbirth or perinatal death, and his or her sensitivity to the parental feelings of anger, loss, confusion, and disappointment. Intervention of this sort can determine the healthy adjustment of some parents (Estok & Lehman, 1983).

Forrest and his associates (1982) have published the preliminary findings of a study on the support of families after perinatal death. Fifty families experiencing perinatal death were randomly assigned to the supportive counseling group or to the control group that received routine hospital care. Assessments were made at intervals of 6 and 14 months after the death, using both interviews and self-rating scales. A number of interesting contrasts were noted between the two groups. The duration of bereavement reaction after perinatal death was judged to be appreciably shortened by support and counseling. The researchers drew certain practical implications from this experience. The value of follow-up discussion between medical personnel and parents is evident. Parents need to verbalize their common questions about what went wrong in the pregnancy and their anxieties and doubts about future pregnancies. They need to review the results of an autopsy if one has been performed and to be assured that everything that could have been done for the child was done. This requires a good communicative relationship between the doctor and the parents.

These and other attempts to extend the hospital's responsibility for bereaved parents have succeeded in identifying some important issues for such intervention efforts. Some of these findings are discussed below.

Parental Grief

Helmrath and Steinitz (1978) have correctly observed that perinatal death is often the first important death experience of a couple. They may not have had any prior personal experience with intense grieving. Therefore, they may be surprised to discover the depth of their feelings and their duration. Because so many of the messages they receive directly and indirectly from family and friends may communicate "It's over; get on with living," the grieving spouses may attempt to mask their true feelings. A husband may want to protect his wife from additional hurt and thus may deny his own feelings. This suppression of feeling inhibits grieving and delays effective resolution of mourning.

Parents need to be helped to realize that their subjective reactions to the loss of their baby are normal and that their feelings are shared in common with many other persons in similar circumstances. They also need to be helped to understand that emotional responses vary. Individual spouses will react differently, expressing their grief in diverse ways. Some women experience the loss in a desire to hold, cuddle, and rock their infants. They may find themselves experiencing intense episodes of sadness and crying. Dreams and fantasies about the baby may interrupt their sleep and they may think that they hear the baby crying in another room.

A husband may find that he is adjusting more quickly to the loss, and no longer feels the intense pain that he perceives in his wife. He may have cried soon after the delivery but finds that he no longer feels the need to do so. He may become a bit impatient with his wife's tears and sobs. This common reaction of husbands not only further isolates the woman in her grief but can be a source of additional stress in the marriage. The husband may discover that his investment in his work intensifies, almost as if he seeks an escape from the pain of loss in increased activity. His absence from the home may extend from early morning until late in the evening.

Each of these behaviors is a common reaction to loss and a normal reaction of grieving parents. One of the most beneficial services that can be provided to parents in the aftermath of a perinatal death is to anticipate some of these grief responses and engage the couple in a productive discussion of their own feelings (Meyer & Lewis, 1979). Such communication between spouses is of paramount importance in determining the ways in which couples will face and resolve their loss.

Replacement Pregnancy

A common strategy of grief resolution is another pregnancy. While this is not an undesirable course of action, the timing of such a decision is important. The consensus of opinion among therapists actively engaged in counseling parents who have experienced perinatal death is that a new pregnancy should be delayed for a least 6 months to 1 year (Pozanski, 1972; Lewis, 1979; Hildebrand & Schreiner, 1980; Mahan & Schreiner, 1981; Sahu, 1981; Harrington,1982). There are some important psychological factors that dictate such advice.

Pregnancy can be a way of avoiding the task of mourning. Lewis (1977; 1979a) believes that a pregnant woman becomes so increasingly preoccupied with the new life that the mourning of her stillborn or deceased neonate is interrupted and that it is virtually impossible to resume that grief work later. Some might argue that this is a positive secondary gain of a subsequent pregnancy, and it may be generally applauded by friends and family. However, it may have adverse psychological ramifications for the new child. Lewis (1979a) has suggested that the new pregnancy may lead to idealization of the child as a reincarnation of the dead sibling, or it may be the genesis of child abuse. These psychopathological responses are thought to have their origin in interrupted or incomplete mourning.

Inhibition of mourning by becoming pregnant is a curious psychological process. The dynamics are still not clear even though some excellent efforts have been made to suggest an explanation for the behavior observed in many pregnant women. Lewis (1979) reasons that during the mourning process the bereaved unconsciously imagines the deceased person as being incorporated into the self and is thought of variously as dead, yet alive within. In pregnancy, the deceased infant and the new fetus both inhabit the mother's mind and body, thus setting the stage for a confusion of her feelings for the fetus with those for the deceased child. Lewis concludes by assuming that the inhibition of mourning serves to protect the new fetus from the threat that such a process might have on its development.

In his study on the motivations for pregnancy, Rabin (1965) offers some interesting theoretical models that can be applied to the specific circumstances of a replacement pregnancy. These motivations are summarized under four category headings: altruistic, fatalistic, narcissistic, instrumental. *Altruistic* motivation springs from an unselfish desire and concern for the anticipated child. It obviously is the healthiest motivation and presumes readiness and conscious choice on the part of the parents. *Fatalistic* motivation derives from the sense of responsibility to the human race to bear children; it is the response to duty. A *narcissistic* motivation stems from seeing child-bearing in terms of self-fulfillment and as a personal expression of the self—making someone "in my image and likeness." Finally, *instrumental* motivation is connected with a utilitarian goal, for example, cementing a problematic marriage or providing additional manpower for a family business. If the decision to replace the deceased neonate or stillborn with another child is narcissistic or instrumental, it can be a source of additional stress to a family, not the solution anticipated. A new pregnancy should never be conceptualized as a way to resolve the crisis represented by a prior pregnancy that ended in perinatal death. Another pregnancy is not a magical solution to a painful loss.

Reactions of Other Children

Many of the psychiatric sequelae to perinatal death or stillbirth have not been carefully studied, although there are numerous case reports that help to identify the issues. One area that is clearly underrepresented is the effect of stillbirth or perinatal death on a surviving older child. A very early study by Cain and Cain (1964) reported that in the case of miscarriage, the surviving child's predominant reaction was confusion and bewilderment. The promised brother or sister suddenly no longer is coming, and parents, immersed in their own grief, find it difficult to share helpful and necessary information and explanations with their other children.

When such information is lacking, the child's imagination can supply a number of explanations that may never become verbal. These imagined reasonings can be frightening and threatening to the child and can catalyze certain destructive reactions, such as assuming some personal responsibility for the loss. Because the birth of a sibling represents an encroachment on one's personal turf, ambivalent feelings toward the unborn are normal. Having verbalized a wish that the baby not be born, the child may judge the outcome of the pregnancy to be the fulfillment of that wish. Guilt is an ordinary consequence of this mental process.

There is much debate about children's abilities to comprehend death. While there is no strong consensus about whether young children have the cognitive structures necessary to grasp the realities of death, it is unquestionably true that they experience the feelings that attend death within the family. Specifically, children sense the grief and confusion of their parents and internalize some of these feelings. They know that things are different as a result of the death, because they see that the parents have changed and, especially, that their parents' behavior toward them has changed. They are often ignored or given over to the care of others. Their parents are often not emotionally tuned into them and responsive to their needs. Their sensed deprivation leads to behavioral change in the children and is manifested, predictably, in acting-out, angry, and destructive displays, as well as in other ways. Enuresis, encopresis, night tremors, and regressive clinging are also common psychological symptoms in such circumstances. Certain manifestations of child psychopathology have their root in the incomplete mourning of a death and in parents' neglect to assist a child to come to terms with the loss of an expected sibling.

Stress in Marital Relationship

The death of an infant can have a profound and continuing influence on a marital relationship. Drotar and Irvin (1979) noted that infant death seems to pose special problems to parents, different from those characterizing other bereavements. For example, these parents tend not to appreciate the differences in their responses to the loss nor, understandably, do they attempt to avoid the intense distress connected with the grief experience. This attempt to avoid the experience may be reinforced by certain other social inhibitors, including the reactions of medical staff and family members.

The isolation experienced in the hospital setting may be intensified in the months following the stillbirth or perinatal death, and may be a major obstacle to the completion of the tasks of mourning. It is entirely normal that parents, especially a mother, search for explanations that answer the question, "Why did the baby die?"(Seitz & Warrick, 1974; Krein, 1979). The mother is extremely vulnerable to self-blame, and may be particularly hurt when her husband might impute responsibility for the death to her. This projection of blame on his part may be nothing more than his attempt to process the loss but, given her vulnerability, it may have more serious effects on the relationship.

Because ambivalence often attends pregnancy, it is not unusual that one or both spouses articulate some doubts or hesitation about the prospect of assuming the responsibilities of parenthood. Should the pregnancy end in the death of the child, these earlier ambivalent feelings can intensify and explode into a burden of guilt. In reviewing the course of pregnancy, every act or choice is material for scrutiny, and each event has a potential to be judged as responsibile for the infant's death. While none of these issues may have a causal relationship to the infant's death, they nonetheless have a powerful psychological hold on the parents' thoughts and feelings and can affect a couple's relationship.

Isolated in these obsessive reviews and susceptible to being hurt by the comments of others, a husband and wife look to each other for support. It is not unusual in these moments of need that sexual desire actually be intensified and that the desire for intimacy increase (Orfirer, 1970; David, 1975). These feelings may be frustrated for two reasons. First, the communication between the spouses may be poor so that neither is able to listen and respond to the other's needs, each seeming locked into a private world of thoughts and emotions. Secondly, parents may be reluctant or guilty to enjoy each other's closeness. Sex may be a continuous reminder of the act that led to their child's death and their present pain (Phipps, 1981). If the sexual relationship was previously experienced as healthy and satisfying, this shift in the pattern of relating may signal a problematic association with the sexual act. Left unaddressed, it can cause further stress in the marriage.

A couple who may be experiencing grief together for the first time may not be prepared for the amount of anger that may be felt and expressed. Not infrequently, they become the mutual recipients of each other's outbursts. This inflicts pain and is not productive, especially since it may not be properly understood. Since much of the anger parents feel is diffused, that is, not directed to any particular individual, it can often end up expressed toward the partner.

These needs, feelings, and reactions can burden a marital relationship already under considerable stress because of the stillbirth or infant death. In routine follow-up care to which the majority of parents are receptive, some of these sources of tension can be addressed and couples assisted to deal constructively with them (Meyer & Lewis, 1979). Parents need to be helped to understand that these intense feelings may be situationally determined and that in time they will begin to diminish. Some parents find participation in self-help groups like A.M.E.N.D. (Aiding Mothers Experiencing Neonatal Death) to be both insightful and supportive. Of course, more intensive psychotherapy may be required if the relationship before the perinatal death was problematic or if the grief in one or both spouses is pathological and unresponsive to simple intervention efforts.

The early findings of Cullberg (1972) note that 19 of the 56 women studied had been treated for some psychiatric disturbance following the death of their infants. While this may not be an alarming statistic, it does point out that parents, especially mothers, are a population-at-risk and that intervention strategies aimed at assisting and strengthening the relationship between spouses are well directed. With better knowledge of the possible psychiatric sequelae to a perinatal death, the health care community can better plan ways to assist parents in such need.

Chernus (1982) reviewed the literature on the psychodynamics of the mourning process and the intrapsychic defenses against it in parents whose babies die. Uncovering numerous difficulties encountered by couples in acknowledging the ongoing significance of the infant's death, this survey found countertransference issues to be particularly important.

Related Issues of Special Concern

Losing an infant is a distinct possibility for every expectant couple. Therefore, attention should be drawn to the educational function and psychological benefit of couples addressing this possibility during their prenatal preparation. Secondly, the particular concerns of parents who must deal with the survival of a less than perfect baby deserve at least brief discussion. Finally, some pregnant women will carry a baby to full term having previously determined to surrender the infant for adoption. This separation involves a loss and engages a set of dynamics not unlike those generated by stillbirths and perinatal deaths.

Prenatal Preparation for the Possibility of Child Loss

Many educators responsible for prenatal preparation of couples for childbirth are ambivalent about including a discussion of the possibility of perinatal death in their curricula. With greater openness to the topic and with an appreciation for the mental health benefits of such preparation, educators are exploring ways to best prepare couples for a possible tragic outcome. Kushner (1979) considers utilizing couples who have experienced stillbirth or perinatal death to return to prenatal class and to share their experiences with the group. Not only might this approach serve the needs of expectant parents, but it might also prove beneficial to the bereaved couple in need of the receptiveness and responsiveness such a group would provide.

Prenatal education does not simply communicate information but aims at preparing the couple psychologically for childbirth and parenting. Many classes place a high premium on enhancing the structures and patterns of communication between the spouses and among the members of the group. In describing her approach, Kushner (1979) comments:

. . . we encourage couples to communicate better, to talk, to touch and to be aware of each other's needs and feelings. We further let them know that we are there to help and support them and nurture an atmosphere of good feelings within the group, helping them to say what is on their minds and to express their fears. If the outcome should be tragic, the couple's awareness of having a warm, supportive group to turn to may help them in their grief as it does in the fearfulness and anxiety during pregnancy. (p. 232)

This openness necessitates informing the group when occasionally a couple suffers a miscarriage during a class series. How this matter is discussed in the class psychologically prepares others for such a possibility, albeit remote.

Peer relationships among members of prenatal preparatory classes may be untapped resources for the care and management of perinatal losses. Since participation in groups of this sort are becoming more common practice among expectant parents, the therapeutic potential of these groups needs to be further explored. By discussing the possibility of perinatal death, these couples can be assisted to see ways in which they can effectively reach out to each other should such a tragic event happen to some member of the group. In examining their feelings about infant death, not only are they emotionally preparing for such possibility in their own lives but they are developing certain skills that may be beneficial in responding to another couple actually suffering loss.

Not all expectant parents will welcome the inclusion of death as a topic in the prenatal program, but with sensitive support and encouragement on the part of the obstetrical educator, couples can be helped to discuss it. Rather than being a source of stress to them, this serves an important preventive therapeutic purpose. Most importantly, they are laying the foundation for a significant human resource and social service.

Newborns with Major Congenital Malformations

When an infant is born with a major congenital malformation or is acutely ill, parents must confront conflicting feelings and often difficult decisions. The overriding feeling is usually guilt for having produced a less than perfect baby. With the ever-increasing sophistication in medical and surgical care of high-risk severely malformed or dying infants, parents are simultaneously faced with a number of complex choices involving the effort to rescue or the decision to allow to die. Klaus and Kennell's (1970) influential discussion of this issue supported the position that parents should have contact with the high-risk neonate, regardless of the extent of the crisis.

Communication with the parents of the neonate after delivery, when a complete report is made on the nature of the difficulties and therapeutic options are reviewed, can begin to address the possible guilt parents feel and serve to reassure them (Slade *et al.*, 1977). As grave as the situation may be, it is important that some measure of optimism be maintained. Parents need to be assured that the infant is valued and will receive the best of care. Discussions with the neonatologist and other staff members give parents critical support and set the groundwork for the life-or-death decisions they may be called upon to make.

Campbell and Duff (1979) believe that in determining the course of care for acutely ill or congenitally malformed infants, parents must have "primary decisional power although the responsible physician usually shares or assumes this in order to help the parents with the burden" (p. 66). To the degree that communication and trust exist between the parents and the physician and staff, they all become partners in the decision-making process. The question has often been voiced whether parents in this crisis situation can make reasoned and informed choices. Campbell and Duff, along with many others, believe they can, provided that adequate time is provided for consultation and reflection. In these circumstances, parents need to experience support and should not be made to feel as though they are making decisions in absolute isolation.

Parents need to be helped to see distinctions in proposed treatment of their newborn child. In deciding for maximum treatment without qualification, it is assumed that the prognosis for such an effort is reasonably good, and that all life-support efforts should be employed. There are other neonates who are not likely to benefit from such extensive intervention. In such cases, the primary goals of treatment are palliative, that is, to ease any possible suffering. Finally, since many of these infants are actually dying, it is important in the judgment of many that life-support efforts be discontinued so that dying is not unnecessarily prolonged.

These complex ethical questions are beyond the scope of the present discussion. They are introduced here because they count among the acute problems facing parents with defective newborns and because they reveal the special sensitivity and skill required to assist them.

Loss by Adoption

Some women choose to carry a pregnancy to term even though they plan to surrender the infant for adoption. In most cases, this decision undergoes much conscious deliberation, and the separation is prepared for psychologically with the help of the supportive counseling available to expectant mothers. Surrendering the child, however, is a form of perinatal loss and involves many of the associated dynamics.

For a long time, it was thought inadvisable to allow mothers who intend to surrender their newborn babies to adoptive parents to see and hold them because physical contact, which intensifies bonding, would increase the pain of separation. Now, given the knowledge gained from experience with other parents who have endured the death of a neonate, it is thought that the deprivation of contact with an infant for adoption is an unnecessary burden for the biological mother (O'Donohue, 1979).

Despite good preparatory grieving, the mother who surrenders her infant for adoption cannot avoid the normal bereavement process engaged by loss. She will have many doubts about the decision she has made and may feel anger and resentment toward those who assisted her in arriving at her choice. She may feel self-hatred for the abandonment of the baby, or hostility toward the biological father who shared some responsibility for the pregnancy. Whatever the constellation of her feelings, it need not be charged with the sense of emptiness caused by not having seen and held the infant, and in most cases, whether or not the mother held her baby is important to the resolution of the grief. What was discussed earlier about seeing and holding the body of the infant in the case of stillbirths and perinatal deaths is applicable here.

Summary

The normally joyful anticipation associated with pregnancy and birth is abruptly interrupted when a stillbirth or perinatal death occurs. Parents as well as many of those who provide care for them are ill prepared for such a crisis. Medical personnel, family, and friends may attempt to be supportive to the couple, but their choice of words may communicate the message that the loss is not important, and they may attempt to minimize it. This can have negative effects on the grieving couple and can account for angry and hostile reactions. Communication between the couple and the physicians who attend them in the postdelivery period can be tense and distorted. It is important that parents be provided with accurate and complete information in an appropriate manner and setting. The immediacy, comprehensiveness, and manner of communication are of paramount importance.

Assistance to parents who have experienced a stillbirth or perinatal death has been rendered more effective through the efforts and recommendations of psychiatrists, nurses, and others who have had extensive experience with people in these circumstances. All seem to agree that it is crucial for the parents to establish the identity of the dead fetus or infant. To help them do this effectively, the "conspiracy of silence" must be broken, and the parents should be encouraged to speak about their dead child. Naming the child and viewing the body are two valuable ways of imparting a personal identity. If parents are unwilling or unable to view the child, photographing the body provides a record of the event the parents may wish to view later. Although parents may not desire to have a formal funeral, they should be assisted in making whatever arrangements they desire for cremation or burial of the baby's body.

Numerous psychiatric sequelae have been noted among parents who have experienced a stillbirth or perinatal death. Physicians are reminded that their responsibilities for the family do not end after delivery but continue during the period of grief and adjustment. It is important to note that parents experience genuine grieving in the wake of a stillbirth or perinatal death, and they have individual needs in effectively completing this process. For many couples, this is the first significant experience of grieving, and they may not understand or recognize the somatic and psychological manifestations of normal grieving. Health care professionals are in particularly useful positions to help couples to deal with these special issues of adjustment.

Replacement pregnancy is frequently suggested by well-intentioned family and friends, and it is often considered by the bereaved parents themselves. Since conception and pregnancy can interrupt the normal grieving processes, couples might be helped to consider postponing another pregnancy for 6 months to 1 year after a stillbirth or perinatal death.

It is just as important that other children in the family be appropriately informed about the stillbirth or perinatal death. Since children anticipate the birth of a sibling and have begun to prepare emotionally for the event, they need information and support as they reconcile the unexpected outcome of the pregnancy. Failure to appropriately involve children or blocking their reactions may lead to psychopathological behaviors.

Stillbirth can place stress on a marriage and on each of the partners. There is a tendency on the part of some women to internalize the experiences of the stillbirth or perinatal death and to blame themselves. The critical event may unleash a whole repertoire of negative reactions a couple may not understand nor be able to cope with. A third party, either an individual counselor or a peer self-help group, may be beneficial to a couple dealing with these sources of tension.

The whole discussion of stillbirth and perinatal death has given rise to the issue of introducing this topic into routine prenatal preparation programs. The records of preventive psychiatry confirm the importance of doing so.

Many of the topics discussed in this chapter have particular relevance to the communication with and the care of parents who give birth to infants with major congenital malformations. The issues surrounding stillbirth and perinatal death bear as well on the circumstances of a woman who surrenders her child for adoption soon after childbirth, and who may experience a number of the psychological reactions associated with perinatal loss.

Stillbirth and perinatal death are early death experiences for many young couples. Even though these deaths share some features in common with other deaths in the human life cycle, the particular circumstances of a stillbirth require special communication skills and intervention strategies if parents are to be maximally assisted in dealing with the crisis of loss.

2
Sudden Infant Death Syndrome

General Definition

Clinical Description of the Syndrome

- General Descriptive Features
  - Gross Examination
- Microscopic Examination

Epidemiology of Sudden Infant Death Syndrome

- Age Distribution
- Medical, Familial, Socioeconomic, and Climatic Variables

Theoretical Approaches to Sudden Infant Death Syndrome

- Apnea Theory
- Psychophysiological Theories

Psychological Issues for Families of SIDS Victims

- Initial Impact of Discovery of a Dead Infant
- Concern for Other Children in the Family
- Impact on Marital Relationship
- Replacement Child
- Population at Special Risk: the Single Parent

Summary

Although there is evidence of Sudden Infant Death Syndrome (SIDS) dating back to biblical times (1 Kings 3:19–20), the modern work of SIDS research is scarcely more than 40 years old (Werne, 1942; Werne & Garrow, 1947, 1953). These early studies challenged the prevailing theories of suffocation, suggesting that some natural mechanism might trigger laryngospasm, the spasmodic closure of the larynx, which causes death. Since then research efforts have intensified and dozens of theories have been suggested, each one exploring a possible explanation for the sudden death of an infant. Today SIDS is recognized as a major medical problem and has become the focus of a federally mandated research effort. Although Congress, the National Institutes of Health, and numerous independent medical researchers have mounted this effort to address SIDS, groups of parents of SIDS victims were the individuals instrumental in calling attention to the social significance of SIDS and the ones who lobbied for more research (Johnson & Hufbauer, 1982).

Despite the intensification of research and debate within the scientific community, the etiology and pathogenesis of this syndrome, which claims the lives of between 8,000 and 10,000 infants in the United States each year, are still uncertain. Two international conferences on the subject (1963,1969) have brought together principal investigators from around the world for mutual exchange of theory and research. Pathologists have taken a lead in the organization of these efforts, which are not only sensitive to the issues of etiology and diagnosis but also seek to identify strategies for assisting families who survive a SIDS crisis.

These discussions have identified a cluster of characteristic clinical features that have been observed in many cases of infant death. The grouping together of these characteristics gives meaning to the term *syndrome* to describe the phenomenon whereby apparently healthy infants die suddenly and unexpectedly. A syndrome refers to a set of symptoms occurring together and serving to describe a morbid state. Because definitive conclusions about the etiology and pathogenesis of SIDS are still uncertain, a formal definition is neither appropriate nor feasible. The Second International Conference on Causes of Sudden Death in Infants agreed on a working description of this syndrome, which has enjoyed wide acceptance in the medical community since that time. This description will serve as an operational definition of the syndrome:

. . . the sudden death of any infant or young child, which is unexpected by history and in which a thorough post-mortem examination fails to demonstrate an adequate cause for death. (*Proceedings of the International Conference on Causes of Sudden Death in Infants*, Seattle, Wash.: University of Washington Press, 1970, p. 17)

Clinical Description of the Syndrome

General Descriptive Features

Infants who die of SIDS are generally discovered by a parent or babysitter either early in the morning or at a periodic check. Instinctively the infant is taken into the arms of the parent or caregiver, who frantically attempts to revive or resuscitate the baby. In cases where the infant has not been moved and emergency help called, the superficial observations are noteworthy. Occasionally the infant is found with its face pressed down and its hands reflect strenuous clutching and intense motoric activity. Beckwith (1973) noted the presence of feces and urine in the diaper of some SIDS infants. He considers this evidence of a reflex discharge suggesting that death was a "cataclysmic agonal event," his words evoking horrible, ominous images of struggle and suffering. Other pathologists are more conservative in estimating the number of instances (about 10 percent) in which the evidence would support such a description. Whatever the evidence, caution needs to be used in describing an infant's death as "agonal." This term refers to the death agony and implies some degree of pain and suffering. Such a label can be an additional burden to grieving parents if they dwell on the supposition that their babies died a torturous death.

While the SIDS literature occasionally makes reference to the appearance of *petechiae*, or bruisings, on the infant who succumbed to SIDS, this is not a common occurrence. This discoloration, when evident, may lead some police and emergency medical technicians who respond to an emergency call from parents of a SIDS victim to suspect child abuse as a cause of death. Petechiae on the surfaces of thoracic organs are known to be the result of sustained *hypoxemia* prior to death (Guntheroth, 1970, 1973). Hypoxemia refers to a deficiency in oxygenation of the blood. Petechiae related to hypoxemia are simple postmortem changes and are not to be confused with ecchymoses, or black-and-blue marks associated with physical injury or assault.

The definitive diagnosis of SIDS is determined through competent postmortem examination. The findings revealed by autopsies on SIDS victims are complex and consistent. A number of excellent summaries have been published, bringing together the major conclusions of pathologists who have studied these findings. Since 1967 Valdes-Dapena has published comprehensive reports of the world literature on SIDS (1967, 1970, 1977, 1980). Another concise presentation of major results of pathological studies has been made by Shaddy and McIntire (1982). This research will be discussed below under two headings: evidence from gross examination and the results of microscopic studies.

Gross Examination

In the majority of cases autopsied, the infants' bodies are generally well developed, even those who might have been premature or low birth weight. It is not unusual to note frothy or blood-tainted mucus in and about the nostrils. Such discharges may be associated with fluid in the lungs or pulmonary edema. As noted above, intrathoracic petechiae are found on the surfaces of the lungs, heart, and thymus and could be understood in relation to sustained hypoxemia (Beckwith, 1977). It is important to stress that in each of these pathological findings, no single lesion is sufficiently pathological to be the cause of death: this is the most important variable in arriving at the diagnosis of SIDS.

Other pathological findings note that blood in the heart is liquid, not clotted. The thymus, which is necessary in early life for the development and maturation of immunological functions, is frequently enlarged but still within normal limits. As expected, the urinary bladder is empty. Hemorrhagic fluid is found in the lungs, and the larynx or trachea often contains a bit of mucoid fluid or some aspirated gastric residue. This datum is noteworthy, as the presence of this gastroesophageal reflux seems to play an important role in apnea, which will be discussed later in the chapter. This reflux is an involuntary regurgitation of gastric contents in the esophagus without vomiting and without the involvement of either the gastric, abdominal, or diaphragmatic muscles. It is thought to cause obstruction in breathing (Pasquis, Tardif & Nouvet, 1983).

Microscopic Examination

Although there may be some histologic evidence of upper respiratory infection, and the number of viral and bacterial isolates may be higher in these babies, in general these are not considered to be present in lethal proportions. In some cases there is evidence of fibrinoid necrosis or cell death in the larynx. However, Emery and Dinsdale (1978) have shown that ulcerations in the larynx are no more frequent in SIDS victims than in properly selected controls.

At the time of autopsy SIDS infants are clearly not normal, yet the pathological variations do not adequately account for their sudden death. The insufficiency of these data to explain the cause of death establishes a diagnosis of SIDS. While competent gross examination of the infant's body can reasonably ascertain SIDS as a cause of death, diagnosis is only confirmed after both gross and microscopic postmortem examinations have been performed. The decision whether to perform a postmortem is the decision of the coroner or medical examiner and in many jurisdictions is a legal requirement. Of course, helping the parents of a SIDS infant understand the necessity for such a procedure is of utmost importance. This topic will be discussed later in the chapter.

Epidemiology of SIDS

With a brief clinical appreciation of the syndrome that claims thousands of babies each year, we may now turn our attention to its *epidemiology*, the study of the various factors determining the frequency and distribution of the disease in a community. Since the 1970s, epidemiological reports have begun to reveal some interesting information on the incidence of SIDS.

Age Distribution

Sudden Infant Death Syndrome is demonstrably not a neonatal syndrome, since it is rarely reported in infants prior to one month of age. The peak incidence for SIDS is 2–3 months, and 90 percent of SIDS victims are under 25 weeks of age. It is unusual to find the syndrome claiming a victim beyond 2 years of age. In this respect, it is an age-specific problem. As such, it is the largest single cause of postnatal mortality, accounting for the deaths in approximately 2-3 per 1,000, or .2 percent, of live births each year in urbanized Western societies who have monitored the incidence of this syndrome and have reported these data.

It is difficult to project accurate statistics on the incidence of SIDS. Although many reports in the United States and abroad seem to indicate a decrease in the number of cases, the figures fluctuate from year to year. For example, Naeye noted an increase in the number of SIDS cases in the United States during the winter of 1982–1983 (Naeye, personal communication, May 12, 1983). Any significant reduction in fatalities may be attributable to better identification of neonates at risk, particularly those with repeated apneic episodes. In some of these cases precautionary hospitalization with cardiac and respiratory monitoring may rescue these infants at risk from becoming SIDS victims.

Medical, Familial, Socioeconomic, and Climatic Variables

As noted above, the early 1970s witnessed the publication of numerous studies that combed case histories in an effort to identify clues to etiology. These studies succeeded in recognizing a number of factors that correlated positively with the incidence of SIDS. In no instance were these seen to be causal, and careful multivariate analysis is still needed to demonstrate the possible interactive and causative effects of certain common factors. The findings have contributed, however, to a more complete picture of the most likely SIDS victims.

It seems that SIDS has a greater incidence among males, particularly those born into lower socioeconomic groups (Bergman, Ray & Pomeroy, 1972). Premature infants (34 weeks of gestational age) and full-term infants of small birth weight (less than 2500 grams at birth) appear to be at higher statistical risk of falling victim to SIDS than their full-term average-weight counterparts

(Lipsitt *et al.*, 1981), as are neonates requiring intensive care after birth and who are discharged from neonatal intensive care units (Kulkarni *et al.*, 1978).

Curiously, this syndrome is less frequent in first-born infants and more prevalent among second children (Froggatt *et al.*, 1971; Peterson, 1972). The incidence of SIDS increases with the number of children in a family because the infection rate likewise increases. Possibly, minor infections brought home by older children trigger the death of the infant sibling. According to Naeye, infection plays a significant role in the etiology of SIDS (Naeye, personal communication, May 12, 1983).

Sudden Infant Death Syndrome is also found among multiple-birth infants, regardless of zygosity (Kraus & Borkhani, 1972). Although this may be related to birth weight, it is an interesting statistic and may lend some additional support to those theories emphasizing the effect of environmental factors.

Another variable repeatedly mentioned in discussions of SIDS is the higher incidence of this syndrome during the winter months, regardless of the ambient temperature of the various geographical regions that figure prominently in the statistics. (Bergman *et al.*, 1972). This variable frequently accompanies evidence of mild upper respiratory tract infection in numbers of SIDS victims (Guntheroth *et al.*, 1980). While these trends have been noted in the United States and similar supportive patterns have been reported in Australia, Czechoslovakia, Denmark, France, Germany, Great Britain, and Japan, the evidence is still inconclusive. Children with apneic spells have more such spells and longer spells when they have an infection (Naeye, personal communication, May 12, 1983).

A number of maternal factors may also have some bearing on the epidemiology of SIDS. The incidence among infants of unmarried women is significant. These women are often young (less than 20 years of age) and many have had little or no prenatal obstetrical care (Bergman *et al.*, 1972; Kraus & Borhani, 1972). Incidence of SIDS among cigarette smokers and drug-dependent women is also notable (Bergman, 1976). Of particular significance is the use of methadone (Pierson *et al.*, 1972). Further, a short interpregnancy interval may have some relationship to the incidence of this syndrome (Lewak *et al.*, 1979).

Whether any of the variables cited in relationship to maternal characteristics are directly related to the syndrome is uncertain. Little recent study has focused on these questions, and most of the information concerning them depends heavily on early research. All of the maternal characteristics cited seem to point to environmental stresses, but these issues alone do not account for a higher incidence of SIDS, since infants in quite opposite conditions fall victim to the syndrome.

One final variable that links the majority of SIDS victims is sleep. Most infants who die of this syndrome are discovered in their cribs. Occasionally there are reports of infants dying in their carriages while being wheeled by a parent, or of infants who succumb while being nursed. Regardless of circumstances, the preponderance of cases involve sleeping infants. Most parents recall no audible outcry in the agonal moment, and death seems to occur noiselessly when the infant is almost certainly asleep. Whether sleep is a necessary component of the syndrome is a central issue about which the major theories and much research revolves.

Theoretical Approaches to Sudden Infant Death Syndrome

Numerous theories have arisen in the attempt to explain the mystery surrounding the timing, circumstances, and environmental conditions of SIDS and the perplexing pathological evidence garnered from thousands of postmortem examinations of infants who have died suddenly. Each of these theories attempts to explain the etiologic and pathogenetic factors related to this syndrome. Although there are literally dozens of theoretical formulations, only the principal thematic approaches will be reviewed.

Apnea Theory

Alfred Steinschneider's pioneering work has been instrumental in stimulating research on the relationship between SIDS and apnea. *Apnea* refers to an interruption of respiratory function or breathing. Steinschneider (1972) reported on several infants who manifested prolonged apneic episodes after several weeks of normal life. These episodes were irregular, but seemed to occur most often during periods when the infant suffered *nasopharyngitis*, or inflammation of the nasopharynx. Some of these infants eventually died of SIDS.

The theory relating apnea to SIDS has gained wide acceptance in the field of SIDS research, and a number of independent sources substantiate it. Because SIDS is at least temporally related to infants who appear to succumb during sleep periods, it is reasonable to look for causal relationships with sleep-related disorders. Many respiratory reflexes may be depressed during *REM-Sleep*, rapid eye movements or active sleep, creating a situation of greater vulnerability to asphyxia (Read *et al.*, 1982). Steinschneider (1972) noted that the periods of apnea were most frequent during periods of REM-sleep.

Such vulnerability to asphyxia in sleep, coupled with subclinical damage to respiratory reflexes, can trigger periods of arrested breathing. A similar phenomenon is seen in adults who display chronic abnormalities in respiration and who characteristically underventilate their lungs during sleep. In both of these situations lung volume and oxygen gas stores are reduced, intercostal muscles are checked, and breathing is maintained by the diaphragm.

Naeye assumes that such characteristic underventilation of the lungs would leave anatomical tissue markers. His research has identified abnormal increases of muscle in the small pulmonary arteries of 60 percent of the SIDS victims he has examined. This, he supposes, was directly related to chronic hypoxemia.

Naeye (1980) has reported on the implications of these observations. The process he describes has a coherent logic. If an infant is chronically underventilating, the number of muscle cells in the pulmonary arterial walls will increase. This condition is identified as *hyperplasia*. The result of this process is the resistance of the vascular system to provide adequate blood flow to the lungs. In turn, this places additional stress on the right ventricle of the heart. The heart responds to this pressure in a way similar to that of the pulmonary arteries, by increasing the amount of muscle in the right ventricular wall. This dual manifestation of hyperplasia in both the pulmonary arteries and heart reduces the level of oxygen in the pulmonary air spaces and in arterial blood circulating throughout the body.

The tissue markers Naeye expected to find as a result of this chronic condition of hypoxemia were identified. In more than half of the SIDS victims he autopsied, abnormal amounts of brown fat had been retained. At birth this brown fat surrounds some vital organs, but in the course of infant development the organelles, or *mitochondria*, are lost and the cells lose their brown coloration and distinctive microscopic appearance.

When infants are chronically hypoxemic, they characteristically retain these fat cells with their brown-colored mitochondria. The implication of this anatomical phenomenon is apparent: such evidence in postmortem examination suggests chronic hypoxemia. Naeye supports his contention by citing other supportive evidence, including the increase in adrenal gland tissue, which produces epinephrine. The secretion of epinephrine may partially account for the retention of brown fat cells.

All of this research lends intelligibility to the relationship of apnea to SIDS and suggests the possibility of some physiological handicap before birth. This continues to be an important research question, as does the reason for underventilation.

David Read (1982) has attempted to further illuminate the mystery of underventilation. His research indicates that respiration control is managed differently in the first months of life than in later life.

Infants spend the major portion of a 24-hour period engaged in sleep. In this early developmental period, the infant may invest 50–80 percent of its average 16-hour sleep in a state resembling REM-sleep. In trying to understand the developmental significance of this characteristic sleep pattern in infants, it has been suggested that REM-sleep may furnish the central nervous system with endogenous stimulation at a time when exogenous stimulation is not that available. REM-sleep in infants would provide stimulation to key sensory and motor areas of the nervous system during this critical period of growth and maturation. Not only may this internal stimulation provide practice to key motor and sensory pathways of the brain, but it may contribute to a form of primitive programming that may be responsible for the integration of instinctive and environmental events.

Read notes in neonates during the first 6 months of life a partial collapse of the lungs during the REM-phase of sleep. This partial collapse occurs because the intercostal muscles cease functioning, creating a condition in which respiration is interrupted and hypoxemia ensues. When this occurs, survival depends on reflex arousal from REM-sleep and the retriggering of those brain-stem mechanisms that control breathing.

The inability to restart breathing once it has stopped may be related to the underdevelopment of the principal artery of the neck, the *carotid*. This small neurovascular structure, the carotid body, contains chemoreceptors that monitor the oxygen content of the blood and helps to regulate respiration.

Naeye (1976) reports that there was evidence of carotid underdevelopment in more than half of the SIDS cases he autopsied. These same infants showed evidence of chronic hypoxemia with the characteristic signs described earlier. Naeye and associates (1976, 1980) have hypothesized that carotid underdevelopment may be directly related to the lack of stimulation to the carotid from the respiratory control centers in the brain stem. A carotid body reflex may be initiated by changes in blood oxygen content acting on chemoreceptors in the carotid body.

To verify this hypothesis is exceedingly difficult given the anatomical and functional complexity of these and other centers that control the activities of diverse vital organs. There is some initial supportive evidence of astroglial fibers in the lateral reticular formation of the brain stem that may result from chronic hypoxemia (Naeye, 1976). This may indicate CNS damage and help to explain dysfunction in the central mechanism that controls autonomic response.

The difficulty in verifying underdevelopment in the centers that control respiration and other vital functioning, as noted above, is related to the structural complexity of these centers and their close association with each other. One might reasonably expect that infants with weakened abilities to control respiration might also display other functional deficits, such as feeding and temperature regulation. Although this is an intriguing avenue of correlative research, it has not been adequately demonstrated that such a relationship does in fact exist in SIDS victims.

Much of the ongoing research seeking to establish a relationship between apneic episodes and SIDS (Harper *et al*. 1981; Stockard, 1982; Camfield, *et al*., 1982; Guilleminault, *et al*., 1984) is uncovering valuable information. In reviewing the world medical literature on this issue, Valdes-Dapena (1980) concluded that "idiopathic protracted apnea, especially during sleep, *may* be part of the pathogenetic mechanism in *some* instances of SIDS." While much of this knowledge positively correlates with postmortem findings in a large percentage of SIDS victims, it does nothing to explain the 30 percent of cases in which such pathological indications of chronic hypoxemia are lacking. In a careful review of the relationship between apnea of infancy and Sudden Infant Death Syndrome, Brooks (1982) has noted several different pathophysiologic mechanisms. Some of these mechanisms are related to abnormal neuroreflex control of cardiac and respiratory functioning and may provide an explanation for the syndrome.

Psychophysiological Theories

In those cases where signs of chronic hypoxemia are not present, the variable of sleep remains constant. Newborns and infants, as noted above, spend more than half of their total sleep time in REM-sleep. As the infant matures, the amount of REM-sleep progressively diminishes (Hoppenbrou-wers, *et al.*, 1982). Researchers who have monitored this developmental pattern think that the progressive reduction in the ratio of REM-sleep to total sleep time relates to the maturation of central nervous system processes. The interactive relationship between carotid bodies and the brain stem, which was discussed earlier in the chapter, is linked to this maturation process. REM-sleep provides an intense source of stimulation to the central nervous system, and thus functionally excites the higher cortical centers—one of which controls respiration. As these centers mature, they may have less need of endogenous stimulation and this may account for the progressive decline in the amount of REM-sleep required.

This hypothetical explanation for the diminution in REM-sleep parallels observations made by some experimental developmental psychologists (Lipsitt, 1979) who have identified the gradual weakening or waning of congenital reflexive activities in neonates and infants. The fact of progress from reflexive to voluntary activity is well established. Lipsitt reasons that as cortical innervation progresses, subcortical control of reflexes probably becomes subservient to newly learned responses. Using this paradigm which identifies certain developmental relationships between congenital reflexive activities and sensory experience, another attempt to understand SIDS has been mounted. In this approach, attention is focused on learned defensive responses, which replace the congenital reflexes that decay with progressive cortical maturation.

In presenting a behavioral hypothesis related to SIDS, Lipsitt builds upon the pioneering work of pathologists and physiologists who have isolated important pathologic indicants, none of which is sufficiently serious to cause death. He moves the research a step further when he investigates the implication these pathologic signs may have for psychophysiological development.

In reviewing some of the aspects of the developmental histories of many SIDS victims, it was noted that prematurity, lowered birth weight, and other perinatal complications are often cited (Lipsitt *et al.*, 1981). If neonates have suffered anoxia, they may be enervated, displaying less motoric and visual involvement. In general, they make less contact with their environment. Since many developmentalists consider environmental contact and stimulation to be critical vehicles for survival learning, an infant who is deprived of this crucial experience is potentially at risk.

Studying insects, reptiles, and mammals, comparative psychologists have documented many instances in which delays in learning and appropriating critical survival behaviors have resulted in the premature deaths of neonates and infants of these various species. It is possible that such a learning disability in human infants can be either a contributing or precipitating factor in their premature and sudden death.

Healthy neonates are born with a repertory of unconditioned responses that are important for their continued learning and survival. As *myelination*, the process of sheathing and insulating the nerve axon from surrounding tissue and fluids, proceeds and dendrites proliferate, these rudimentary reflexes change markedly and are replaced by learned responses. It may be reasoned that this period of accelerated development of the neonate's neurophysiological function is directly related to the accretion of specific learned responses, and that some of these must be appropriated during this time (Lipsitt, 1979). It is as if these learned responses must be in place by the time the unconditioned reflexes are programmed to decay and are rendered dysfunctional.

Lipsitt, Sturner, and Burke (1979) suppose that the neonate who does not respond reflexively and aggressively to threats of respiratory occlusion may be an infant-at-risk for SIDS. This supposition undergirds Lipsitt's hypothesis: "If the newborn does not have a strong defensive response to threats to respiration or head restraint, however, it is possible that the appropriate voluntary operant behaviors will not become learned which must ultimately supplant this congenital response by 2 to 4 months of age" (Lipsitt, 1979, p. 35).

Given much of the data already discussed about the histories and pathology reports of SIDS victims, this learned-response hypothesis has some merit. According to it, infants who have not learned to engage in responses necessary to clear airway passages threatened with blockage will be in special danger when the unconditioned protective reflexes no longer ensure the safety of the organism. Lipsitt would argue that crib death is the consequence of the interaction of "minimal congenital deficiencies with environmental conditions that fail to ameliorate the basically organic deficit" (Lipsett, 1974, p. 36).

Until very recently it would have been purely speculative to assume that the brain anatomy could be affected by experience. Neuroscientists have now demonstrated that variations in sensory and social aspects of the environment of the neonate can affect both the gross and fine structure of the brain (Greenough, 1975; Greenough, Wolkmar, & Fleischman, 1976). Enriching the environment of the newborn can have pronounced metabolic and structural effects. Such plasticity of the cortex might reasonably be expected to serve some adaptive function. Since normal cortical development prepares for voluntary defensive reaction as neonatal reflexes decay, it is plausible that with appropriate stimulation, an infant-at-risk could be helped to learn responses that will later ensure survival, particularly if these responses are not forthcoming.

These theories attempt to reconcile the data gleaned from clinical observation, pathological studies of SIDS victims, and epidemiological reports. Not only are they important supports to ongoing SIDS research, but they can provide useful information to those medical and psychological practitioners who must face the task of interpreting these same data to grieving parents who mourn the premature loss of their baby.

Psychological Issues for the Families of SIDS Victims

Sudden Infant Death Syndrome is one of the most traumatic crises parents may face. The infant's death is so unexpected and explanations about cause so unsatisfactory that survivors are ill prepared for such a loss. The particular circumstances of the infant's death place the family in a situation of special vulnerability, and efforts to intervene may actually exacerbate the grief (Smialek, 1978). Many excellent efforts to understand the particular constellation of feelings of SIDS survivors have aided professionals and other service personnel to be more effective in their combined efforts to assist parents and families who experience such a tragic infant death (Bluglass, 1981; Chernus, 1982; Crawshaw, 1978; DeFrain & Ernst, 1978; DeFrain, Taylor, & Ernst, 1982; Emery, 1972; Krein, 1978; May & Breme, 1983; Williams & Nikolaisen, 1982).

Many of the studies of SIDS survivors identify a common set of reactions. Although some of these reactions are related to a more general set of responses to loss, the particular circumstances of a sudden infant death without apparent cause does merit a special discussion of these reactions. In addition, it is the consensus among many practitioners in the fields of medicine, nursing, and mental health that the impact of SIDS upon surviving parents and family members may be more problematic than that occasioned by other losses and other circumstances of death. Although this would be difficult to prove, ample evidence supports the position. Several of the relevant findings will be examined and some implications for intervention with SIDS survivors will be explored.

Initial Impact of Discovery of a Dead Infant

Many SIDS victims are discovered in the course of a routine supervisory check by a caregiver. The shock of finding a cold and lifeless body in the crib or carriage plunges the parent or guardian into a numbing panic. Instinctively the adult may attempt to revive the infant, shaking the infant's body and engaging in frantic mouth-to-mouth breathing. When efforts of this sort fail to resuscitate the child, police and emergency medical resources are summoned.

It was early in the morning when I went to check on Karen. Her crib was a horror to behold. The blankets were in a mound in the corner and my little baby was tangled up within them. Frantically I picked her up and knew immediately that she was dead, but I would not let myself believe it. In rage I threw the blankets on the floor and began to scream for help. John came running in from the bathroom where he was shaving. 'What are we going to do?' I cried. John was already on the phone; I stood there sobbing, holding my dear Karen in my quivering arms.

—A Massachusetts mother

Police and hospital emergency room reports frequently describe the parents or guardians of the SIDS victim as visibly shaken, in a trancelike state. This extreme manifestation of denial can last for hours, and is often punctuated by formulaic statements of personal culpability: "It's all my fault; I let my baby die." Denial is a normal and anticipated response in these traumatic circumstances. It is not unusual that parents speak of the deceased infant in both present and past tenses. From the moment the infant is discovered, a rapid series of interventions is set in motion that overwhelms the grief-stricken parent or parents. The momentum created by these events has been described by some SIDS parents as a nightmare from which they never fully expect to awake. Certain aspects of reality interpose themselves, forcing the surviving family members to accept the fact of the infant's death. As this truth is gradually assimilated and denial becomes a less effective defense, it is replaced by a variety of expressions of guilt (Krein, 1979). DeFrain, Taylor, and Ernst (1982) report a Kansas mother's reflections a year after the sudden death of her daughter (p. 18).

Immediately after the death was a feeling of depression, loss of goals and overall confusion. It still does not seem like our baby has been gone for over a year. At times I wonder if we did everything possible or whether we did something wrong; but then I remember how happy our little one was, and the good times we had and I remember her smile and laugh.

I frequent the gravesite to gaze upon the grave, look to the sky for hope, faith and strength and to think and to maybe give myself peace of mind. In my heart I know we were not at fault, but little things remind me of her and I wonder.

The parents likewise become victims of the syndrome that has precipitously claimed the life of their infant. Because no cause can be immediately identified to them, nor the possibility of neglect or negligence ruled out as a contributing factor, the parents are vulnerable to their own self-blame. Although police and other related service personnel may have no intention to impute blame or culpability, their behaviors or interrogation may communicate suspicion. In situations of grief, a spouse may accuse the other, or both may be ready to blame the pediatrician who did not diagnose whatever caused the death to happen, or the emergency medical personnel who did not succeed in resuscitating their child.

When the police arrived, one of the officers grabbed Karen from my arms and began mouth-to-mouth resuscitation efforts. The other officer tried to calm John and me; he began to ask some questions, but I was unable to respond. John got angry with the police, asking why they did not send an ambulance with oxygen. The officers were both patient with us and helped us to regain some control and we accompanied them to the hospital. . . .

—A Massachusetts mother

Aware of the extremely disruptive circumstances in which a family finds itself, those who deal with the parents and family need to be particularly sensitive. The quality and competence of early contacts with the bereaved parents and family can have a potentially significant impact upon the course of their readjustment and recovery.

Support to the family begins with the first contact (Stevenson, 1981). In no sense should efforts be made to block the ventilation of feelings. Parents will often want to accompany their infant to the hospital emergency room. They should be afforded whatever privacy is available. This is not always an easy thing to provide, but some attention should be given to this need. As soon as possible they should be given some information about the suspected cause of their child's death. Since an autopsy will be necessary to definitively diagnose SIDS, parents will need to be prepared for this legal procedure.

It is to be expected that parents will frequently be engaged in what Freud termed an "obsessional review" (Freud, 1917). They will aimlessly retrace all of the events that led up to the discovery, looking for any clue or sign which they might have missed. This process may appear to be counterproductive, but it can aid in their acceptance of the reality of the death, even though it frequently can contribute to an increase in the sense of personal guilt. Nurses and physicians can help the grieving parents by suggesting that there may be a more rational explanation for the infant's death than the premature cause they may have settled upon. The postmortem examination can contribute to this understanding.

   While we were sitting in the hospital waiting room, John and I kept going over everything we had done with Karen the day before. We kept reviewing every movement and every sound we could recall, looking for some clue that might help us to understand why she died. John had put her back in her crib after the two o'clock feeding. He remembered placing her on her stomach, with her head gently turned toward him. He covered her with the lovely blanket his mother had crocheted for her, with pink tea roses. His last memory was bending down to kiss her head. "Maybe I shouldn't have put her on her stomach after giving her a bottle; maybe I didn't burp her right. . . ."

—A Massachusetts mother

Entering the phenomenal and grief-stricken world of parents at this time to inform them that a postmortem examination is to be performed is a difficult task for many professionals. Two ineffectual approaches are common in medical practice. The first is detached, dealing quickly with the suspected cause of death and informing parents of the legal requirement of an autopsy in a matter-of-fact manner. The other is a hesitant bridging of the question, communicating as little as possible to the parents, avoiding mention of the autopsy. This procedure is crucial to the diagnosis, even though certain of the superficial characteristics of a gross examination of the deceased infant might lend strong support to the suspected diagnosis of SIDS. There is much merit to an approach that patiently works to gain parental understanding of the value of the autopsy without communicating in either a cool, indifferent manner or in a way that skirts the issue entirely.

Because guilt feelings of parents are often quite intense at this time, it is understandable that they might initially be opposed to the autopsy even though it is legally mandated, but there is no substitute for the time that is required to assist them in understanding the necessity and purpose for such a procedure.

The professional needs to be prepared for the unleashing of both physical and verbal abuse when the topic of an autopsy is raised. It is a final acknowledgement that the child is dead. This form of catharsis is helpful to the parents, although it requires a significant degree of understanding and control on the part of the attending professionals. It has been the experience of many nurses and physicians that parents usually accept the necessity of an autopsy even when they were initially quite forcefully opposed to such a procedure.

Parents may require some personal medical attention themselves. For example, if the mother was nursing the deceased infant, she will require medication to suppress lactation. Also, the emotional expenditure of the couple is intense, and they may request some mild sedation. However, many physicians are too quick to offer tranquillizers to grieving parents. Rather than proving beneficial, drugs of this sort may inhibit normal grief and appropriate mourning. Frequent contacts with primary care personnel during these early hours of the crisis are of incalculable benefit to the parents and survivors.

As soon as the postmortem examination has been completed, it is desirable that the results be communicated to the parents. Although it places an additional burden on the pathologist to meet with the parents, it is a worthwhile investment of time and trouble. As the individual who has performed the autopsy, the pathologist is in a key position to provide accurate information to the parents and to gently counter false explanations the parents may be using to blame themselves. Because guilt feelings are generally high among SIDS parents, they have a strong need for reliable information (Lowman, 1979).

The ambiguous nature of SIDS may make physicians uncomfortable in communicating with bereaved parents, but the content and manner of their communication is crucial to the psychological recovery of parents and families. It is admittedly an art to translate pathology findings into language non-medical persons can understand. The essence of this communication must be that the parents in no way caused or could have anticipated or prevented what happened to their infant. This may need to be repeated a number of times since grieving persons do not always hear what is being said to them.

Apart from the presentation of factual evidence that supports a conclusive diagnosis of SIDS, the physician needs to be prepared to listen to the parents and to respond carefully to the questions they inevitably pose. Frequently these questions will provide rich insight into the ways in which they are experiencing the loss and may guide future planning of resources to assist them.

Concern for Other Children in the Family

A frequent concern identified by parents is their relationship to their other children (DeFrain, Taylor & Ernst, 1982; Nikolaisen, 1981; Williams, Lee & Polak, 1976). In the emotional upheaval within the family, other children are vulnerable. Some parents find it difficult to speak openly with their other children about the deceased infant, and they become increasingly upset when they note behavioral changes in them. Reports of nightmares, enuresis, problems in school, crying, and withdrawal are not uncommon among the siblings of SIDS victims. These normal grief reactions in bereaved children are not assisted when they are met with uncharacteristic emotional responses in parents, especially anger, impatience, and volatile tantrums (Williams, 1981). These and other concerns about the siblings of the SIDS victim may be raised in conversation with the physician or visiting nurse who may follow up with the family (Stevenson, 1981).

Because the circumstances of the infant's death are cloaked in mystery, it is understandable that the whole experience may be relegated to the realm of secrecy (Cepeda, 1981). A more direct approach may be necessary to elicit concerns from parents about their other children. It is not unusual that parents may need assistance so that they can talk productively with their surviving children about the death of an infant sibling.

Parents try to adjust their communication to the cognitive level of the child. In doing this they are prone to use euphemisms and circumlocutions that skirt the fact and reality of the death. It would be interesting to trace the effect of certain of these false communications in early childhood and their contribution to the development of phobias in later life. Simple, direct communication is always preferable to tales of fantasy. Cepeda (1981) suggests clear statements like: "He died; he will not be coming back." Young children are far more capable of understanding death than was once thought. Although this understanding may be primitive, certain cognitive aspects of it being proper to their particular stage of development, young children nonetheless can grasp the notion of death. Little is still known about the ways in which children relate to the death of an infant sibling (Black, 1978). However, some common concerns frequently are voiced.

The death of an infant sibling may excite in a child a concern for his or her own well-being. "Am I going to die too?" is the voiced concern of numbers of bereaved children. This question is difficult for parents to hear, and touches a point of particular vulnerability. Parents need to know that SIDS is an *infant* syndrome, rarely affecting a child more than a year old. They must thus reassure their children.

We know that in early childhood the mind is comparable to a sponge capable of absorbing everything in its environment. In addition to their own personal feelings of loss, children absorb the feelings and emotional reactions of their parents. They interpret protective and overprotective behaviors by parents as causes for concern and alarm. Perhaps they feel as if they too might die just as their infant brother or sister did. They see the parents' behaviors toward them as attempts to prevent this event from happening.

Parents need to be helped to develop greater insight into the complex constellation of feelings that form the inner world of the surviving child, and be
encouraged to listen and talk with the child. Peer support groups of other
SIDS parents have proven to be the single best resource for helping parents
to bridge the topic of death with surviving children. The personal experiences
of these other parents are invaluable assets to recently bereaved parents who
feel ambivalent about what to say to surviving children. Discussions among
peers often uncover excellent ways for parents to respond to the important
needs of their children.

Just as parents require some rational explanation for the infant's death, so
children will often ask: "Why did he die?" Although parents have asked this
question many times and the best answers available have been given to them,
there is no completely satisfactory answer to the question. Most parents are
prone to answer the child's query with: "I don't know." It is important to underscore the complete acceptability of this answer. There is honesty and integrity in not having an explanation.

Older children who conceptually grasp the notion of cause and effect may
initially be unsettled by such a reply. Given the nature of SIDS, for which no
single cause can be pinpointed, the lack of an identifiable cause itself must
serve as an explanation for death. This is admittedly difficult for many children
to grasp; many adults have difficulty understanding this themselves. The most
important point to make is that the child's question is an excellent opportunity
to engage communication between the parent and the child. The question
may be masking other pressing concerns that need ventilation. Communication of this sort may be somewhat distressing and awkward, but it can also
be extremely therapeutic for parent and child alike.

Impact on Marital Relationship

Any major crisis can place stress on the marital relationship. Whatever
areas of vulnerability may exist in the relationship may be heightened by the
emotional sequelae of a sudden infant death. Spouses are individuals and
have different life experiences and different styles of coping. If these patterns
are essentially different or conflict with each other, they place additional stress
on the relationship.

For many couples the loss of an infant may be their first personal encounter with death (Nikolaisen, 1981). Because of the circumstances, they are
frequently unprepared for such a stress and are unskilled in understanding
their own feelings as well as the feelings of a grieving spouse.

Women seem to be at somewhat greater psychological risk and their grief
may be prolonged. The particularly close maternal bond so necessary to human survival is ruptured, leaving a mother open to a wide array of feelings.
The death of the infant has interrupted the rhythm of her life and has broken
the routine that governed her activities. Bereaved mothers occasionally report
experiencing hallucinations, believing that they hear the baby crying in an
adjoining room. Some women acknowledge preparing food or bath water as
they ordinarily had done when the infant was alive. These experiences not only

revive the painful memories and loss but they frighten mothers, who may quickly interpret them to mean that they are losing their minds.

Self-confidence suffers a significant blow, and many women report doubts about their abilities to care for children. These self-doubts can be reinforced by the implications and innuendos that may be inadvertently communicated by physicians, nurses, spouses, or other members of the family. They are internalized to such a degree that the conclusion is certain: "I am not a good mother." This process of self-depreciation can be a significant factor in the depression that preys upon many SIDS mothers.

Recrimination and scapegoating within the extended family is a defensive attempt to deal with the devastating aspects of the loss. However, frequently the mother of the deceased infant becomes the object of this projection of blame. Grandparents can contribute to this difficulty by masking their own grief and attributing carelessness to their own children. This can be particularly true of in-laws who adhere to strict sex role stereotypes and directly or indirectly assign culpability for the grandchild's death to their daughter-in-law.

It is interesting to note that the bereaved mother attracts the most attention. The father escapes notice for several reasons, but this should not be interpreted to imply that he is not at risk. In fact, many of the external clues that signal rapid adjustment may be camouflaging pain and uncertainty. One significant source of marital conflict is the inability of one or other of the spouses to talk about his or her pain. Some men find it exceedingly difficult to share their pain.

Some men feel a responsibility to protect their wives from what they judge to be unnecessary additional pain (DeFrain, Taylor & Ernst, 1982; Hawkins, 1980). This reasoning leads them to mask their own hurt and sense of loss. However, the well-intentioned effort to protect the other has destructive consequences on both individuals. The protected one feels emotionally isolated at a time when open and shared feelings are needed. The protector is prevented from access to normal channels for ventilation of feelings and the working through of the grief occasioned by the loss. In the course of their extensive research of SIDS families, DeFrain, Taylor, and Ernst received numerous written replies. The men, they report, were less frequent respondents and when they did reply, wrote less. One Nebraska father was more verbal and summarized his feelings and perceptions quite well.

I sensed people were telling me it was all right for me to have cried immediately following Jennifer's death, but now my mourning must stop and I should be able to repel those strong emotions and be a man for my wife, family and society. My wife was allowed a period to not be herself, but I was expected to go back to work upon our return and function as though nothing had happened. My tender defense emotions quickly turned into a feeling of hostility toward society in general as it somehow told me I couldn't really be myself, I couldn't cry anymore, I must be strong, I must be a man. (DeFrain, Taylor & Ernst, 1982, p. 25)

Husbands ordinarily do resume their normal occupations quickly and this reengagement of daily routine may have certain therapeutic benefits. Although ambivalent feelings may be present, as the case above shows, the resumption of ordinary routine tasks can ease the psychological adjustment. Women, on the other hand, if they were primarily occupied with care of the deceased infant, experience a profound void. Frequently men do not sufficiently appreciate the emotional lacunae wives describe. Women find it difficult to help their husbands understand that these holes in their lives are not simply filled by taking on many activities.

Discussions of these kinds of issues can rupture the thin membrane separating many fathers from their own grief and some men respond defensively. They try to propose facile solutions to their spouses, and these very efforts can contribute to a growing alienation between the couple.

Efforts to support grieving parents need to include ways of contacting both of the partners. Ideally, conjoint interventions are the most useful since they provide opportunities and supportive structures to assist both individuals in expressing their feelings. More importantly, such interventions help to establish communication between the spouses that is crucial to many future decisions about surviving children and future pregnancies.

Replacement Child

A recognizable strategy many people employ to deal with loss is to seek replacement (Bluglass, 1981). Applied to the situation faced by parents bereaved by the sudden death of an infant, this basic psychological principle may appear to be an invalid solution. However, it is not unusual that bereaved couples will choose to begin a pregnancy soon after the death of the infant, and the decision is generally welcomed by family and friends.

The psychological liability of such a choice can, in fact, be considerable. Grieving is a taxing process that requires a significant psychological and physical investment of energy but is productive when properly assumed and allowed to proceed along its charted course. It has been estimated that grief work requires several weeks of concentrated effort but is diffused through the first year following the loss. Replacement pregnancy may halt this process, delay it, or abort it altogether.

Pregnancy is sufficiently fraught with anxiety, even in the most healthy circumstances. It is quite understandable that a couple who have lost a child to SIDS will experience some additional anxieties as they prepare themselves emotionally to give birth to and care for another child. Information they may have assimilated from their own research of SIDS or from data presented to them by nurses and physicians may inadvertently fuel this anxiety. Many such parents worry about predispositions to the syndrome in their new baby, and many become excessively vigilant. Some develop phobic reactions and express doubts about their abilities to care for a newborn. The following passage illustrates the heightening of anxiety that can occur as a parent attends the birth of another child.

> Two months after Chris died I found out I was pregnant but it had to be within days of Chris' death. I wasn't trying to replace Christopher but I knew I wanted to have more children. I wasn't sure if I was emotionally ready.
>
> I didn't realize what the birth of Benjamin really did for all of us until a few months after he was born. There was fear, incredible fear, but along with that came a great healing process. Much of my anger was leaving me and to be able to love and be loved by another human being was wonderful. I was once again feeling good about myself and my life.
>
> By the end of the pregnancy, I didn't think that this baby was going to solve any problems at all. I felt that maybe there were going to be a whole lot of problems. I really thought I was going to become a mental case; that it was going to be a constant worry. I wasn't going to be able to sleep; I was going to make this baby crazy with overprotection. . . . (DeFrain, Taylor, & Ernst, 1982, p. 77)

Obstetricians and providers of prenatal care need to be particularly sensitive to both the issue of incomplete grieving and the possible intensification of anxiety in pregnancies following a sudden infant death. Openness in exploring both of these problems with parents can be very beneficial to parents and can enhance the pregnancy experience.

As far as a replacement child is concerned, it is wise to allow parents to decide this question on their own. Those who may counsel parents of a SIDS victim need to be helped to come to terms with the fact that another child will never replace the one that has been lost, since each child is unique. If a first-born child becomes a SIDS victim, the second pregnancy may create problems that are psychological in nature, including fears and night tremors. However, the existence of several children in a family at the time of a SIDS death often mitigates the problems of a subsequent pregnancy. All of these issues need to be considered when counsel is engaged with SIDS parents exploring the question of another pregnancy.

Because overprotection is a natural reaction in parents who have experienced a sudden infant death, some further counsel may be necessary. Parents report difficulties in sleeping and find themselves checking the infant on dozens of occasions throughout the day and particularly during the night. If the newborn, given the recent family history of SIDS, is judged to be at some risk because of recurring apneic episodes, the use of a monitoring system may be suggested. An apnea monitor measures thoracic movement and signals any cessation of movement.

It must be recognized that such a preventive device, while allaying some fears in parents and providing them some measure of control, can at the same time increase their anxiety. The parents of infants who are placed on apnea monitors will need help in using such an apparatus and in learning to perform cardiopulmonary resuscitation should an actual emergency occur. More crucial than teaching the simple mechanics involved in these procedures, however, is addressing the natural anxieties and apprehensions of the parents, who usually report feeling relieved when the critical period of the first year has passed. The apnea monitor issue is very complex and requires discussion beyond the scope of this chapter. The literature on this question is extensive and merits a careful review.

Population at Special Risk: the Single Parent

The entire discussion of SIDS has assumed an intact family situation comprised of two spouses and frequently an older sibling. While this in fact may describe the normative population affected by SIDS, it excludes another group that may be at even higher psychological risk. There has been an increasingly higher number of births reported among single parents. Since demographic and etiologic data place some of these births in categories of additional risk for SIDS, this subgroup requires special attention.

Many of the ordinary support systems that assist monogamous couples may not be available to a single parent. Many SIDS-related situations involve a single woman, usually in her late teens or early twenties, and an interplay of certain socioeconomic and psychological factors.

Women who are attempting to raise an infant in situations of inadequate food and shelter may be at greater risk for SIDS. These same women, because of their immaturity, lack of educational opportunities, and economic disadvantage may not have benefited from proper prenatal care and routine pediatric follow-up for their babies. Should sudden infant death claim their children, they may prove to be more vulnerable than their married counterparts.

Single mothers more easily fall prey to the suspicions of neglect and abuse as contributing factors to the sudden and unexplained death of an infant. The generally impoverished conditions in which some of these people live tend to reinforce these suspicions. We have already discussed at some length the reactions of the average couple to the investigation and interrogation of police and other service professionals in the routine follow-up of a sudden infant death. The grief of a single parent is compounded when she is alone and has little or no social support upon which she can depend.

For many such single persons, this may be the first major adult crisis they have had to face and the first time they have had to turn to social service personnel for advice and support. They may not have the skills to use these social services well, and may prematurely disengage themselves from the support process. Because the trauma of loss is intensified by the environmental circumstances in which a single parent finds herself, all of these factors require special care and attention in planning, coordinating, and delivering support to her.

Summary

The sudden, unexpected, unexplainable death of a baby occurs approximately twice in every thousand live births in the United States, averaging between 8,000 and 10,000 deaths of children between 2 to 24 months. More than 90 percent of these deaths occur before 25 weeks of life. Sudden Infant Death Syndrome represents one of the most serious human crises a young family may have to face. This chapter has examined various aspects of this syndrome, including the ramifications of SIDS upon the families of its victims.

In an effort to provide a description of SIDS, some of the common features of the syndrome were identified. Since this is frequently a sleep-related death, the victims are often discovered wrapped in their crib coverings. As a result, some parents conclude that their infant suffocated and are ready to assume blame for negligence. Because SIDS has been described in such terms as "cataclysmic agonal event" (Beckwith, 1973), some families have borne the additional burden of thinking their infants suffered excruciating pain. However, the latest research indicates that the death of a SIDS baby is "sudden" and without agony or pain. The greatest suffering is sustained by the parents and families who survive the infant's death.

Immediate physical examination of the dead baby's body may suggest an early diagnosis of SIDS; however, a definitive diagnosis can only be made after a thorough postmortem examination, including gross examination and microscopic studies. Although few SIDS victims reveal identical evidence, the similarities in the evidence are significant. The most common evidence points to hypoxemia, a reduction of oxygen supply to tissue below physiological levels, despite adequate perfusion of the tissue by blood. Another common symptom is the presence of gastroesophageal reflux, or the regurgitation of stomach contents into the esophagus. This reflux can obstruct breathing and, if the child is unable to clear this obstruction, can contribute to his or her death.

Microscopic studies identify many related variables, including histologic evidence of upper respiratory infection and cell death in the larynx, but none of these factors alone adequately explains the cause of death. For this reason, the working definition of SIDS describes the syndrome as "the sudden death of any infant or young child, which is unexpected by history and in which a thorough post-mortem examination fails to demonstrate an adequate cause for death" (*Proceedings of the International Conference on Causes of Sudden Death in Infants*, Wash.: University of Washington Press, 1970, p. 17).

Epidemiological studies of SIDS in various parts of the world are drawing greater popular attention to this problem. One of the benefits of these investigations has been to identify infants at high risk for the syndrome, particularly those who experience apneic, or interrupted breathing, episodes. In addition to breathing problems, particularly during sleep periods, these careful epidemiological studies have identified other related variables, including a higher incidence of the syndrome among males and in children with low birth weight. Premature infants are also at greater risk, and birth order and multiple births may have some bearing on the syndrome. There seems to be a strong link between the presence of infection—most prevalent during the winter months when these viral and bacterial isolates are most communicable—and the vulnerability of some infants to this syndrome. Certain maternal factors have been strongly linked to the syndrome, concerning young mothers who have not had good prenatal medical care and those who are drug-dependent. Another contributing factor is a short interpregnancy interval. Although there are strong positive correlations associating all these factors with the incidence of SIDS, it is impossible to establish a causal link between these variables and the syndrome.

The inconclusiveness of all of these sources of investigation and evidence has given rise to numerous theories that attempt to offer some rational explanation for Sudden Infant Death Syndrome. Since sleep and breathing continually surface in the presenting symptoms of SIDS, it is not surprising that apnea theories have attracted the most attention in the field. The pioneering work of pathologists like Steinschneider and Naeye have helped to articulate the relationship of chronic apnea and SIDS. They have yet to answer the question why hypoventiliation, or underventilation, of the lungs takes place. Respiration is automatically controlled; when the brain mechanisms controlling this function do not work properly, alveolar hypoventilation occurs, resulting in acidosis and in vasoconstriction of the pulmonary arterioles. The autopsies of many SIDS victims present evidence of asphyxia and underventilated lungs.

Certain other scientists are tackling this problem, the research of which has targeted the important role that REM-sleep seems to play. It has been suggested that REM-sleep may furnish the central nervous system with an internal source of stimulation at a stage in human development when external stimulation is not available. This inner stimulation may play an important role in "programming" developing cortical functions. Crucial to this line of reasoning is the function of the carotid body. The carotid is thought to mediate the oxygen content of the blood and respiration. The fact that carotid underdevelopment has been documented in numerous autopsies performed on SIDS victims has strengthened the supposition that this may be an important causal factor in the development of SIDS.

The psychologists who have been involved in this type of biomedical and developmental research have been tackling the issue on closely parallel tracks. Their principal studies have likewise been investigating the interactive relationship between REM-sleep and the stimulation it provides to higher cortical centers, one of which controls respiration. Lipsitt and his colleagues have proposed a behavioral hypothesis linking vulnerability to SIDS with the developmental task of learning certain defensive responses that replace the congenital reflexes that decay with progressive cortical maturation. If these important life-supporting behaviors are not appropriated during the critical acquisition period, the child will be weakly defended when the unconditioned reflexes decay according to the neurophysiological timetable. The intriguing aspect of these psychophysiological theories is the attempt they make to bridge the chasm between neuroscience and the world of sensation and environment in explaining the neurological development of the infant. It may be in this type of research that a breakthrough may occur not only in the understanding of the syndrome, but in designing strategies for prevention.

The most serious problem facing the caregiver who is involved in a SIDS case is that the first symptom the parents must confront is death itself. In most cases, there has been no warning, no prior indications. This chapter has surveyed some of the psychological issues confronting parents, families, and the health care providers who work with them.

The ways in which the first hours of the intervention are managed are of great significance. Panic and guilt color many of the initial responses and reactions of parents. It is correct to note that parents themselves become victims of this syndrome. As support is provided to a family in these circumstances, nothing should prevent the expression of their ambivalent feelings, nor should efforts be made to protect them from their growing realization that the baby has died and cannot be resuscitated. Efforts to help them understand the syndrome begin with the initial communication about the child's death. This process will necessarily continue through the next several weeks and months as the family processes the information offered and their own personal feelings. Although some professionals are uncomfortable with this process, their role in it is indispensable. What they say and how they say it is crucial to the psychological recovery of the family.

This is a family syndrome, affecting a family's entire network. Among the most vulnerable victims in this constellation are other young children whom parents might try to protect from the painful realities associated with the loss. Parents may need some assistance in addressing the questions older children may ask or harbor within themselves. Since children, even very young children, can understand death, it is important that communication on this subject be truthful and shared with a child as befits the child's age.

Death of a child, particularly one resulting from SIDS, can place great stress on a marital relationship. The divorce rate among SIDS parents is higher than the national average. For many young couples, this may be their first personal encounter with death, and their needs as individuals must be considered. Grief is a personal experience, and not everyone expresses emotion in a similar way. Self-help groups of parents who have experienced a SIDS death may be a useful resource to couples involved in grief work. Physicians and nurses, particularly those who were involved in the crisis of the discovery of the dead child, can also be helpful intermediaries in facilitating the communication between spouses in the course of their bereavement and adjustment.

One important issue is the frequent desire on the part of SIDS parents to have another child. Though the word *replacement* may never be used in describing this desire, replacement is often a strong unconscious, if not conscious, motivation. Counsel to parents should not discourage this decision, while suggesting that the pregnancy not be attempted too soon. Grieving demands time and psychological energy; a replacement pregnancy might seriously interrupt this process. This could have important consequences for the new child as well as for the bereaved family.

Finally, since many of the epidemiological studies isolate single parents as a population at special risk for SIDS, particular attention needs to be directed to the care and support of these women. For many, some of the ordinary social supports available to their married counterparts may be lacking. Professionals working with this special population need to be sensitive to the individual needs of these mothers, and some extra support and resources may be necessary to help them adjust to this crisis.

Research has yet to answer the question "Why?" to the mystery of Sudden Infant Death Syndrome, but it has opened many doors to the solution. As we have seen in this chapter, diagnosis and prevention may prove to be something complex, or very simple. Work with many families who have experienced this crisis has helped to identify important ways of coping with this syndrome. Many parents of SIDS victims have become a powerful lobby in supporting federal investments in the necessary research into the causes of this syndrome. These same parents have become the most important supports to other parents who have lived through this nightmare. Together they have been the best teachers of the professionals dealing with SIDS victims.

3

Childhood Bereavement

Children and the Experience of Death

Children's Understanding of Death

- Piagetian Developmental Phases

- Maria Nagy and the Child's Conceptual Awareness of Death

- Recent Research and Theories

Children's Fear of Death

Grief and Mourning

Adjustment to Parental Death in Childhood

- Analytic Theories of Childhood Mourning

- Surviving Parental Efforts to Protect Child from Reality of Death

- Children's Guilt Reactions

Traumatic Aspects of Parental Death

- Variability and Extent of Trauma

- Psychological Outcome of Childhood Trauma

- Normal Responses of Children to Trauma of Parental Death

Therapeutic Considerations

Summary

Children and the Experience of Death

The death of a parent can be one of the most traumatic events in a child's early life. As for adults, the extent of psychological impact of death on a child depends on numerous social and environmental factors as well as the child's own coping resources. Yet children, by reason of age and experience, have limited powers. Their cognitive development may preclude adequate understanding and processing of the information, be it already limited, that is provided to them. Their emotional immaturity may make it difficult for them to fully appreciate their loss. All of these age-related, developmental factors contribute to the way in which a child relates to the premature death of a parent and affect the course of adjustment.

Children's reactions to parental death have not been sufficiently explored as a topic in the scientific literature. Yet, based on certain actuarial tables, it is estimated that approximately 6 percent of the child and adolescent population in the United States experiences the death of one or both parents before they reach young adulthood (age 18 years). This statistic underscores the importance of efforts on the part of health care professionals to gain greater understanding of the particular dynamics of childhood grief. If children are to be assisted in the work of bereavement proper to their own age and developmental level, then those who help them need to appreciate the particular ways in which children relate to death, especially parental death.

Mental health research in this area has sought to determine a relationship between premature parental death and depressive illness in later adult life (Birtchnell, 1969, 1970, 1971, 1972, 1974). The emphasis on a causal nexus between childhood bereavement and adult psychiatric morbidity (Birtchnell, 1975, 1978, 1981) may have eclipsed the equally important issue of understanding the ways in which childhood grief may be qualitatively different from the mourning processes of adults. Epidemiological research is of limited value (Birtchnell, 1974) because of the inherent difficulties of inadequate methodology. Reviewing the psychiatric literature, Tennant, Bebbington, and Hurry (1980) conclude that the findings are quite inconsistent and that in even the most rigorously controlled studies, no causal effect was found between childhood parental bereavement and depression in later life.

From a clinical perspective, one would be reluctant to posit a causal relationship between the event of early parental death and psychiatric morbidity in later adult life (Birtchnell, 1970a, b; 1972a). The intervening years and the effect of the many experiences and events that color those years weaken the possibility of balancing a cause-and-effect equation. However, this is not to deny how parental death and the ways in which it is managed may contribute to the later emotional health of the bereaved child.

This chapter will explore the popularly held assumption that children have little awareness of death and little fear of it. The experiences of a bereaved child whom the author saw in psychotherapy will serve to illuminate whether bereaved children are psychologically capable of grieving as well as how the tasks confronting bereaved children are similar to or different from those of adults. Discussions investigate the traumatic effects of parental death on children and the coping strategies they use. A critical examination of these various issues will contribute to a better understanding of how bereaved children mourn, and will be beneficial to those professionals who may assist the child and a surviving parent during the important phases of adaptation and adjustment.

Children's Understanding of Death

Piagetian Developmental Phases

One of the earliest and most influential formulations of a child's cognitive developmental process is attributed to Jean Piaget. It is scarcely possible to overemphasize the influence of Piaget on researchers who have attempted to apply his insights to the question of a child's ability to grasp the meaning of death. Piaget succeeded in demonstrating how the thinking processes of a child differ from those that characterize adults. Because of the importance of Piaget's work, it is useful to review the major stages of his theory.

Although Piaget identified certain normative ages at which a child progresses through the four basic phases leading to adult cognition, he acknowledged that children may reach these stages at different times. Variability is due in great part to environmental influences—an important point to keep in mind because it bears significantly on the impact a parent's death may have on a child's understanding of death. The cross-cultural research that has tested this theory over the past 60 years has tended to support the universality of the progression Piaget identified.

The *sensorimotor stage* spans the period from early infancy to 18 months and has certain characteristic features. It appears that infants do not perceive permanence in objects, behaving as though objects lose their existence when they are no longer in sight. Gradually this perception modifies, the evidence being that children actively begin to seek lost objects. Certainly by the end of the first year of life a child emotionally reacts to separation from a parent.

Another major acquisition of this first phase of cognitive development involves the notion of causality. Infants begin to perceive the relationships that exist between certain behaviors and specific effects. Also, they begin to situate objects within space. Progress is noted in the change from a perceptual process dependent almost exclusively on sensorimotor stimuli to one that relies on notions of object permanence, causality, and space. The appropriation of these concepts is the basis for all other cognitive growth, and with the ancillary ability to mentally represent objects, they move on to the next phase of cognitive growth.

The *preoperational stage* spans the years from 18 months to age 6 or 7. The work of this stage involves the developing abilities to use symbols, including language and play. Symbolic functioning means that children, alone and without external stimuli, are able to produce symbolic representations and are capable of manipulating these symbols. The characteristic feature of this thought process is its egocentricity; all reality is somehow seen only in terms of its relationship to the child and according to the child's requirements. Nowhere is this more evident than in a child's play, where inner thought finds an effective medium for expression.

Concrete operations characterize the years from roughly 6 or 7 to 11 or 12. During this stage of cognitive development the child begins to shape notions of class, relations, and number. The quality of thinking is less dominated by the egocentric reasoning of the previous stage and more able to grasp relations and constancies among objects and experiences. Piaget concluded that during these years children understand the laws of conservation of matter and volume and the principles that govern transformation. These developments are considered to be the direct result of the coordinaton of mental operations. Although children appear to internally process many experiences, they are still not capable of purely abstract reasoning.

The final phase of cognitive development is called *formal operations*. This period of development begins around age 11 or 12 and extends until age 14 or 15, or the period of early adolescence. The child displays a quality of thinking that is adult in nature. In addition to the demonstrated ability to reason logically, the adolescent is capable of abstract thinking. This process has often been described as "thinking about thinking." These developed abilities permit the adolescent to penetrate more deeply into the ethical and philosophical levels of issues and is considered by some developmentalists to be the basis for the identifications and commitments young adults make to certain moral and social ideals.

Maria Nagy and the Child's Conceptual Awareness of Death

Nagy, a Hungarian psychiatrist and a follower of Piaget, researched the application of cognitive developmental stages to children's understanding of death. Her 1948 publication, reporting on the outcome of work with 378 children living in Hungary, became a bench mark for subsequent research. She detailed three age-related stages of the child's awareness of death.

Stage One

Similar to what Piaget described, Nagy found that children under 5 years relate to death in egocentric ways. They consider death to be reversible, subject to the same magical power which they think governs many other physical phenomena. While they might accept the fact that an individual has died, they nonetheless attribute animistic qualities to the dead person. They consider that the dead person "lives" in ways that are comparable to the way he or she lived before death. The child senses the pain of separation, and may be actively engaged in seeking behaviors, including inquiring about the person and asking when the person will come back.

Stage Two

During this stage, which is solidly rooted in the middle years of childhood (5–9 years), Nagy observed that children tended to give death a personality. Death is acknowledged as permanent and conceptualized in concrete terms, yet as something external to the self.

Stage Three

Nagy concluded that children after age 9 have realistic knowledge about death as an inevitable and irreversible human experience that has its genesis within the body. They grasp the finality of death. With this understanding, children display more affective responses to death than younger children characteristically exhibit.

Although this formulation has been widely cited in discussions of children's understanding of death, it has also been criticized for its methodological inadequacies. Common to critiques of Nagy's theory is the claim that it does not sufficiently take into account the roles of environment, culture, and experience as contributing factors to a child's understanding of death.

Recent Research and Theories

Kane (1979) has conducted a study of 122 middle-class American children, ages 3–12. She did not find evidence of Nagy's "personification stage" (Stage Two) in her research. Her study, like Nagy's original work, depended on the theories of cognitive development proposed by Piaget. Kane describes three stages in the child's awareness of death that correlate closely with the last three stages of Piaget's schema.

Stage One

From age 2 until the age of reason, the child relates to death structurally, that is, it is real and there is actual separation. Recognizing that the dead person is immobile, the child may rely upon certain magical and animistic mental processes to understand the way dead people "live." In the same way, the child may be prone to believe that magical thinking might cause death, for example, a child's angry outburst, "I wish you were dead."

Stage Two

During the years comparable to Piaget's concrete operations (7–12 years) the child appreciates that death has two essential sources: one that is internal (disease, old age) and another that is external (murder, accident). These "causes" produce an irreversible result.

Stage Three

During the final stage of cognitive development (the early adolescent years) the child exhibits the ability to establish more accurate relationships between cause and effect. The most striking change is the abstract and speculative way in which children of this age think about death.

A significant challenge to how "stage theory" attempts to describe children's awareness of death is offered by Bluebond-Langner (1978). In her sensitive book describing the private world of terminally ill children who ranged in age from 3 to 9 years, she states that each of these children came to an adult's understanding of death. The process by which this knowledge was gained was not contingent upon cognitive development *per se*, but depended rather on the experience of being ill and on being in the company of other children who were similarly ill, some of whom died. These children described death as a "mutilating experience" that causes final separation from family and things. Although Bluebond-Langner describes "stages," these are not to be understood as formal. The "staging" of the awareness of death correlates with the staging of self-perception. This staging is similar among all dying children, regardless of their age. The basic schema is as follows:

Self-Perception	*Stage of Awareness*
1. I am seriously ill	1. Illness is serious
2. I am seriously ill, but I'll get better	2. Acquires knowledge of drugs involved in treatment
3. I am always ill, but I'll get better	3. Understands the goals and purposes of treatment
4. I am always sick and will never get better	4. Comes to appreciate diseases through a series of relapses and remissions
5. I am dying	5. Understands death as the culmination of a series of relapses and remissions

Dr. Bluebond-Langner observed the close relationship between the acquisition of knowledge about the scope of a disease and the related perceptions applied to the self. Reaching an understanding of death resides in the ability to integrate and digest cognitive developments. Earlier we made the point that for Piaget experience and environmental conditions were significant variables exerting influence on how and what a child at a particular age might understand. It is evident from Bluebond-Langner's studies that terminal illness and exposure to other terminally ill children at various stages of dying contributes to even very young children's awareness of death. This awareness is not subject to the kinds of limitations that other stage theorists have suggested. The personal involvement of a dying child in experiences shared with other dying children creates a milieu in which a realistic awareness of death can be acquired. She concludes that terminally ill children know they are dying even before death becomes imminent.

This research has generated a renewed interest in the questions of what a child understands about death and when. Bluebond-Langner's conclusions throw into question the assumptions that have dominated the field of inquiry for many years, namely, that until approximately age 10, children are not generally aware of the nature and implications of death. The close personal experience of death concretizes for terminally ill children what death is all about, even though their thoughts may exhibit some ambiguity about what happens on a philosophical or biological level. While Bluebond-Langner's conclusions are tentative, her research has indicated that children are more aware of death at far earlier ages than many cognitive developmentalists have considered possible.

Unawakened by immediate personal experience, children's awareness of death appears to be tied to the normal processes of cognitive maturation. However, the personal exposure to death may impress upon a child a sophisticated awareness of death at an earlier age than normal development would anticipate. For those children, even very young ones, who have lived in an environment in which a parent or sibling was terminally ill, one might expect that the awareness of death may be keener than may have been considered possible (Koocher, 1973).

Children's Fear of Death

In a frequently cited psychoanalytic study of the fear of death, Zilboorg (1943) remarked that a child's intrapsychic world, because of ego immaturity, is vulnerable to terror, helplessness, and guilt. In this inner world in which children live, there is little possibility of exerting control over a hostile and threatening environment. It is not difficult to imagine that death would have some place in the structure of this inner world, and be a legitimate fear with which children must contend. For a long time, assuming that young children have little cognitive grasp of the concept of death, some psychologists were reluctant to consider that fear of death is a problem children face.

Mitchell and Schulman (1981) have explored the hypothesis that the innate fear of death in the human being is universal and that the child, least of all, is immune to death fear and its symbolic representations. They maintain that death fear knows no boundaries of age or developmental level. As Rheingold (1967) stated earlier, death is fantasized and felt, not thought, and it is this emotional experience that gives death its meaning. In other words, a child has an awareness of personal extinction and an emotional reaction to the prospect of extinction before he or she has any cognitive understanding of mortality. In some respects, then, it makes more sense to argue about when a child has a cognitive grasp of the concept of death—the awareness may be there before thought catches up to it.

The literature on children's understanding of death supports the conclusion that youngsters entertain primary concerns about losses, endings, and separations. It is axiomatic that the more a person understands phenomena, the more able he or she is able to deal with the consequences of such realities. In the case of children, immaturity in age, understanding, experience, and ego defenses may leave a child more vulnerable than an adult to the threat or fact of death. Among adults, death places those with less stable ego functions at greater emotional risk than those with secure ego strengths. If this is true of older persons, it follows that children may have insufficient armor in their psychic arsenal to adequately defend themselves against the threat of death.

In existential situations in which significant adults deny a child's understanding of death and in which the child suffers inner experiences and fears of death alone, the child frequently seeks solace in defensive fantasies. The evolution of these fantasies is tied to cognitive development. The animistic and magical qualities of preoperational thought are reflected in the ways in which children attempt to marshall defenses against death fears. It is not surprising that many of the fantasies that support children's play involve the attribute of omnipotence. Children picture themselves able to fight off monsters and beasts of gigantic proportions, much in the vein of the biblical David in combat with the mighty Goliath. This dependence upon fantasized power and strength is a primitive defense that a child may use to cope with the subjective threat of death.

The popular Walt Disney children's television show was introduced by a theme song that opened the gates of Fantasyland. The lyrics maintained that "when you wish upon a star your dreams come true." This declaration accurately translates a psychological reality for children. Wishes are endowed with magical power, for good and for ill. The negative and destructive potential of these wishes, particularly those expressing death threats, explains the guilt reactions they produce in children. In situations of anger and frustration, children may entertain and verbalize destructive wishes, directing them toward parents, siblings, or others. Should one of these individuals subsequently die, the surviving child may conclude that death was caused by his or her powerful wish.

Mitchell and Schulman (1981) correctly note that reality for a child exists within his or her thoughts or feelings. Death is never considered to be merely a natural occurrence or chance happening. It is caused by something, and the child, within a certain cognitive perspective, can see himself or herself as the primary agent of a death within the immediate family. Guilt, therefore, is a common way children respond to death, particularly that of a parent, sibling, or close friend. Children may harbor these inadmissable feelings in an inner world that is ill-equipped to process them. The nightmares and phobias of childhood may be little more than evidence of the failure of their immature

ns to support and consolidate the experiences and fears associated
The issue of children's guilt will be treated more extensively further
chapter.

Grief and Mourning

Grief is the psychological pain that accompanies a major loss. The processing of this loss is the work of *mourning*. Freudian models of grief and mourning and those of more contemporary analytic authors have been applied to the question of whether children grieve and mourn, but since these models are intended to guide an understanding of the normal grief processes of otherwise healthy adults, it is not surprising that when applied to children, they yield the conclusion that children neither grieve nor mourn.

The following case, drawn from the author's psychotherapeutic practice, will provide a focus for a discussion of childhood grief and mourning. The child was age 7 at the time of his mother's death. Three years later, at the suggestion of the family's pediatrician, the child was referred for psychological assessment and treatment. The presenting repertory of problems outlined by the father all centered around David's apparent inability to communicate his feelings effectively. David frequently cried when he was unable to cope with certain tasks or situations, was cold to the woman his father was dating and whom he was intending to marry, and made excessive demands on his father's time and affection.

David is the youngest of 3 children born to Elizabeth and Derek Steiner. The first child, a boy, died 3 months after birth. A year after this sudden infant death, Karen was born. She is 3 years older than her brother David. Chronic arthritis was diagnosed in David's mother around the time of his birth and Elizabeth had difficulty reconciling herself with this illness.

The family lived in New York City at the time of the tragic death of their first-born son; a year later they moved to Chicago. When David was a year old the family moved again to St. Louis; 3 years later the family relocated to a suburb of Boston. Mrs. Steiner was hospitalized for a serious, but noncritical, illness. In the routine course of that period of hospitalization and treatment, she contracted a serious staphylococcus infection that quickly and unexpectedly caused her death.

The family was significantly disorganized by this crisis. David did not think his mother was sick; Mr. Steiner told both children of their mother's death, and David recalls feeling sad and crying. He felt very lonely. The funeral took place the following week in New York, where the Steiner's families still lived. David viewed his mother's body and attended the nonreligious funeral service.

After the burial, he stayed with his paternal grandparents for several days. Since the death occurred in the early part of the summer, David was sent to spend the remainder of the summer with an aunt and her family who lived on a farm in rural Pennsylvania. His sister, Karen, spent the summer with a maternal aunt in New Jersey. The family was reunited around Labor Day, just prior to the reopening of school. There was virtually no familial discussion of Mrs. Steiner's death.

Mr. Steiner spent the summer months trying to regroup his own energies. Although he had initially thought of moving from the family's suburban home, he postponed that decision for one year. After David completed third grade, the family relocated to a renovated townhouse in Boston.

David did not seem to adapt to his mother's death. While he continued to do well in school, his teachers consistently reported that he was withdrawn and sad. His relationship with his sister Karen was not good, although they had often been left alone to care for themselves during the years after the mother's death. In a number of ways, Karen tried to assume many of her mother's former nurturance roles, and David appeared to resent her attempts to "mother" him. David was most dependent upon his father, although the father did not find much time to give to his son. The demands of his very successful professional life, coupled with his personal investment in building a relationship with a divorced woman, made him emotionally less available to David.

It might appear from this brief overview of the Steiner family dynamics, that David was not able to grieve his mother's death. As will be shown later, the inhibition of grief and the postponement of mourning contributed to many of the symptoms that his pediatrician identified and that suggested psychotherapy might be advisable for him.

One of the most prominent proponents of the theory that children are unable to mourn is Wolfenstein (1966). She concluded from her studies of bereaved children that they seem unable to "mourn" until young adulthood. Her reasoning, apart from cognitive developmental issues, hinges on the assertion that the separation-individuation tasks of the adolescent period are essential to the ability to mourn. In commenting on her thesis, Palombo (1981) suggests that Wolfenstein's consistent and orthodox analytic position may have colored her observations. Within that frame of reference, children are too reliant on parents for gratification of their needs. If a parent dies during these early years, a child defensively scrambles to repair the narcissistic wound and restore delivery of emotional needs. Wolfenstein and others argue that a child is not able to love others as objects distinct from self, and as such do not mourn.

Freud (1957) described mourning as a decathexis of object representation. Wolfenstein found that this release of libido does not appear to be possible in adolescents and children. She explains this position by observing that children may tend to idealize the deceased parent. Although they may acknowledge and verbalize that the parent has died, they hold on to the fantasy that the parent is "alive" in some ways. On the other hand, the deprivation they feel as a result of parental death may be expressed in hostile and retaliative behaviors directed at the surviving parent. This rudimentary defense, which partially denies that a parent is dead, makes grieving an impossibility for children.

Other researchers have theorized about children's capacities for mourning and have supported the position that Wolfenstein proposed. The immaturity and undifferentiated state of the child's ego, problems with reality testing, awareness, recourse to denial, and the reversal of affect can effectively block mourning. Forceful as these arguments may be, the counterposition is equally strong.

The grande dame of child analysis and childhood bereavement, Erna Furman, is not content with the superimposition of the adult model of grief and bereavement on the child. Rather, she attempts to conceptualize childhood mourning as something discrete from adult dynamics. In her conceptual scheme, once a child has reached a stage of development wherein object constancy has been achieved (as early as one year of age, but more commonly thought to be acquired by age 3), mourning is possible. In addition to the concept of object constancy, the principal mental processes that engage mourning are perception and memory. She argues that children do emotionally survive the death of a parent and are willing to allow others to provide for them in ways in which the deceased parent did. She interprets this behavior to mean that there is a degree of autonomous investment of self of which even very young children are capable (Furman, 1974).

When David was first seen for diagnostic evaluations, he was invited to participate in a projective expression of three wishes. His answers were quickly produced and showed an interesting relationship. He wished for a horse, more time with his family and finally for a farm on which to live. It is important to recall that David spent the summer immediately after his mother's death with his relatives on a Pennsylvania farm. One of the most serious concerns of his father in seeking psychological help for his son is the child's persistent clinging behavior, the degree of resentment and rejection he shows for his father's fiancée, and his withdrawal at school and at home from peer activities. The only thing that seems to satisfy him is time spent exclusively with his father. It appeared to the father that David would not allow anyone else to satisfy his emotional needs—a task which the father felt poorly disposed to meet.

Mourning, or emotional decathexis, depends on the level of maturity and ego development of the child. The dynamics of this process in children may resemble its adult counterpart in general while differing from it in certain particulars. Birtchnell (1969b) summarized the conditions permitting childhood mourning. These include the following:

1. attitude of remaining parent or other adults
2. recognition of and tolerance for the anxious and hostile ways in which children react to the death of a parent
3. the denial mechanisms and defenses of the surviving parent
4. the oedipal significance of the lost parent for the child and the effect of this on the relationship with the surviving parent
5. the availability and consistency of a replacement parent figure

In the Steiner family's adaptation behaviors, Derek Steiner maintained a significant degree of denial about his wife's death. He mistakingly read David's silence and apparent success in his academic work at school to indicate normal adjustment. He absorbed himself in his work and substitute relationships as an antidote to his own grief. The message given to the children was "life as usual" and discouraged any family processing of the mother's death. David's consistent behavior showed a desperate reaching out for his father, who physically and emotionally was so often absent. As will be shown later, the inhibition of mourning forced David into substitute behaviors that not only inhibited adjustment but were regressive.

His case demonstrates what many people today believe—that children are capable of grief and do have mourning tasks to perform which are linked to both developmental and environmental conditions.

Adjustment to Parental Death in Childhood

Analytic Theories of Childhood Mourning

In conceptualizing the process of human development, Freud asserted that in the early months of an infant's life, all libidinal energy is self-directed, a condition that he termed **primary narcissism**. Basic and fundamental needs are satisfied and the child forms attachments with his or her caregivers. At times these caregivers prove to be unreliable and fail to supply certain satisfactions. Casual observation of an infant's behavior can demonstrate how the child responds to the temporary withdrawal of attention. The child appears to rage at the caregiver, and revert to a primitive posture of seeking gratification in the self. Attachment to a parent teeters between a love for the parent rooted in need gratification and a love independent of functions supplied.

Freud and others have seen this defensive maneuvering to be essential to healthy ego development, since survival will ultimately depend on the person's ability to assume responsibility for the provision and management of functions once provided by parents or parental surrogates. Emotional maturity is measured by the degree of autonomy a person achieves in this process. The final outcome of this process depends on the ability to make a net distinction between the attachment to the need-satisfying dimensions of a parent and the intrinsic value of that person.

Palombo (1981) prefers the psychoanalytic formulation of Kohut (1971). Kohut hypothesized that the human infant is born into the world with a relatively cohesive sense of self. Parents and other adult figures provide an environment that nurtures and encourages this individual self to grow. They complement the infant's development by becoming **selfobjects**, which the child incorporates and internalizes. An interruption of the relationship of the child with a selfobject can be disruptive of normal development, and can in some instances threaten survival.

Building upon this psychoanalytic psychology of the self, Palombo (1981) has suggested that the death of a parent might be understood as **narcissistic injury**. In considering a child's reaction to parental death, attention needs to be focused on the ways in which the deceased functioned as a selfobject and how the child perceived the relationship. Within this framework, sense of loss is proportionate to the degree of attachment and the degree of injury to the self.

David was able to identify the ways he often feels. The word he constantly uses is "lonely." He misses not having his mother at home. Not having her there makes him feel sad. Linked to these feelings is the complaint that his father is often absent from the home and that he does not have more time to do things with him.

David's perceptions are clear and he is able to remain focused on a discussion of these feelings. His facial expression translated his reports of feeling sad; rarely did he smile in therapy sessions. However, he did become quite responsive when he sensed a particular interest in him and in his sketching and artwork.

He would comment on how his mother used to like his drawing. This hobby now had become a solitary activity; his father rarely inquired about his art work and showed little interest in what he might have produced.

David, as a 10-year-old, was becoming a loner who was ambivalent about being alone and being with other people. He was overly attached to his father, but showed no attachment to anyone else. The only exception to this seemed to be his positive responsiveness to any adult who showed an interest in his work and who praised him.

It is not enough to look at the emotional bonds that may have existed between a child and the deceased parent. Of equal importance is an appreciation of the ways the parent was a selfobject. Palombo has redefined the scope of childhood mourning in light of this dual focus. Mourning does not involve simply the processes of withdrawing libidinal investments from the deceased and the undoing of the object representation. It likewise involves addressing the imbalance in self-esteem the loss of a selfobject causes. This perspective is useful because it attends to two related, but distinct, objectives of childhood mourning. Responses, therefore, can be expected at both the level of object attachment and at the level of injury to the sense of self (Palombo, 1981).

Of all of the possible ways in which a child is likely to experience the death of a parent, the most significant affect is linked with the agonizing sense of abandonment. *Separation anxiety*, inextricably linked to a child's sense of his or her own fragility and dependence, dominates the mourning behaviors of many children.

Children mourn parental loss in different ways. We will now consider some of the characteristic patterns of adjustment found in childhood bereavement.

Surviving Parental Efforts to Protect Child from Reality of Death

One of the attributes often credited by children to their parents is omnipotence. The "my daddy's stronger than your daddy" pattern is familiar in children's games. This attribution provides a secure environment for the child in which to go about the task of building ego strengths. When the powerful parent dies, the child is faced with the fact that a selfobject proved to be not as powerful as the child had previously thought. The child may respond to this perceived defeat with rage, anger, or disillusionment. The surviving parent, engaged in his or her own personal grief, may contribute to an intensification of this response. If the surviving parent's grief is intense and expressive, the child may feel even more insecure.

Some surviving parents attempt to shelter and protect the child. They may find it difficult to talk with children about the death, and thus they avoid reference or discussion of the event. Becker and Margolin (1967) reported this common reaction among surviving parents. Children, in their efforts to adapt, will seek their own reasons to explain the loss. These explanations are often rooted in fantasy and magic. Some may derive from certain religious explanations of afterlife, or exhibit some other imagery furnished by a parent or another adult. Sometimes children assimilate information from their peers and incorporate the data into their explanatory formulations. Becker and Margolin found that parents in their study group were reluctant to correct or modify their children's theories. The therapists reasoned that parental promotion of their children's fantasies may be related to the surviving parent's own difficulty in gradually withdrawing libido from the deceased. The tacit approval of childlike explanations may function as a displacement of the personal conflicts parents address in their own mourning.

This insulation of the child has two principal effects. First, it may inhibit mourning. Some children, observing the surviving parent's reactions, conclude that it's not right to talk about the deceased parent and may consider such discussion to be taboo. This repression can engage a whole constellation of other fantasies and feelings that because of their relationship to the deceased, cannot be processed through appropriate channels.

When Mr. Steiner spoke about his concerns about David, he noted that the boy spent most of his time in his bedroom, playing with pet gerbils and stuffed animals. In therapy it became quickly apparent that David was compensating for the lack of suitable object relationships with parent and family by seeking some gratification in these associations. In fact, his whole fantasy life was deeply invested in these relationships with pets and toys. His drawings always pictured escapes to the countryside; frequently he pictured himself and his father riding together.

Although his father was inclined to dismiss his son's preoccupation with the country life as a rebellion against his decision to relocate the family in the city, it seemed reasonable to think that David may have fixated on that traumatic summer spent in the country following his mother's death; he yearned for the opportunity to talk with his father and to be reassured of his support and presence.

When David was asked what kinds of things he discussed with his pets and stuffed animals, he quickly answered, "I tell them how sad I feel and how much I miss my mommy."

A second effect of this kind of insulation is the hardening of denial. Some parents in the Becker and Margolin (1967) research withheld telling their children of the death for several hours, in some cases days or months later. These same parents acknowledged difficulty in sharing the information with their children. This behavior can block any efforts to come to terms with the finality of death, and engage those processes that are necessary to achieve healthy adaptation to such loss.

Children may be excluded from participation in the cultural rituals that aid adults in coming to terms with a loved one's death. Deprived of these socio-cultural supports, a child can be blocked in his or her need to grieve and to mourn. If we acknowledge that children are aware of death and respond to it, then it is understandable why a position that discourages young children from participation in the mourning process may not be in the best mental health or developmental interests of the child.

Children's Guilt Reactions

When a parent dies, a child is very vulnerable to feeling guilty. In describing children's *guilt reactions* to parental death, Gardner (1977a) noted that such reactions are often inappropriate. A reaction is judged inappropriate when a person believes that he or she is responsible for something for which he or she is in no way accountable. Gardner discusses the psychodynamics of this reaction.

When a child is left alone to process a parent's death, the child will often seek solace in guilt. Guilt can be one way to attempt to gain control over the uncontrollable. The child will search the memory looking for some thought, word, or deed that can supply a rationale for the parent's death. The output of this search may be inconsequential, but a trivial datum can become the focal point of an obsession that has but one conclusion: "I am responsible for Mommy or Daddy's death." Gardner cites numbers of factors he considers operative in this delusion of guilt. The conclusion a child reaches—"It is my fault"—signals an effort to gain control. With preoperational children, the confession of guilt may be a magical attempt to reverse the situation. For example, if daddy died because I said "I wish you were dead," then the act of being sorry for saying that will bring daddy back to life. Even in older children whose cognitive level would not entertain such reasoning, the vulnerability to guilt remains a constant. They hold on to the obsession and struggle not to repeat the destructive behavior lest another loved one also die.

Gardner points out that guilt reactions of this sort are unprecipitated and stem from a child's efforts to gain some mastery over the confusing experiences of the death. However, he observes that some familial environments that place strong emphasis on searching out and assigning blame can fuel the child's natural inclination to blame himself or herself. Verbal reassurances may not be too useful since there is a certain security in the delusion of guilt. In terms of self-esteem the child is struggling with the power-impotence issue; children need to learn how the power they do have can be marshalled in service of their need to mourn. Bereaved children need to experience success and gratification in this area if they are effectively to surrender obsessional guilt.

Those who work with bereaved families often comment that children seem to react less dramatically to death than do adults. Erna Furman (1974) confirms this observation by underlining the more positive affects exhibited by bereaved children. This optimistic behavior may be nothing more than a child's defensive attempt to deny the painful realities associated with the death. This is the analytic interpretation Furman offers to explain the otherwise inappropriate response of children to parental death. Play is the normal conduit through which many intrapsychic conflicts seek resolution. When children's play is carefully observed, including attention to their art and storytelling, one would not readily conclude that children are immune to strong affective responses to death.

In the course of treatment, David was often invited to draw. Since he had a natural interest in sketching and a certain talent for it, he was most responsive to this suggestion. His drawing not only tended to relax him, but it provided a rich source of important material for discussion.

On one occasion he was invited to do a sketch of his father. Selecting a black pen, he drew a large wing chair placed at the far extreme of the page. He pictured his father enveloped in that chair, with blank expression and a drink in his hand. At the other extreme boundary of the paper he drew a television set with extended antennae. There was no other detail provided in this drawing and no color.

When asked if he would like to follow up this drawing with a picture of his mother, he somewhat reluctantly agreed. He drew his mother in a full-length dress, without facial expression, standing at the kitchen stove. The only evident activity in the picture is a tea kettle on the back burner, vigorously boiling, emitting billows of steam.

While drawing this picture, he began to cry and clung to me while he sobbed, clearly needing to be held. Apart from the obvious grieving which this activity precipitated, it was interesting to note that this portrait of the mother pictured her in a long dress. It was learned that Mrs. Steiner had been buried in a long gown and that her casket was fully opened. David's last picture of his mother saw her clothed in this way.

Because their defenses function differently from adults' and responses are apparently so diverse, children themselves may feel guilty that they did not love the deceased parent sufficiently. This conclusion may be based not only on subjective experience but on comments they receive from adults. A surviving parent may remark: "If you really loved Daddy, you wouldn't do this or that." While this statement may be nothing more than an attempt to foster compliance, the bereaved child may misinterpret it to mean that there is a questionable deficiency. This can contribute to intensified feelings of guilt in the child.

Finally, children may feel ambivalence about the parent's death and their own continued existence. This is a common experience among adults who confront the issue of personal mortality each time they are faced with another's death. The reaction "better him than me" is recognized not as a callous, detached response, but as a way of dealing with the disquieting emotions that the death of another mobilizes. Children, not yet able to benefit from abstract reasoning, but subject to reactions similar to those of adults, can feel guilty about being glad that it was the parent who died, not themselves. While the "better him than me" reaction is common, it is not ordinarily verbalized to other persons. Children may be ashamed that they feel this way and are unable to express their embarrassment.

In each of these experiences, children can benefit enormously from intervention that both recognizes the potential source of the guilt reaction and responds appropriately to relieve the child of the unnecessary burdens it causes. Professionals who have access to the child, including teachers, school nurses, pediatricians, and clergy, can be resourceful in this respect. These same professionals may be helpful to the surviving parent as together they coordinate efforts to assist the child in need.

Traumatic Aspects of Parental Death

The thrust in childhood bereavement research has been to establish a relationship between early parental death and psychopathology in later life. Although, as earlier noted, the intervening variables make it virtually impossible to establish cause-and-effect relationships, this type of research has illuminated some of the ways in which children experience a parent's death. A better understanding of the impact and significance of the event can assist caregivers in lending the best support to the bereaved child and in mitigating certain long-term negative sequelae.

Psychological trauma is an emotional shock that makes an indelible impression on the mind, especially on the subconscious mind. The event is numbing to the extent that the ego and the executive functions it normally performs are rendered temporarily ineffective.

Variability and Extent of Trauma

In discussing events that are potentially traumatic it is important that emphasis be placed on the ways in which the person experiences the event, and not simply on the external reality itself. Palombo (1981) has outlined a number of variables that distinguish the event of a parent's death and contribute to the measure in which such a death might be traumatic.

One child may watch a parent deteriorate through the course of a long terminal illness. Another may be confronted with an accidental or suicidal death. Still others may have witnessed the violent death of one or both of their parents. While the external event is the same for all of these surviving children, the circumstances surrounding it determine the degree and kind of traumatization.

A lingering terminal illness threatens the basic order and function on which most families depend. The anticipated death of a parent disrupts the dynamics of a family, and to some members it may signal the dissolution of the family. While a crisis of this magnitude need not be so catastrophic, it may be perceived as such, particularly by younger children. Given the uncertain course of many terminal illnesses, the intensity of the crisis may wax and wane over weeks or months, and the emotional hazard posed by the crisis may be difficult to assess. Regardless of the particular circumstances within a given family, it is safe to conclude that it may not be the death that is so traumatic for the child, but the prolonged and extended disturbances which attend the whole process of a parent's dying.

A suicidal death creates a distinctly different familial environment. Cain and Fast (1966) noted that the child whose parent committed suicide is more likely to develop guilt feelings than the child whose parent died from other causes. Secrecy frequently shrouds the family discussions, and children are often shielded from the truth. If they are told, strong restrictions are placed on the child, and he or she is forbidden to share this information with anyone. The aura of mystery and silence surrounding a parental suicide can actually intensify the trauma for the child. The distortions, innuendo, and confusion in familial communication may increase the pain of loss and fuel the trauma a child experiences.

There are unfortunately too many cases of children who have witnessed the brutal and violent deaths of parents. While these frequently occur in the heat of domestic argument, they can also be the result of other criminal acts. Whatever the circumstances, most therapists who treat these children are agreed that such experiences imprint a lasting image in the child's memory. Lebovici (1974) concludes from his psychotherapeutic treatment of children who witnessed the violent death of a parent that the notion of traumatization is very ambiguous, though no one would doubt its existence. Not only is trauma difficult to assess, but it is likewise not easy to treat.

Trauma may be conditioned by factors such as which of the parents dies, mother or father. The particular parental relationship may also contextualize the death: a child may relate differently to the death of an adoptive parent, a stepparent, or a foster parent than to the demise of a natural, biological parent. Analytic authors consider the sex, age, and developmental stage to be significantly related to the sex of the deceased parent. Oedipal issues, identification, role modeling, and role substitutions can each contribute to the way in which the death is organized in experience.

Becker and Margolin's research (1967) asserts that the timing and manner in which children are informed of the parent's death can contribute to the degree of trauma. This communication extends not only to the fact of the death but to the ways in which the reasonable and anticipated questions and concerns of the child are encouraged and answered. The information shared with children should be as accurate and factual as the children's ability to comprehend dictates. As pointed out in the discussion of guilt, surviving parents report that communication of this sort with their children is very difficult and, not uncommonly, avoided if at all possible.

Johnson (1982) studied the variability in surviving parents' and children's perceptions of family closeness and communication and in children's experiences following the death of a parent. Confining her study to children aged between 6 and 12 years, she compared bereaved children and their parents to a matched control group. Children differed markedly from surviving parents on the issue of discussions of death within the family circle. Children overwhelmingly reported that parents did not talk about death, whereas parents felt that they had prepared children to understand death. Parents reported that after the death had occurred, children initiated discussions of death, although the children all seemed to agree that parents brought up the subject. Many of the children seemed uncomfortable with the number of death-related conversations within the family. Communications among bereaved children and their surviving parents seem confused, and mixed messages appeared to be common.

David's crying episode was a turning point in his treatment. It opened the way for more direct and useful conversation concerning his feelings about his mother's death. He said that his father "never wants to talk about it." He confessed that his father always said, "You'll get over it; I have and you will."

David very much resented the woman whom his father was intending to marry. Even in this regard he displayed his characteristic ambivalence. On the one hand, he readily admitted that "She is very nice, kind of like my Mommy." However, whenever he was with her and her two children, he felt that "she bossed me around." In fact, he frequently got angry and hostile toward her, a behavior that disturbed Mr. Steiner very much. When he reprimanded David, the youngster cried and withdrew.

When therapy provided a way to talk about these things, David said, "I don't want another mommy; I want my daddy." Until he felt secure in his father's protection, he was not able to entertain someone else replacing his mother and taking his father further away from him. Curiously, his father admitted that he never considered that this might be at the root of the behavioral protestations and resistance.

The relationship that the child had with the deceased parent is an additional traumatic factor, which was shown earlier to figure significantly in the development of the selfobject and its relationship to the child's self-esteem. Some parents develop very close relationships with their children, and the loss of one such parent can be devastating to the child. An incomplete understanding of what happened to this loved object may increase the degree of trauma.

Each of these variables, and many others as well, contribute to the impact parental death may have on a child. Within a family, siblings may react differently to the death of the same parent. In the Steiner family network, it is easy to see how these variables combine to determine how each child will experience the parent's death. Karen showed fewer adjustment problems and seemed to adapt to the changes in family life. David, on the other hand, was severely regressed in his emotional development, even though he was able to continue to do well in his school work. The intrapsychic state of an individual child determines the extent to which a parent's death is traumatic.

Psychological Outcome of Childhood Trauma

Palombo (1981) proposes that the trauma related to the discrete event of parental death has positive and negative effects. The positive effect involves recalling the painful event. The repetitive recollection and reliving of the experience helps the child to regain control over the event that has temporarily immobilized the ego. This resumption of control entails conscious processing, including talking about the event and actively working it through. In the case of children, as noted earlier, this is normally accomplished in play.

David began to talk more spontaneously about his recollections of his mother, and began to ask more direct questions about her death. He needed explanations about why she died and why the doctors could not fix her up. Therapy provided a way to explore feelings and fears that had not previously found an appropriate vent.

Mr. Steiner was able to become an active partner in this process and his willingness proved to be effective. He began to note a change in David's behavior, and this improvement not only was gratifying to him, but it helped his relationship with the woman he was preparing to marry.

As therapy moved toward its termination, David found himself less invested in his solitary play activities with his pets and toy animals. He began to develop a friendship with one of the boys in his class and for the first time showed an interest in the soccer team at school.

The negative effect of the death of a parent may dispose the child to psychopathology. If the trauma is ignored and conscious processing is inhibited, as we have seen in the Steiner case, then the conflict may seek resolution in maladaptive behaviors, including compulsive and ritualized activities, character disorders, and other neurotic displays. Repression exacts its cost in some symptomatic behavior, either soon after the parent's death or at some later time.

A surviving parent is sometimes relieved to find that the child appears to have survived the traumatic event and has recovered. This child apparently did not require any discussion of the death or any specific efforts to aid mourning. In fact, the denial and repression may be so complete and effective that, to all outward appearances, no apparent changes can be observed. It is this situation that has led research in adult psychopathology to look for relationships between emotional and behavioral dysfunctioning and childhood parental loss. Delayed grief reactions are not uncommon among children who seemingly made easy adjustments to a parent's death. It is reasonable to expect that children will grieve and mourn. If circumstances and environmental conditions inhibit this need, the child may resort to denial and repression, which can pave the way to future psychopathology.

Normal Responses of Children to Trauma of Parental Death

In searching for some adequate understanding of trauma that would be sufficient to describe the way in which a child experiences and relates to parental death, trauma was defined in terms of the temporary immobilization of ego functions. The course of development accounts for the fact that the child's ego is still immature and reliant upon the selfobjects in the phenomenal world, of which parents are among the most important. One of the crucial functions these selfobjects provide for the maturing ego is protection against flooding or overstimulation by internal as well as external forces, by unconscious as well as environmental pressures. This gatekeeping function ensures the child the safety and equilibrium essential to normal development.

The traumatic aspect of a parent's death for the child is the loss of this selfobject and children's inability to assume autonomous ego functions for themselves. Specifically, this means that the child may experience the death of a parent as being left vulnerable to a world in which he or she feels powerless. The degree of trauma is contingent on the extent and intensity of the child's reliance upon the deceased parent, and the specific ideations the child entertained about him or her. Not only is this important in terms of the child's relationship with the deceased parent, but it is also important in assessing the relationship with the surviving parent.

The surviving parent is emotionally involved in his or her own grief feelings and may be unable to fully care for dependent children. Simultaneously deprived of the ego protection the deceased parent as well as the surviving parent once supplied, the child may be immobilized and regress in search of some security and safety. To best assist a child, it is crucial to gain some concrete understanding of how these selfobjects are understood by the child, and what disruptions their unavailability have created.

To mitigate the short- and long-term effects, the goal in intervention is the restoration of a selfobject that can assume the protective functions lost through the death of the one parent and the temporary inability of the other to supply necessary assistance. Too frequently, in the wake of a death within the family, the children are cared for by other relatives or friends. Siblings may be separated during this time. The intention may be to provide the surviving spouse with some respite, apart from children. Allied to this purpose may be the unspoken assumption that it is better that children be protected from the emotions and experiences associated with death.

Many therapists share the judgment that children's adjustment is aided by maintaining constancy in their environment. The negative effects of the loss are offset to some degree by the security to be found in familiar places and routines. It is within this environment that effective reconstructive work can be undertaken in the family. Each person in that network has special needs and requirements. The child's world, like that of adults, has been disrupted by the death. While healthy adults have other ego supports to fall back upon in this time of crisis, children are not so well defended. It is essential that children be assisted in regaining lost selfobjects and the important functions they formerly supplied so that they can continue in a normal, unbroken course of development.

Therapeutic Considerations

Unless a bereaved child is permitted and encouraged to work through the feelings he or she is experiencing, grief work may be postponed and somatic and psychologic disturbances may ensue. For these reasons, it is important to conclude this treatment of a child's reactions to parental death by drawing together some suggestions for facilitating a child's grief work.

The most important step in a child's grief resolution is the acceptance of the death. Erna Furman (1974) advises that the child be encouraged to express whatever he or she may feel. Although children may initially resist efforts to encourage expression of their feelings, they will generally respond. This expression takes varied forms and is not restricted to verbalization. Adults need to be patient with the child in this process. Expression of feeling is predicated on trust—the very trust that may have been shattered by the death. The poignancy of a bereaved child's experience is resumed in the question the child is likely to ask: "Why did Daddy die? Didn't he love me enough to get well?" (Salladay & Royal, 1981). Plank and Plank (1978) observe that children will test out the waters to determine if it is safe to reinvest and trust again. So many of their challenging and testing questions need to be understood in this light.

David had an opportunity in therapy to deal with the feelings of grief and separation precipitated by his mother's unexpected death. His feelings of loneliness and fear of being left behind by his father also needed to be addressed. David responded very well to these interventions and left treatment showing good evidence of being able to continue to deal with related issues.

In a posttherapy followup meeting with David and Mr. Steiner, it was clear that things had improved dramatically in the months since termination. Not only had a great burden been lifted from David's shoulders, but the process had helped Mr. Steiner talk more openly within the family about his own feelings about his deceased wife, and his hopes for the future.

Acceptance of death depends on appropriate communication of factual information. Euphemisms and magical explanations may introduce more anxiety and confusion into a child's inner world than a more simple statement of fact. Metaphorical explanations, while intended to be soothing and reassuring, may not have their anticipated effect. They can trigger lasting fears in children. Salladay and Royal (1981) cite as an example the common explanation that "God reached down and took Daddy to heaven while he was sleeping." Such an image can make a child fear going to sleep, lest God reach down and take him or her. The origin of certain phobias can be traced to such explanations.

The fact of parental death necessitates a child coming to terms with it. The challenge to a parent or other counselor is to help children grasp the meaning of this experience in terms they can cognitively process. Efforts must be made to reconcile whatever previous understandings a child may have entertained about death with the current work of integrating the personal experiences associated with a parent's death. If the child has been allowed adequate contact with a terminally ill parent, then some useful groundwork may have already been laid. If death was sudden, accidental, or suicidal, the difficulties may be compounded. Nevertheless, specific efforts must be undertaken to assist the child in grasping the significance of death on a level appropriate to the child's development and experience.

This process is best engaged in in an environment that is familiar and secure. In the earlier discussion of trauma, emphasis was placed on the necessity of reestablishing, as soon as possible, the normal environment of the family. For some bereaved parents, this is difficult to manage, but it is to be encouraged since it is in the ultimate best interest of all the family members. It is within this normalized environmemt that the most useful and productive grief work can be mounted within the family. Children are more likely to proceed with their own grief work if they perceive the environment to be inviting and receptive.

Rosenthal (1980) comments that occasionally a family may require the assistance of a professional who can act as a facilitator in helping the surviving parent and other family members to participate in the child's grief and help to finalize mourning. Apart from the parent's comfort in inviting the child to share memories of the dead parent and entertain questions about the death, the child needs to sense the security of the environment in which such important issues are raised. The more normal and natural the environment, the more likely the child will feel safe in pursuing these important tasks.

It might be said that death is untimely, regardless of when it interrupts relationships among persons. This statement has particular significance to a young child who loses a parent to death. Since children are more able to understand death than adults might have previously considered to be possible, they are as vulnerable as adults to grief and mourning, albeit in a way distinct and proper to their own level of development. Parents and other caregivers have a significantly urgent task in assisting them in the normal resolution of grief.

Summary

Some old beliefs about children die hard. One of those myths is the notion that what the child does not actually see or hear he or she will not know. This assumption has guided some adults in their attempts to shelter children from the experiences and realities of death. While the motivation and intention to protect a child from pain and suffering are noble, contemporary developmental research and clinical experience have begun to reveal the futility and even the harm in such efforts. Children do understand death and, like adults, need to confront death and to grieve. Bereavement and separation are now recognized as important variables in the repertory of childhood behaviors, even though it is more difficult to assess the role these early experiences play in later adult life, particularly the influence they may exert on adult psychopathology.

Most mental health professionals who work with children would agree that parental death is perhaps the most traumatic loss a child may sustain. In the United States it is estimated that about 6 percent of the population under age 18 face this loss; if the losses suffered through divorces were added into these statistics, the percentages would increase dramatically. This chapter has attempted to identify and discuss some of the more interesting and important aspects of childhood bereavement.

Until recently, psychologists assumed that children had little concrete understanding of death. This assumption relied heavily upon theoretical explanations of a child's cognitive development, in particular those of Jean Piaget. Piaget offered a four-stage theory of the development of thought processes from infancy through adolescence, focusing on the characteristics and quality of the child's thinking.

This scheme greatly influenced the applications that the Hungarian psychiatrist, Maria Nagy, made in the 1930s of Piaget's theory to the ways in which children understand death. She concluded from the case studies she gathered in Budapest with children of various ages that it is not until around age 9 that a child begins to have some concrete and realistic understanding of death.

More recent researchers have continued to apply Piaget's theories and have found correlations between his stages and the ways in which children appear to understand death. Kane (1979) has utilized interviews with children to propose such a paradigm. In these more contemporary researches, the role of cognitive developmental level, tied closely to chronological age, dominates the theory-building effort.

Bluebond-Langner has challenged the principle that children's understanding of death is dependent upon the level of cognitive development. Although she accepts a notion of "stages" of awareness and understanding of death, she understands stages in a less structured sense than would Piaget. Bluebond-Langer views a child's understanding of death more in terms of a particular child's *experiences*, rather than of chronological age or stage of cognitive development. Experiences mediate understanding. Therefore, even very young children can understand death—both their own dying, and the death of another. Her research, conducted with terminally ill children, has provided a different focus on the issues involved in a child's understanding of death and dying.

A child is vulnerable to a wide repertory of fears. For this reason, adults have tried to protect children from fears associated with death. However, practitioners in the field of child psychiatry now suggest that the fears associated with death are innate and that the child least of all is immune from the fear of death and its symbolic representations (Mitchell & Schulman, 1981). Utilizing the Piagetian categories discussed earlier, they have linked children's fears, fantasies, and defenses to the ways in which a child *thinks* about death.

It is not surprising that traditional psychology has long assumed that children neither grieve nor mourn. Wolfenstein (1966) concluded from her research that bereaved children seem unable to mourn until young adulthood. Orthodox psychoanalysis would strongly support this conclusion. However, that position has been challenged by others who are unwilling to superimpose an adult template on a uniquely child experience. Furman (1974) has suggested that children, as early as 1 year of age, but certainly by age 3, have made a sufficiently autonomous investment of self to render them capable of grieving when important objects are lost to them.

Among important analytic theories of childhood mourning, the neoanalytic formulations of Kohut (1971) have particular relevance here. Kohut suggested that the infant enters the world with a relatively cohesive sense of self. Those who assist this child to grow, mature, and develop become **selfobjects**, and these complementary individuals are incorporated and internalized by the child. Disruptions in the relationships with selfobjects, among whom parents are principal representatives, can interfere with the normal course of development and can threaten the child's survival.

Palombo (1981) has made interesting applications of Kohut's theories. He underscores the importance of assessing the ways in which the deceased adult (or sibling) functioned as a selfobject for the child in order to understand the significance of the loss. Childhood mourning, according to Palombo, involves not only the classic notion of withdrawing emotional investment from the lost object (decathexis), but also addressing the level of injury to the self, precipitated by the loss of an important selfobject. Separation anxiety, however, may be more important than guilt as a factor in childhood bereavement.

Adults' protective instincts try to shield children from the pains associated with death and bereavement. However, efforts to shelter them may be ineffectual. Loss is perceived; it is felt. Children respond as adults with a full range of emotions, including anger, rage, and disillusionment. The surviving parent, involved in personal efforts to manage grief, may find it difficult to communicate with his or her children about their common loss. Isolation in a personal world of grief can be problematic for an adult; for the child, the ramifications may be more serious than many would suspect. The inhibition of grieving for a child can trigger behavioral reactions as well as intrapsychic conflicts.

Guilt is one of the more serious problems in the inhibition of normal grieving. A child is extremely vulnerable to assigning blame for a parent's death to himself or herself. The child may attempt to work through some of these inner conflicts in play. This is one vehicle through which a child seeks release from the burden of guilt and the conflicts associated with death. Any intervention with a bereaved child seeks to relieve some of the potential sources of guilt.

Death within a family is traumatic. The particular vulnerability of a child to death cannot be overemphasized, despite the impression that some children give that they are mildly affected by the event. The extent of trauma is determined to some degree by the ways in which the child experiences the event and the ways in which he or she is assisted in the mourning process. By definition, a psychological trauma temporarily immobilizes the normal functioning of the ego. Since a child's ego is still immature, he or she is particularly vulnerable to the effects of early parental loss. Children cope with the traumatic aspects of this loss in various ways.

All of the issues relating to childhood bereavement have special relevance for intervention with children whose parents have died. The insights of recent research can be beneficial to surviving parents who are often uncertain how best to assist their children in the process of a family's regrouping and adjustment to death. Finally, this chapter's discussion can be particularly valuable to a pediatrician or family practitioner who, by virtue of his or her longitudinal involvement with children and families, is in a privileged position to provide guidance for a family in which a loss has taken place. The case study utilized throughout this chapter has emphasized the importance of effective and timely interventions and, occasionally, the necessity of referral to psychological professionals for appropriate diagnosis and treatment.

4
Childhood and Adolescent Cancer

Overview

Acute Lymphocytic Leukemia: The Disease and Its Treatment

- Description of the Disease
- The Diagnosis of Leukemia: First-stage Treatment
- Neurological Complications of Chemotherapy
- Central Nervous System Irradiation: Second-stage Treatment
- Maintenance Modalities: Third-stage Treatment

Psychological Issues in the Care and Management of Pediatric Cancer Patients

- Loss of Control
- Separation
- Therapeutic Aspects of Play Activities
- Normalization of Hospital Life
- Primary Nursing Care
- Hypnosis and Relaxation Techniques
- Children as Mutual Resources
- Reentry to Home and School

Relapse and the Problem of Terminal Diagnosis

Anticipatory Grief and Death

Summary

Overview

Significant advances have been made in the diagnosis and treatment of malignancies in childhood and adolescence. Until recently these diseases were invariably fatal. Today treatment protocols successfully produce not only disease-free states in many children suffering from cancer but what is termed a cure in a significant number of cases. *Cure* commonly means "disease-free for 5 consecutive years." Encouraging as these trends may be, they do not mean that significant numbers of children still do not die from the whole range of leukemias and various solid-mass tumors. Although accidents and suicides are the leading causes of death among children and adolescents, among disease categories, cancer is the principal cause of childhood death. However, survival rates for childhood and adolescent cancer are steadily improving and this accounts for the modern trend of describing cancer as a *life-threatening disease* rather than a necessarily *terminal* one.

Although sarcomas, carcinomas, lymphomas, and other solid-mass cancerous tumors are common occurrences in children and adolescents, these are well beyond the scope of this survey. In the following discussion of the broad topic of childhood and adolescent cancer, the focus will be on leukemia, beginning with the issues involved in its diagnosis. This background is essential to the understanding of some of the psychological problems encountered in assisting pediatric and adolescent cancer patients and their families. Not only do most families come to know and understand the biomedical issues related to leukemia, but the afflicted children themselves become quickly socialized to these realities. As will be seen in the extensive case report of a 14-year-old relapsed leukemia patient, children learn many of the technical details about their diseases and utilize some of these data as a way of exercising some control over their cancers. Much of what will be said of the leukemic child and his or her care is easily applicable to other forms of childhood and adolescent cancer. Although there are hundreds of discrete cancers that may afflict a child or adolescent, there are certain physical and psychological characteristics that are common to these different diseases, not the least of which leukemia.

The American Cancer Society (1983) reports that remission rates are as high as 90 percent, particularly in the treatment of *acute lymphocytic leu-*

kemia (ALL). This is the most common form of leukemia affecting children, constituing more than 60 percent of childhood leukemias. The specific characteristics of this disease will be explored later. For now, it is sufficient to define ALL as a progressive, malignant disease of the blood-forming organs.

The 5-year survival rates of children diagnosed and treated for leukemia are very impressive, ranging between 50 and 75 percent. Some of these children do eventually succumb to the disease or some other complication. It is important to stress the fact that the overall survival rate differs with respect to the type of leukemia. For acute lymphocytic leukemia (ALL), the survival rate is at least 50 percent, while the rate is between 30 and 40 percent for acute myelogenous leukemia (AML). Improvement in these statistics is inevitable, given steadily increasing skills in diagnosis and treatments, coupled with ever expanding knowledge about the nature of leukemia. It is optimistically projected that these advances may contribute to longer periods of remission in the majority of properly diagnosed and treated children. Complete cure may be achievable in a third of children afflicted with ALL (Sallan & Weinstein, 1980).

Acute Lymphocytic Leukemia: The Disease and Its Treatment

Description of the Disease

Leukemia results from a rapid and steady proliferation of immaturely formed blood cells. When we speak about leukemia, we are referring to an abnormal production of *lymphoblasts*, or the immature white blood cells. The cause for the rapid multiplication of these lymphoid cells is still uncertain and remains an important question in current research. Some methods currently being used include the use of immunologic cell surface markers and a biochemical assessment of cytoplasmic content of the leukemia cells. In the study of the chromosomal patterns of these cells, a reappraisal of the shape and cytochemical differences between the cells has aided in determining the problematic cell of origin (Sallan & Weinstein, 1980).

The *bone marrow* governs the production of blood cells. This production involves three distinct kinds of cells: red blood cells, platelets, and white blood cells. Leukemia develops from the latter of these three groups of cells. Whatever normally controls the maturation process of the *white blood cells (WBC)* becomes dysfunctional in the bodies of leukemic children. Rather than maturing and assuming their proper function in the total body's chemistry, they remain immature and quickly multiply.

There are three principal classes of WBC: *lymphocytes*, which aid in warding off infections; *monocytes*, which destroy alien materials; and *neutrophils* which combat bacteria. The goal of leukemia treatment is to destroy these *blasts* which accumulate in the bone marrow and threaten the normal blood cells developing there.

Leukemia, as we earlier defined the disease, is a cancer of the blood-forming tissues. These tissues release millions of cells into the body's two circulatory systems: the cardiovascular system and the lymphatic system. When leukemia is present, millions of lymphocytes are released into these systems. The immaturity of these cells interrupts the performance of their principal function, namely, the warding off of infection. The proliferation of the abnormal immature white cells prevents normal, healthy cellular production to check infection (white blood cells) and prevent anemia (red blood cells). The high number of these immature cells interrupts the production of platelets, whose chief role is to aid in blood coagulation and prevention of hemorrhaging.

Leukemia is understood in different ways by children. An 8-year-old whom the author interviewed describes the disease in this way:

> There's like a war going on inside my body. The white cells are killing the red cells, or the red cells are killing the white ones. I'm not exactly sure, if that's right. Anyway, what the doctors want to do is to stop the war and let the dead cells grow again.

A 14-year-old relapsed AML patient, Geoffrey, whose case will be monitored throughout the chapter, spoke of his disease in vivid and emotional detail.

> I'm really scared. . . of dying. I've got a thousand platelets; that's pretty bad. My blood work is depressing—up, down, up, down, down, down!. . . I'm frightened when I wake up and there's blood all over the place and I've got wicked headaches and am freezing and running a high temperature; I think, this is it—I'm dying. That makes me really scared. This leukemia is the pits.

The body gives evidence of the dramatic upheaval taking place in the bone marrow. Because the blasts interrupt normal blood cell production, certain effects can be noted. If the red blood cells, *erythrocytes*, are in short supply the child may appear to grow pallid and listless. Since *platelets* control clotting, a deficiency of these cells may cause bleeding problems as well as spontaneous bruising or *petechiae*. Finally, if certain white blood cell production is inhibited by the abnormal blasts, then the child becomes vulnerable to a whole range of infections.

The Diagnosis of Leukemia: First-stage Treatment

Because the first indications of leukemia can be confused with symptoms of many other ordinary childhood illnesses, parents and pediatricians may not always suspect leukemia. Error in early detection is the cause of much guilt in parents who may have minimized the seriousness of any one of the early signs. The only definitive way in which leukemia can be diagnosed is by analysis of the blood. Initially an examination of the peripheral blood may be made, but the results must be confirmed by a biopsy of the bone marrow. While the peripheral blood may only evidence a small number of blasts, the bone marrow provides the definitive picture of lymphoblastic activity.

The biopsy involves a procedure known as *bone marrow aspiration*. A needle is inserted into the hip bone and tissue samples are withdrawn. Blood analysis looks for an excessive number of abnormal white cells. Once diagnosis is made, the treatment is rapid and aggressive if it is to be successful in stemming the proliferation of abnormal cells.

Antileukemic chemotherapy sets as its goal complete remission, which is simply defined as the cessation or absence of those symptoms by which the disease was initially diagnosed. In addition to the suppression of symptoms, remission involves return to normal of the white blood count, hemoglobin, and platelet count. This treatment aimed at remission ordinarily requires the hospitalization of the child for an average of 2 weeks and outpatient treatment for at least a year. The actual time it takes to achieve remission is judged to be significant in determining prognosis. Sallan and Weinstein (1980) report that children who enter remission within a month after treatment is begun are statistically at less risk of relapse than those who require 2 months of chemotherapy to achieve remission.

The treatment protocols for leukemia are aggressive, routinely involving chemotherapy and irradiation. Chemotherapy attempts to interrupt the normal development of the leukemic cells and ultimately to destroy them. In achieving this objective, chemotherapy can also affect normal, healthy cells and cause many stressful and unpleasant side effects.

Chemotherapy interferes with the bone marrow's ability to produce normal blood cells. Because of this, the child in treatment needs to be monitored for three specific complications. If his or her platelet count is low, there is danger of intravascular leukocyte thrombi and intracerebral hemorrhage, which would necessitate platelets transfusion and administration of heparin either intravenously or subcutaneously. A second complication is anemia due to the fewer red blood cells being produced. The third complication is the vulnerability to infection due to the lowered white cell count. Care must be taken in chemotherapy to avoid rendering the child neutropenic and thus unable to deal with these life-threatening complications of treatment.

Many of the drugs used in cancer treatment require intravenous or intramuscular administration. Some are able to be taken orally, and some few others are injected directly into the spinal canal (intrathecal). It has become routine procedure in many patients to surgically implant a direct line in the chest cavity connecting with the vena cava. Through this line, all intravenous medications can be pushed, providing the patient's veins with some respite and reducing some of the anxieties that can attend repeated intravenous (IV) punctures. Geoffrey (the 14-year-old relapsed patient referred to at the beginning of the chapter) speaks about this procedure:

A couple days ago, I had a line put in. This was the first time I'd had this done. The surgeon came and talked to me about it and explained how it worked. You learn a lot with this disease, like protocols, the risks. . . . You don't know what it's like to be constantly tied to an IV pole. You don't know what it's like to have to draw your IV wherever you go.

Chemotherapy generally involves a combination of antineoplastic drugs, rather than a single drug. Protocols of treatment have been developed to address specific leukemias, and are adjusted with respect to an individual child's tolerance and response.

The most common drugs included in these protocols include Adriamycin, ara-C, cytoxan, L-asparaginase, 6-mercaptopurine, methotrexate, prednisone, and vincristine. A person visiting an outpatient cancer treatment clinic who is unfamiliar with these drugs, would be surprised how well acquainted children and their parents are with the names of these drugs and the specific side effects associated with their use. There are dozens more drugs that are also in use, some of which are investigational or experimental. Many of these drugs have common side effects, which include nausea and vomiting, bone marrow depression, hair loss, mouth ulceration, and diarrhea.

Neurological Complications of Chemotherapy

Many of the drugs mentioned above that are routinely used in leukemia treatment are especially **neurotoxic**, that is, they are poisonous or destructive to nerve tissue. The treatment team is acutely aware of the risks and benefits of such intense and prolonged treatment. Use of these drugs and other experimental agents must be reconciled with the long-term effects of their administration as well as with the consequences of possible alteration of the blood-brain barrier by CNS filtration (Hanefeld & Riehm, 1980).

Because treatment is aggressive, a number of neurological complications have been reported in various studies (Soni *et al.*, 1975), ranging from generalized focal grand mal seizures to symptoms of somnolence or lethargy, often referred to as the "apathy syndrome" or the "somnolence syndrome" (Freeman, Johnston & Voke, 1973; Ch'ien *et al.*, 1980). Reports of **neuropathy**, or functional changes in the nervous system, in leukemia patients are frequent and these include manifestations of muscle loss, muscle spasms, double vision (**diplopia**), facial paralysis (**diplegia**) and voice changes to higher pitches. Peripheral neuropathy can also affect the way children walk. The diminished tone of the skeletal muscles (**hypotonia**) and muscle weakening of the plantar flexors and dorsiflexors are contributing factors to the external manifestation of such neuropathy (Hanefeld & Riehm, 1980). There is likewise the possibility of neuropsychological sequelae following intrathecal methotrexate and cranial irradiation, although there is need for further research to determine in what specific ways these drugs and procedures affect the quality of life and the ability to function (Moss & Nannis, 1980).

Central Nervous System Irradiation: Second-stage Treatment

A second-level strategy in leukemia treatment involves the irradiation of the *central nervous system* (*CNS*). In monitoring the course of relapses after initial remission has been achieved, leukemic infiltration of the central nervous system has been noted. In many treatment centers children are routinely treated by prophylactic CNS irradiation. This is considered by many to be a crucial staging in the treatment of leukemia, and is mounted as soon as remission has been achieved. Where this has been done, it has been judged to be successful in stemming the tide of relapse and CNS involvement.

The central nervous system is impermeable to many of the cytotoxic agents used in the treatment of leukemia. As such, it is vulnerable to leukemic infiltration. *Craniospinal irradiation* is by far the most common method of providing CNS prophylaxis. This aggressive prophylactic treatment is not without its risks and consequences. Irradiation of the CNS has a direct effect on the nervous tissue and increases the blood-brain barrier permeability. As a result, antileukemic substances may gain passage to the CNS. While the irradiation procedure may be useful in combatting leukemic infiltration of the CNS, therefore, it also creates a potentially serious barrier disorder. This issue is receiving the careful attention of many cancer researchers and clinicians (Ch'ien et al., 1980; Eiser, 1978; Moss & Nannis, 1980).

Treatment of this sort is preventive in nature; it is difficult to assess its factual effectiveness in forestalling relapse since hematologic remissions are not long-lived. Where cranial irradiation is not included in the treatment plan, it is not unusual that some other precautionary measures are taken against CNS relapse. Intrathecal injections of drugs like methotrexate or ara-C have been used to provide protection for the CNS against leukemic invasion. Sallan and Weinstein (1980) report prescribing infusions of ara-C on a regular schedule for some of their patients, although they are uncertain whether such a procedure will prove to be a successful prophylactic in the long term.

Maintenance Modalities: Third-stage Treatment

Treatment in the maintenance mode may continue for a year or more after initial remission has been successfully achieved. Continuing medical monitoring and treatment seeks to destroy any leukemic cell that may have survived the initial remission induction treatment. The goals of this third stage in the treatment process are not simply precautionary in nature. Maintenance therapies are considered to be imperative, since decisions in the past to abort treatment efforts prematurely have resulted in quicker relapses for many patients. With careful regard for toxicity and a child's tolerance, multidrug combination chemotherapy is the most ordinary approach to maintenance therapy.

The strategies for treating leukemia are a major subject of ongoing research and discussion. A combined treatment of antileukemic chemotherapy and cerebral irradiation is the most common method. For the children for whom treatment successfully irradicates the disease system, the long-term effects of the treatment of the brain and nervous system are not so easy to predict, and their long-term survival poses special concerns. As might be expected, there is always the lurking fear that termination of drug treatment might precipitate relapse (George, *et al.*, 1979; Tiller, Ekert, & Richards, 1977).

The ever-present danger of relapse needs to be reconciled with the equally real danger of the combined negative effects of long-term administration of the powerful antineoplastic drugs. Some of these effects were alluded to earlier in regard to nervous system reactions to irradiation and intrathecal administration of antileukemic agents. Issues concerning the quality of life for long-term survivors of leukemia are necessarily a part of the development of maintenance treatment programs (O'Malley, *et al.*, 1979).

Psychological Issues in the Care and Management of Pediatric Cancer Patients

The psychological care of the leukemic child and his or her family is as important as diagnosis and medical treatment. The ways in which children and their parents understand and respond to medical treatment does affect its course and must be given due consideration (Adams, 1978; Cotter & Schwartz, 1978; Fife, 1980; Johnson, Rudolph & Hartmann, 1979; Oury, 1981; Ross, 1979, 1980; Wright, 1974).

Cancer remains a stigma in our society, despite the fact that we know much more about diagnosis and have achieved a modest success in efforts to treat it. This section will examine some of the issues concerned with the fear of cancer and its internalization by society, and consider ways in which children and their families might be helped to deal with these issues.

Loss of Control

Cancer is frequently described as a powerful enemy that ravages the body and defies efforts to contain it, and the whole experience of diagnosis and treatment tends to reinforce this caricature. Many children feel as if their bodies have become a battlefield where physicians and technicians are mapping out a strategy and waging war upon a fierce and often elusive enemy. This imagery was evident in the transcript cited earlier of the 8-year-old's description of her leukemia. Cancer children's art frequently shows sketches of beasts and monsters consuming innocent victims. Adolescents' poetry uses verbal imagery to communicate the same message (Adams, 1976; Hodges, 1981). Depending on their particular stage of cognitive development, children are perhaps even more liable than adults to perceive their experience of cancer in terms of combat and warfare.

The language of cancer is foreign. The word itself is threatening, its diagnosis bringing parents to tears. Regardless of the vocabulary or nosology chosen to describe the disease, the child seems to perceive that something is seriously wrong. Although he or she may not fully understand much about the treatment or prognosis, the child does relate to the seriousness of the situation, not necessarily as a result of direct and simple communication by parents or a doctor, but more often by rather sophisticated assimilation of many nonverbal cues from the total environment.

Families feel a loss of control because treatment is begun so rapidly once diagnosis is made. Aggressive treatment and hospitalization spell loss of control to the children as well. Observational studies of hospitalized children often comment on the ways in which children attempt to compensate for this loss of control by manipulating parents, siblings, and hospital staff (Bruneau, 1981; Flaherty, 1978; Katz, Kellerman & Siegel, 1980; Pfefferbaum & Lucas, 1979). Another behavioral reaction is more difficult to recognize and manage: withdrawal. The withdrawn child seems to express the feeling that the combat is unequal; some small amount of security is found in retreat. Both manipulation and withdrawal represent subtle efforts to regain a modicum of control in the face of overwhelming threats.

Cancer disrupts the normal course of the child's developmental pattern. In his attempt to describe the course of human development, Erik Erikson placed a high premium on the child's progressive mastery of the world in which he or she lives. This mastery is achieved as a child explores, initiates, and succeeds. Cumulative gains contribute to the emerging sense of self and the child's sense of control. Catastrophic illness presents certain serious challenges to the direction in which this process is moving and signals the contrary message that one has lost the ability to control.

The aggressive treatments that are a routine part of intervention with a diagnosed child can involve considerable discomfort and pain, and the side effects of these treatments can also be quite disruptive. Bone marrow aspirations and lumbar punctures are frequently repeated procedures during initial treatment and follow-up maintenance therapies. While children become quite familiar with these procedures, they do not seem to adjust to them. Geoffrey, the 14-year-old relapsed AML patient we have been interviewing, recalls his initial treatment for leukemia, and the circumstances of his relapse.

It took ten months to treat me. I was in the hospital initially for a month and then I had to keep coming back to the clinic for LPs [lumbar punctures] and bone marrows [aspirations]. I got really mad at the doctors; I must have had at least 50 of them and I never got used to them. . . .

I knew I was relapsing. I started getting drowsy, angry. . . no petechiae, no bruising—I was glad no bruising. When I relapsed I went into shock, because after two and a half years off treatment, you know, you have a horror about the treatments. The thought of going back to that pretty much blew my mind.

I'm real good friends with the doctor. When I saw him he said: "You either have a virus or you've relapsed." I had relapsed. He took us in the room and we all broke up crying.

When I relapsed I went and got a haircut—the last haircut before I entered the hospital. . . . I'm glad I've got a private room because I couldn't take all the crying—I have enough trouble sleeping as it is. Since I've been here, I've been really depressed, drowsy, scared.

It is clear that for at least some young cancer patients these medical procedures come to represent a life they cannot control. Geoffrey's own analysis of his depression saw it linked with beginning another painful series of treatments. His knowledge about the course of his particular leukemia made him wonder aloud whether it was worth the suffering.

Since so much of communication depends upon nonverbal messages, many children rely heavily for information upon what they infer from the attitudes and behaviors of their parents, nurses, and physicians. In perceiving adult fears, anxieties, and ambivalence, these children understand the seriousness of their illness. However, children do not seem to interpret from these nonverbal clues that the disease itself is out of control.

The child who has been gradually assuming greater autonomy and control in his or her life, now is faced with retrenchment. Not only are the familiar markers of home, school, routines, and activities disrupted, but they are replaced with a world that is totally unfamiliar and unmanageable. Witness Geoffrey's despair:

I'm really down in the dumps. You know that you are in here; you know that you're going to become more weak, there's nothing to do. Your parents come in, your relatives come to see you . . . but you're just going to get sicker. Look, my hair's starting to come out already. I lost it four times the last time.

Efforts to manipulate this environment or the psychologic withdrawal from it may be viewed as ultimate attempts to regain minimal control. Regression is not an uncommon psychological retreat in the face of these two options, and this presents a most serious challenge to both treatment and day-to-day management.

Separation

Physical separation from families and the distancing that children perceive on the part of some relatives and professionals enable children to comprehend the seriousness of their illness. Approach-avoidance conflicts of parents and medical staff may further isolate the child, who may sense the conflict without understanding it. Spinetta, Rigler, and Karon (1974) have reported on the issue of isolation. In a doll house that simulated a hospital setting, children were asked to position dolls representing parental and health care individuals. The children placed the dolls in what has been described as interpersonally distant positions, clearly demonstrating feelings of isolation and loneliness.

Separation is an issue closely related to those of isolation and loss. Separation, even in adult life, presents certain challenges to emotional adjustment. For a child this creates a particular set of problems. The kinds of separations necessitated by hospitalizations, and by chemotherapeutic and irradiation treatments engage the anxieties of children. The regressed behaviors and management problems noted above derive from feelings of isolation, loss, and separation. Night terrors are but one common behavioral response to separation (Kellerman, 1979). Hospital personnel acknowledge difficulty in dealing with the clinging behaviors evident in so many children. However, the natural reaching out to a parent or primary nurse may be an important vehicle in helping the child regain some sense of security. Initial consultations with a hospitalized pediatric cancer patient not only need to consider the stresses being experienced by the child and family but must also seek ways to coordinate available supports (Koocher, 1980; O'Malley & Koocher, 1979).

Results from projective test protocols of children in situations of separation reflect a pervasive state of anxiety. Children's stories are frequently laden with descriptions of destruction and defeat that can easily be understood as veiled allusions to death (Spinetta, 1977). While these references may be oblique and death not specifically mentioned, it is clear that the child's inner psychological life is actively engaged in processing what he or she clearly perceives to be serious and life-threatening. The child reflects a need for support as he or she tries to find some assurance of security.

Being here again really scares me. I think that I'm going to die. This scares me the most. All my friends and all my stuff—none of my friends are dying! It's like I'm not going to be around the next fifty years and they will. I can't get married, can't have kids. . . . I'm tired. You know, what shocks me the most is when I get a high temperature, and there's blood all over the bed—it scares me. And I think, "Well, Geoff, that's it."

Therapeutic Aspects of Play Activities

Those who routinely deal with pediatric oncology patients are sensitive to the dynamics described above. Pediatric cancer centers are acutely aware of the psychological problems encountered by children with life-threatening illnesses. Margaret Adams (1976) describes a structured therapeutic group-play program that she facilitates at Memorial Sloan-Kettering Cancer Center in New York City. Her program assists children in expressing feelings of separation and loss while providing them with opportunities to regain a sense of mastery and control. Not only are these experiences important for the period of hospitalization and initial treatment, but they seem to influence adjustment in the posthospital environments of home and school.

Play is therapeutic for the hospitalized child because it provides a release valve for many conflicts. In addition, play provides an opportunity to work through emotional problems and encourages the child to gain mastery over them. In the hospital environment the child is relegated to the predominantly passive role of a recipient. Play reengages the child in an active process, which affords opportunities for cathartic relief, reality testing, and insight development. All of these psychological activities can restore some sense of control in the midst of overwhelming challenges.

Opinion varies among activity and play therapists as to the value of hospital-related play for cancer patients. One position sees the play room or activity center as a safe haven away from the world of often painful hospital procedures. Activity coordinators of this persuasion believe the child needs some legitimate escape from the world of medicine and its related procedures, and do not allow recreation to include the reenactment of these experiences. Another school of thought believes that such hospital-related play is an important component in the integration of experience and an important vehicle in assisting the child in his or her efforts to cope with the catastrophic impact of hospitalization and treatment.

Each position has its own merit. Since many children seem naturally drawn to explorative play involving aspects of their disease and its treatment, it would seem beneficial to allow the child to pursue this need in structured and nonstructured activities. Although some children may reluctantly enter group play of this sort, many adjust quite rapidly to the other children and become active participants. Some activity therapists make available to these children much of the paraphernalia used in the ordinary hospital routine. In addition to stethoscopes and reflex hammers, the children have access to the more specialized materials used in chemotherapies: syringes, needles, intravenous tubing, and bottles. Obviously care is taken so that the children do not accidentally injure themselves or others, and some supplies are modified according to safety standards.

In using these supplies in the context of play, the children profit in two important ways. Group-play of this sort tends to educate children to the nature and treatment of their diseases through the sharing of peers' insights and their experiences in coping with illness. Secondly, by observing and monitoring the content of and affect displayed in these activities, staff and parents can better understand how a child is relating to his or her illness, and can better plan the course of future interventions on their part.

Brunnquell and Hall (1982) note that life-threatening illness throws the child's emerging sense of self-worth and competence into disarray. In addressing the psychological consequences of this developmental trauma, parents and medical staff need to identify areas wherein some sources of control may be regained by the child. The hospital play program is one specific strategy that is being successfully utilized in many treatment settings. Its immediate advantages are evident, since it provides a ready source of information to the child about the nature, symptoms, treatment, and side effects of his or her illness.

The activity program at Children's Hospital and the Dana-Farber Cancer Institute in Boston recognizes the positive effect that self-expression can play in coping with the fact of hospitalization and treatment. An in-house newspaper provides patients with an opportunity to submit creative efforts in the form of poetry, short stories, or art. This outlet for expression has proven to be very beneficial for some children, especially adolescents who may not wish to participate in other activities. For example, a patient like Geoffrey would be reluctant to be involved in play programs in which younger patients might be participating. He was glad to be in a private room apart from these younger children. The needs of an adolescent cancer patient are distinct from those of a younger child; an activity program that invites creative expression of this sort can provide a wonderful vehicle for communication (Fochtman, 1979). A patient like Geoff who is verbally inclined can benefit enormously from an activity program encouraging reflection and expression. The activity therapist is in a special position to become part of the communication effort and to help the child or adolescent who may wish to share some important feelings.

Normalization of Hospital Life

Children hospitalized in the oncology unit are ordinarily encouraged to get dressed in their own clothing each day and to follow some semblance of a normal routine, which includes in-house school and other recreational activities. This is all coordinated to maintain some continuity with normal life and responsibilities. The objective is not always realized, since the presence of discomfort and pain and some negative reactions to treatment may prevent a child from effectively participating.

Health care providers and the families of hospitalized children recognize the need to psychologically engage the child. Even small gains are beneficial. Children in isolated and restricted hospital situations can be given opportunities to assist in their treatments. They feel more in control if they can help in changing tape and dressings. With some assistance they can monitor intravenous treatments, as could Geoffrey:

Would you mind if we stop this discussion for a minute? I've got to get the nurse in here. My IV needs to be flushed. She should have noticed this herself. Good thing I'm on the ball or the whole thing would get fouled up. Sometimes they forget to turn an IV on, or forget a medicine. They're supposed to know these things. I'm sure they do.

Although these activities appear of little consequence, they nonetheless have their place in helping restore some sense of control to the child, and they may be all that is needed to engage an otherwise regressed or withdrawn child.

Primary Nursing Care

Very closely related to the issue of psychological engagement are the interpersonal dynamics which are at work in the relationships between the child and parents and between the child and staff. A child is vulnerable to the multiplicity of contacts with those charged with his or her care. In many cancer centers that primarily treat children, efforts are made to ensure primary relationships in the treatment program, but these are not always achieved.

Primary nursing care attempts to minimize the negative effects of hospitalization and aggressive medical treatments. Primary nurses become important liaisons to families in crisis and contribute significantly to the family's psychological adjustment to the diagnosis and treatment. While this philosophy of nursing care is intelligible and of demonstrated benefit to child and family alike, it is not without its costs to the nurse who elects to participate in such a program of care. Oncology nursing is already demanding; primary nursing care makes additional personal and professional demands on the practitioner. For this reason, it is not unusual that there is considerable turnover in oncology nursing staff.

It is critical that children be helped to understand each of the procedures to which they are subjected, especially when these involve discomfort and pain. Nursing plays an important role in mediating this understanding. Children are particularly subject to fantasize, and their fantasies often tend to be more ominous and dire than the reality these are based on would justify. The time invested in preparation and explanation not only calms fears but also allows the child to maintain some control. Knowledge of medical procedures does not erase the pain, but it does help to ease the psychological burdens that accompany these painful treatments.

Hypnosis and Relaxation Techniques

Psychologists assist in this process in a number of ways. In addition to the recreational activities described above, staff psychologists may engage the child in play therapy to work on some specific problem or conflict. Individual consultations with a child, group meetings with a number of patients, family therapy sessions, or staff consultations are all services that a psychologist may be called upon to provide. Because of the anxieties experienced by many hospitalized children, or the pain created by repeated injections, or the nausea resulting from chemotherapy, hypnotherapy is often quite useful in assisting children to learn relaxation techniques that can lessen the sources of distress (Miller, 1980).

Some children respond well to hypnotherapeutic treatment. Dash (1980) has observed that children make the best hypnotic subjects because of their trust, vivid imaginations, and openness for new experiences. He conceptualizes hypnosis with a child in terms of "teaching" a child a way to control his or her own discomfort. This coincides with the child's developmental need to establish mastery and, in these particular circumstances, to regain control. Some good results have been noted in reducing anxiety and the negative impact of certain stressful components of the treatment protocol (Sacerdote, 1970). Geoffrey himself underwent hypnosis:

That man with the glasses [a clinical staff psychologist] came in to see me the other day and hypnotized me. He did a good job in putting me out. I was tired all day—it felt good. But I was scared though. . . . I'd just like to be warm one day, like on a raft on a sunny day. I want to be at home, at school, with my friends, in gym. . . I want to sleep. Could you help me like that other guy to relax?

Children are taught a variety of inductions and deepening techniques; certain techniques work better with one child than with another. Although pain and anxiety reduction was the principal therapeutic goal in introducing this clinical technique with pediatric oncology patients, a secondary gain derives from learning the skills of self-hypnosis—a sense of mastery—which gain may actually be more important to the child (Miller, 1980).

Children as Mutual Resources

Children continually demonstrate enormous resourcefulness and resilience in adjusting to the realities of their diseases and their respective treatments. The relationships they establish with other children in similar circumstances are extremely important to their adjustment. Some implications of these peer interactions were discussed in relation to play, but they serve even more important functions.

Children learn from the experiences of other children and find much needed support in sharing them. Although there are obvious liabilities in forming relationships—the most evident of which is the possibility of the relapse and death of a cherished friend—they nonetheless provide a child such as Geoff with many of the ingredients for healthy adaptation and accommodation.

I've known a lot of other kids who have had what I have—Jim, Glen, Steve, Kathy. I could give you a whole list. They've all died, except one good friend who hasn't died yet. She didn't relapse. I didn't think I was going to relapse. I thought I had this thing licked. . . and I relapsed.

Friendships are an important counterpoint to the disorienting events that accompany the diagnosis and treatment of life-threatening illness.

It has been generally noted that children must be allowed to express their apprehensions and fears about death, physical disfigurement, and the impact of their disease on family life, school, activities, and sports. It is imperative that they design strategies and acquire skills to deal with these and other related issues associated with cancer (Gogan, *et al.*, 1977). Some children seem to adopt an aggressive posture in addressing these issues, and develop appropriate and helpful methods of coping with their illnesses; others find the challenges too difficult and painful and appear to retreat from engagement.

The loss of hair (***alopecia***) can become a symbolic field on which the battle for readjustment is waged. As Brunnquell and Hall (1982) note, hair loss is a persistent reminder of the life-threatening illness and in fact separates the child from disease-free peers. The way in which a child negotiates this visible hurdle often reflects his or her measure of adjustment. Some cancer patients demonstrate unusual resourcefulness in addressing this question and assist fellow patients to explore ways in which they too can succeed.

Reentry to Home and School

Transitions from hospital to home and school routines become difficult for many children who enter remission (Kagen-Goodheart, 1977). Despite many complaints, children eventually acclimate themselves to a hospital routine and find some security in it. When they return home some children find it very difficult to resume ordinary life again, as did Geoff.

It was hard going back to school after I left the hospital before. Kids are cruel, but now they're not. I stuck up for myself. I punched the kids out. They pulled my wig off; I didn't wear a wig any more. I wore it for a couple of days, but I didn't like it. So, a kid in class pulled it off. I laced him in the side of the head with my fist. He went to the hospital. They don't understand cancer. They should teach them. . . .

The teachers treat me differently. One of my teachers who is a coach used to be pretty mean to me. He wants to push me. He called me on the phone and was really nice to me. He might come down to see me.

Christine Eiser (1980) discusses the ways in which life-threatening illness affects a child's participation in school. Even though at home, children frequently return to the hospital for ongoing chemotherapy and radiation treatments. This necessitates interruptions in attendance at school. Because these can continue for a few years while maintenance therapies are in progress, a certain degree of social difficulties and impaired self-esteem is not surprising (Burns & Zweig, 1980).

Eiser reported that teachers described special difficulties in dealing with leukemic children, and their expectations about performance were significantly modified because of the child's illness. This report noted that most teachers surveyed had a reasonable knowledge about leukemia, including information about treatment and its sequelae. Despite the adequacy of this information, the majority expressed a desire to be more knowledgable. We might interpret this to mean that they wished to be better equipped so that they might assist in the total care of the child. Teachers are an enormous asset in health care efforts responding to the multiple needs of seriously ill children.

Teachers often express doubts about what reasonable goals they might set for a child involved in maintenance treatment. While most would favor a normalization of the school routine for the returning child, they frankly admit that this objective is not easily realized (Sachs, 1980). Although the disease is understood as life-threatening and not necessarily terminal, many teachers relate to it as if it were terminal. If this is the unexpressed and nonverbal understanding, it is reasonable that teachers are more permissive, less demanding, and more solicitous toward the leukemic child. But the ramifications of these responses for the normal development of the child need to be understood. Overprotective attitudes can hamper the child's development and prevent the normalization parents and teachers both desire. Teachers at the other extreme refuse to acknowledge or are unable to account for the special needs of the leukemic child. These teachers maintain unrealistic high expectations of the child's performance. Neither of these extremes is helpful to the child.

The better the communication triad between parents, school, and hospital, the more effective can the classroom teacher be in supporting the reintegration of the child into the school environment (Katz, 1980). The hospital can provide the technical consultation many teachers desire as a supplement to their general knowledge about childhood leukemia.

Many pediatric cancer centers invite teachers to symposia organized at the hospital to provide open discussion of the issues of cancer care, and many teachers welcome such opportunities for continuing education. More importantly, these conferences can provide teachers with release valves for the feelings triggered by close association with a child victimized by leukemia. The more these feelings are addressed and processed, the more resourceful an ally the teacher becomes in the total care of the child. Although the scant research on this topic (Grave & Pless, 1974; Holdswirth & Whitmore, 1974) fails to identify any significant negative adjustments of cancer children to the school environment, explorative conferences with teachers seem to indicate that more can be done to tap the hidden resources of the school in promoting adjustment. This type of consultation activity, in which the hospital can play a key role, can yield enormous benefits for the child who ultimately becomes the beneficiary of informed and coordinated participation by the teacher and school community.

Relapse and the Problem of Terminal Diagnosis

From the beginning of this discussion we have spoken of leukemia as a life-threatening illness. With careful diagnosis and competent treatment, many children enter remission and a significant number of these remain in complete remission. As noted at the beginning of the chapter, a generally accepted definition of *cure* is a state of remission for at least 5 years. Some scientists reason that the actual risk of relapse decreases as the length of the period of remission increases (George, *et al.*, 1979). The termination of antileukemic chemotherapy is an anxiety-filled decision. Although it is a liberating decision and one based on good prognosis for indefinite remission, it is nonetheless a cause of real concern to parents and physicians alike.

From the physician's point of view, there is always the possibility of relapse, but this reality must be balanced over and against the accumulated physical and psychological effects of prolonged treatment. On the medical level, issues concerning organ toxicity and the possible reduction of effectiveness of the blood-brain barrier must be negotiated in electing to terminate chemotherapy. The long-term psychological effects of prolonged treatment are still a matter for research.

Although interim reports do not seem to note any significant differences in intellectual development between children receiving extensive chemotherapy, including CNS irradiation, and those who do not, there is some evidence that certain learning capacities may be negatively affected (Eiser & Landsdown, 1977; Eiser, 1978, 1979).

Parents are also vulnerable when chemotherapy is terminated. Some parents report difficult adjustment problems with the child and their other children (Iles, 1979; Kalnins, Churchill & Terry, 1980). Underlying many of their expressed and unexpressed feelings lurks the anxiety that the child will relapse and the disease will not remit. This is a realistic fear and one that needs to be explored with parents (Koocher & Sallan, 1978).

The initial treatment phase, as we have already discussed, throws the entire family system into significant turmoil. Many of the ordinary day-to-day activities and responsibilities of the family are temporarily suspended. To a limited extent, the family has been attempting to resume normal functioning while the child is in the maintenance chemotherapy period of treatment. The termination of treatment becomes an index for families signalling that they should finally resume full normal functioning. In a sense, the family moves out of a "crisis management mode" into routine life or a close approximation thereof. Some parents find this transition to be difficult and report problems in returning to ordinary responsibilities. The period following the termination of all treatments has a crisis quality of its own.

If the child does relapse, a different set of family dynamics is set in motion. Exposure to other children and their parents over the extended course of treatment educates families to the significance of relapse. Although a second remission might be achieved relatively soon, it often is the beginning of an ominous series of relapses and remissions. Parents and children begin to relate to the disease more as a terminal illness than simply a life-threatening one.

Children with leukemia and other life-threatening illnesses develop, along with their parents, subtle medical sophistication in regard to their disease.

This is clearly seen in Geoffrey's case. Geoff accurately diagnosed his relapse. He not only interpreted his chills and fever, but he was tuned in to other warning signs.

I've lost so much weight. I used to be 150 pounds; now I weigh 135. I lost these 15 pounds in just a couple of weeks.

As shown earlier, on numerous occasions Geoff would speak about his fatigue and his persistent hemorrhages. He would seem quite elated that there were no petechiae or bruises "this time." He would be greatly concerned about his platelet count and anxious about getting infused so that he could blow his nose without risking serious nose bleeds. On balance, Geoff was inclined to view all of these danger signals as signs that he was losing the battle with cancer.

In his work with leukemic children, Spinetta (1977) notes that younger children seem to be acutely aware of the seriousness of their illnesses, even though they may be unable or unwilling to discuss this in adult language. By this he means that children facing multiple relapses and remissions may not directly use the language of death and fear of death, but nonverbal and other symbolic expressions give substantial evidence that such awareness clearly has a place in the child's inner life. From his own clinical experience, the author recalls the following vignette that provides a clear example of a young child's awareness of death.

The case involved a 4-year-old boy hospitalized with ALL. His teenage babysitter was visiting him on the pediatric oncology unit where he was undergoing remission induction treatment for his leukemia. During her visit she was wheeling him up and down the corridor of the unit in a stroller. He fell asleep. When he woke up, his sitter had gone and he was quite agitated. He asked his mother: "Where did Jeannie go?" His mother explained to him that he had fallen asleep and Jeannie had had to go home, but that she would come again to visit him. Without hesitation he responded: "I won't see her anymore, 'cause I'm very sick." Quite unexpectedly, he died that night.

Children in these extreme life-threatening situations show an amazing capacity to cope. This capacity manifests itself in three basic ways: (1) they seem to deal appropriately with their anxieties, (2) they maintain as much as possible a semblance of normality in their relationships to family, friends, and social responsibilities, (3) they take assertive positions vis-à-vis their illness and frequently become precocious philosophers, seeking to find some ultimate meaning in their life situations. Such characteristics contribute to what is judged to be effective coping, and these traits prove to be the rule rather than the exception with many terminally ill children.

Cancer treatment continues to be a frontier of experimental medicine. In cases where the child does not respond to conventional therapies, the family is confronted with a new set of decisions. When relapses are more frequent than usual and normative treatments ineffective in achieving remission, parents are frequently asked permission to try experimental research drugs. The dynamics governing this decision-making process are interesting and important.

Openness is the key to the whole process. Many believe that this openness, appropriate to the age and psychological development of the child, must be fundamental to the whole diagnostic and treatment approach. That the child should assume an active part in discussion represents a shift in philosophy for many physicians, yet it seems normative today in most cancer treatment programs. Children seem to reflect family attitudes in their reactions to the seriousness of their illnesses and the last-hope nature of the proposed experimental drugs or procedures. Their reactions to the honest communication of their physicians span the entire spectrum of emotional response, from quiet acceptance and compliance to assertive opposition. Relationships with physicians and those responsible for the long course of their treatment can dispose the child to want to please these providers, and they readily consent to do whatever is asked. Their greatest anxieties come from fear of more pain and distressing side effects. Many children seem to be disposed to fight the disease, although occassionally one encounters a child who seems to have lost the will to fight and shows resignation to dying.

Parents find decisions about experimental drugs and procedures and the decision to suspend aggressive curative treatments among the most difficult to make. During the long process of diagnosis and treatment of the disease, they have vicariously experienced the physical and psychological pains of their children. While they often voice a desire to do everything possible to conquer the enemy ravaging their child's body, they recognize that the child has limits in what he or she should be expected to tolerate. It is difficult for parents to differentiate their own feelings from those of their child. However, it seems that most parents can intellectually distinguish between their selfish desire to try everything until there is nothing more to try and a concern for the well-being and personal good of the child.

Finally, the physician experiences a most difficult role conflict. As a primary scientist, he or she is dedicated to the goals of research and welcomes any opportunity to push ahead frontiers of treatment toward the primary goal of cure. Yet this may oppose the role of the physician as advocator, who attempts to counsel and support the patient and his or her family in this most difficult personal choice to use experimental drugs.

Nitschke, Wunder, Sexauer, and Humphrey (1977) described the "final-stage conference" that takes place when such a crucial decision is made. In reporting the outcome of a number of cases in which experimental drug treatments became an option, they concluded that parents and their children generally came to the same conclusions. They reported that the most difficult role in the process belongs to the physician. Each case, even though similar to others, is necessarily unique and must be treated as such. Sensitivity to the child and parents and respect for their needs as they move toward decision are of paramount importance. The open communication at the heart of this interaction is very much appreciated by parents, but especially by the affected children.

The decisions children and parents make at this critical crossroad vary. Some will elect to submit to research drug treatments and other experimental procedures. Others will reasonably refuse any additional treatments. From a human and psychological perspective, the well-being of the child and his or her parents depends on the way in which the whole decision-making process is engaged.

Anticipatory Grief and Death

The kind of decision making described above is often a catalyst to the preparation for proximate death. Lindemann (1944) first used the term *anticipatory grief* to define the dynamics of preparation that a family engages in during the weeks and months preceding death. These dynamics principally revolve around the process of disengagement, physical and emotional. This process obviously is not without its difficulties, since a terminally ill child is particularly vulnerable to any separations at this time. Lindemann noted that the process of disengagement frequently may prove more helpful to the survivors than to the dying patient. Earlier mention was made of the child's sense of emotional and physical distancing in the early stages of cancer treatment (Spinetta, 1972, 1977; Spinetta & Maloney, 1975). More systematic research is needed to understand the complex interactions at work during the terminal stage.

The realization that death is inevitable is a new shock to parents. Although this has perhaps always been a hidden fear, the circumstances of the child's unresponsiveness to conventional or experimental treatments confronts parents with incontrovertible evidence. Parents often face a conflictual set of feelings: the desire to be with the dying child and the desire to disengage. Physicians and nurses sense these same feelings as well, although in ways different from parents. Conscious of their own feelings, hospital staff need to help parents work through many ambivalent feelings. Together they must be as accessible as possible to dying children.

Geoffrey's mother, a registered nurse, talks about her feelings as Geoff's condition deteriorates.

When Geoffrey's leukemia was initially diagnosed, I fell apart. My husband was the strong one. He was right here with him, trying to encourage me. I've been with a lot of sick people, and I've always been able to help them. It's very different when it's your own child.

Now the situation is reversed. My husband can't face the facts now. He comes here only on weekends, but he calls every day. He doesn't seem to want to know how serious Geoff's relapse is. He tells me that I understand all that medical jargon and he doesn't. He keeps saying: "Geoff's a strong young man; he'll pull through just like he did before." I feel so tired and so helpless and so alone. . . .

If it weren't for the staff and the other people at the Ronald McDonald House [a place where out-of-town families can stay while children are being treated for cancer], I don't know what I would do. I find it so difficult to leave here at night, particularly when Geoff says: "Mom, stay! stay!" I have stayed with him in his room a couple of nights, but I have to get some sleep sometime. After all, I'm the only one here for him.

Geoffrey found the attitudes of some of the hospital staff to be frustrating. This is how he described his feelings.

It stinks around here [the hospital]. You don't understand. You get to walk around without a pole, without things stuck in you. I mean, I can't take IVs any more. . . . I'd just like to be warm one day. . . .

It's hard, boy. They don't know how it is—always shake, always don't feel good. And then the jokes—"You'll be OK, don't worry about it." The nurses and everybody says it. You *have* to worry about it. It doesn't help me when someone tells me not to worry about it. It helps me a lot when somebody is willing to talk to me about it.

When the child dies, most parents do prefer to see the child's body and to spend some time in the presence of the body. This opportunity should always be provided, and great care taken to ensure whatever degree of privacy is possible to family members. The members of the health care team who were so important to the family during the long course of treatments and hospitalizations are frequently most welcome in this intimate gathering. It seems most appropriate that they share this experience with families. Follow-up studies of families who lost children often speak about how important this time was to them (Kreuger, Gyllenskold, Pehrsson, & Sjolin, 1981). Many attribute the positive direction their mourning took to the sensitivity shown them in allowing contact with the body of the deceased child.

The responsibilities of the physician and hospital staff do not terminate with the death of the child. Many parents relate how important a part of their lives the hospital environment had become, and how connected they feel with not only staff but with the other families with whom they had shared so much. It is not unusual that families will maintain some contact with the hospital for a while. They may become invested in some volunteer projects, or participate in ongoing social service programs aimed at assisting them in their grief work. Hospital staff are acutely aware that their contact with the families extends significantly beyond the treatment of malignancy, reaching as it does into the depths of a family's whole life. Being with a family throughout the entire course of this crisis requires insight, compassion, and commitment. The author's heartening experience has been that all of these ingredients typically characterize the philosophies and policies guiding the care programs of pediatric cancer treatment facilities.

Summary

The words *cancer* and *leukemia* may initially mean very little to a child who first hears this diagnosis. To anxious parents, the mere mention of these words is enough to generate fear and a sense of powerlessness. In the course of treatment, however, these attitudes change. Children come to a remarkably sophisticated understanding of the meaning of the disease. Their parents gradually discover that great strides have been made in the effective treatment of the full range of childhood cancers, especially leukemia.

This chapter has addressed the multiple aspects of childhood and adolescent cancer by focusing on one specific disease: leukemia. Leukemia is a progressive and malignant disease of the blood-forming organs. The etiology of leukemia is still unknown, although research is close to finding the answer.

Whatever normally regulates the maturation of the white blood cells is dysfunctional; these lymphoblasts multiply rapidly. The blasts accumulate in the bone marrow and threaten the normal blood cells that develop there. In addition, the lymphoblasts are unable to perform the normal bodily functions assigned to them, principally that of fighting infection. The significant presence of these immature blasts interferes with platelet production and may lead to hemorrhaging. The principal goal of treatment is the destruction of these lymphoblasts.

Some of the alterations in blood chemistry produce external physical symptoms. A child may look pale because red blood cells may be in short supply. Spontaneous bleeding or bruising may result from the lowering of the number of platelets in the blood. Or the child may become susceptible to a broad range of infections. Some of these symptoms are associated with other normal childhood illnesses and initially may not be accurately diagnosed.

A routine blood analysis might reveal a higher than normal number of white blood cells and may give support to a tentative diagnosis of leukemia. Definitive diagnosis, however, requires bone marrow biopsy and analysis. Once confirmed, treatment begins immediately. The normal treatment program includes a multidrug protocol, with routine monitoring of any lymphoblastic activity in the bone marrow. Initial remission is often achievable within weeks after treatment commences. The amount of time required to achieve remission is considered to be one measure of risk for subsequent relapse.

The drugs currently in use in leukemia protocols utilize all the various routes of administration. Some may be taken orally, others are injected into muscle tissue or into a vein. Some are injected directly into the spinal column. These drugs are powerful cytotoxic agents and produce a wide range of unpleasant side effects.

Many of these drugs are potentially neurotoxic; prolonged use of certain of them can precipitate certain neurological and psychological dysfunctions. The damage to the nerve tissue of long-term survivors who use some of these drugs is difficult to assess. One reason for the difficulty is that many of these drugs are experimental.

Used as a protection against relapse, a prophylactic irradiation of the central nervous system (CNS) is often a second-stage strategy in leukemia treatment. The CNS does not allow many of the cancer-destroying drugs past its barrier. Some drugs, as noted before, are intrathecally injected into the cerebrospinal fluid. CNS irradiation and the prolonged use of cytotoxic drugs both pose an important problem: how to weigh the risks of such treatment against the anticipated benefits.

Maintenance programs for children in remission are generally targeted for a year or two. The child is able to resume a fairly normal routine, although the stigma of cancer and the necessity of regular clinic visits for monitoring and daytime treatments makes adjustment difficult for some children and families. This is particularly true for children above the age of 5 and adolescents. Younger children (preschoolers and elementary school children) have fewer problems with reintegration.

The psychological issues associated with the care and management of pediatric and adolescent cancer patients have been extensively reviewed. Psychological problems can become more pressing in situations in which a child relapses or when the disease does not appear to respond to various treatments. Particular sensitivity and competence are needed in caring for the child with cancer. This does not simply refer to technical and scientific matters but must embrace the often complex psychological dynamics associated with a life-threatening illness.

Control is a common problem in many forms of illness. As a sense of being in control is essential to a person's well-being, this must be considered in planning strategies of treatment and care. A patient, regardless of age, desires to be an active partner in the therapeutic objective. Withdrawal and depression may be signs that a patient's participation in this objective has been ignored. A number of practical ways in which children can be helped to remain active in curative treatment efforts have been reviewed.

Hospitalization necessitates a certain degree of physical separation of children from their families and ordinary routines. In addition, the seriousness of a diagnosis can prevent some people—parents, siblings, other relatives, and certain medical personnel—from important interpersonal contact with the sick child. These two forms of separation—physical and psychological—can compound the problems of children, families, and caregivers. Most pediatric hospitals are sensitive to these problems and have developed approaches to mitigate the negative effects of separation.

In an attempt to normalize the hospital environment, play rooms have been introduced into pediatric units. The therapeutic aspects of play for a child with cancer include recreational as well as psychological benefits. Diverse hospital activity programs have been devised. Clearly the activity therapist is an important resource person on the health care team, since much important communication with a child or adolescent is mediated through play and related structured activities.

In hospitals that have adopted a primary nursing care model, the nurse becomes the most important individual to the patient and family. Between them and this principal care provider, communications are strong as trust builds through prolonged contact. The chapter looked at the assets and liabilities implied in such a humanistic concept of nursing.

The psychologist plays an increasingly important role in pediatric oncology units, both as a direct provider of clinical services and as a consultant. Hypnosis is an example of a specific behavioral treatment used to manage leukemic children's anxieties and physical complaints. Children are responsive to this type of intervention and benefit from the techniques they are taught.

One of the most important resources in the task of social adjustment cancer children must face is contact with peers who have similar illnesses. Children educate one another and help each other to appropriate the skills that enable them to cope with their illnesses and treatments. Bonds of friendship are important vehicles for acquiring information and ventilating frustrations and doubts.

Adjustment to home life and school after initial remission has been achieved is a personal, familial, and social problem. In this adjustment, the hospital staff plays an important role as mediator and educator.

Although the prognosis for childhood cancer patients is constantly improving, numbers of children still die from the disease. The chapter concludes with a look at the dynamics of a situation involving a terminally ill child and shows how dying children display remarkable resilience and coping abilities as well as knowledge about their condition. Also discussed is the ethical dilemma faced by numbers of parents in choosing whether to commence experimental chemotherapies when the disease is no longer responding to conventional treatments. Preparation for death sets in motion the function of anticipatory grief.

In Solzhenitsyn's *Cancer Ward*, the author speaks about the treatment of cancer as a wall rising between the world and the patient until the latter remains alone on the other side. In this discussion of childhood and adolescent cancer, we have attempted to weaken the wall that separates and strengthen the fortress that supports the child, family, and health care providers who together face the challenge of disease, cure, and possibly death.

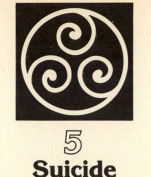

5

Suicide
in Adolescence
and Young Adulthood

Some Demographic and Statistical Data

Etiology of Adolescent Suicide

- Genetic Predispositions
- Biochemical Factors
- Emotional Disorders
- Familial and Sociocultural Determinants

Suicidal Behaviors

- Intentional Suicidal Behaviors
- Marginally Intentional Suicidal Behaviors
- Accidents Raising the Suspicion of Suicidal Intent

Diagnostic and Treatment Issues

- Recognition and Identification of Symptoms
- Hospitalization
- Psychotherapy
- Psychopharmacological Treatment

Prevention of Suicide

- Primary Prevention
- Secondary Prevention
- Tertiary Prevention

Summary

Some Demograhic and Statistical Data

Nothing so effectively marshals the defensive posture of denial in the Western mind as does the topic of adolescent suicide. Suicide may occur at any time throughout the entire human life-cycle, but it is most distressing when children and adolescents take their own lives (Walker & Mehr, 1983). The suicide of youth is an appalling human phenomenon, yet our society has shown itself reluctant to engage in concrete efforts to understand and address the problem. Suicide is a calamity many families must bear. Some learn to cope with this human tragedy while at the same time defending themselves against the social stigma attached to suicidal death.

Research into suicide has been thwarted by conscious efforts on the part of family members and others to mask the true cause of death in order to protect the survivors. It is difficult to plot accurately the incidence of suicide in the United States because it is suspected that more than one-quarter to one-third of all cases go unreported. If these figures are accurate for the adult population, underreporting of adolescent suicides may be even greater (Garfinkel & Golombek, 1974; Cohen-Sandler, Berman, & King, 1982 a,b).

Given discrepancies in the available information on suicide in the general population and on adolescent suicides in particular, the statistics are nonetheless alarming. Every research report in the past 10 years has noted an upswing in the rate of adolescent suicide that parallels an increase of suicide in the total population. Close study of the statistics reveals a number of specific trends (Hollinger, 1978; Hollinger & Offer, 1981).

For example, it appears that the risk of suicide is greater for male than for female adolescents though the statistical gap between the sexes is rapidly closing. While the rate of adolescent male suicides is maintaining a steady rate, the number of adolescent female completers is increasing.

The racial variable also commands attention. The ratio of nonwhites to white suicides among youth is 3 to 5 (Frederick, 1978). However, the rate of nonwhite adolescent male suicides has increased significantly in the past 10 years, surpassing the rate of increase in the total population for the first time since records of these mortality trends have been kept (Seiden, 1981).

Discussion here will focus on the cohort of young people, ages 15–24. In recording and reporting mortality statistics, the Division of Vital Statistics uses

5-year distributions in classifying groups. Suicidal deaths are virtually nonexistent before age 5 and are rare in the age group of 5–9 years. In fact, the policy of the Division does not report the deaths of children under age 8 as suicides, regardless of what data may have been entered on a given death certificate. The classification used for these deaths is "other and unknown and unspecified causes." Therefore, it is extremely difficult to assess the incidence of suicide and any trends that may be present in the 5–9 age group. Suicide is similarly uncommon in the cohort of children, ages 10–14, wherein approximately one death in two hundred thousand children occurs. A noticeable shift marks the age groups 15–19 and 20–24, where the suicide rate jumps dramatically (Hollinger & Offer, 1981).

These statistics do not reflect a society out of control. Depending upon which years are used as bench marks, one can note increases or decreases in the incidence of suicide among the youth of the nation. For example, when current statistics are compared with those for the depression years of the 1930s, the current suicide rate seems significantly lower. However, such a comparison does not justify complacency. The facts are that the absolute number of deaths among adolescents is at its highest level and that many of these deaths are suicides.

In trying to make sense out of all the statistics that are available, it is important to keep in mind that these figures only reveal the tip of the proverbial iceberg. Early researchers attempted to project estimates of suicide attempts in the United States based on cross-sectional and random sampling of various populations (Dublin, 1963; Mintz, 1970; Weisman, 1973, 1974). These early reports concluded that incidence and potential incidence were far greater than the statistics would ever indicate.

Suicide is judged to be the third most prevalent cause of death in the adolescent and young adult age groups (15–24 years of age). Accidental death and homicide assume first and second positions in the ranking. The large number of accidental deaths among adolescents each year has led some medico-forensic specialists and suicidologists to assume that many of these deaths are intentional or subintentional suicides. This issue will be discussed later in the chapter.

The prevalence of homicides among adolescents is also notable. In a classic article on the subject, Wolfgang (1959) suggested that some homicides of adolescents may in fact be suicidal. He coined the term "victim-precipitated" homicides to describe behavior that is intentionally self-destructive. An example of this behavior would be seen in a youth who ventures into an area controlled by a hostile gang, who provokes armed confrontation with that group, and who is murdered in the encounter. The psychodynamics of this behavior will be discussed later. Given the suicidal motivation behind such a death, it is evident that the incidence of suicide among adolescents may be more prevalent than the statistics reflect.

Considering that the number of true suicides may be grossly undercounted, it is reasonable to assume that suicide is a principal cause of death in the adolescent and young adult cohorts. Apart from neoplasms and other fatal child and adolescent diseases, the major causes of youthful deaths are all unnatural: accidents, homicides, and suicides.

Etiology of Adolescent Suicide

Genetic Predispositions

It is not unusual to find a family history of suicide in the backgrounds of some adolescents who attempt and complete suicide (Pfeffer, 1981a). This has led some to speculate whether there may be a genetic predeterminant for self-destructive behavior in these offspring, but there is no evidence as yet to support this biological hypothesis. In fact, the few studies that have explored the relationship between completed suicides and a family history of suicide have found negligible correlations. The largest sample was reported by Patel, Roy, and Wilson (1972), who investigated 764 cases of suicides of all ages and found only 2 percent had familial histories of prior suicides. As will be shown later, the fact of a family suicide may subtly influence an adolescent's decision, but there is no evidence to suggest that such tendencies are genetically transmitted.

Biochemical Factors

It has already been noted that the suicide rate of youth shifts dramatically with the onset of puberty. Setting aside psychological factors, some researchers have wondered what role purely biochemical changes might play in the vulnerability of some adolescents to depression and suicide (Ostroff *et al.*, 1982). Part of the so-called "stress and strain" of adolescence is inextricably linked to endocrinological changes.

Beginning in the 1960s, research has attempted to study the possible relationships between the production of adrenal steroid hormones (17-hydroxy-corticosteroids [17-OHS]) and stress. Until now, analysis of these steroids and adrenal cholesterol concentrations in suicidal persons have yielded inconsistent and inconclusive results (Bunney & Fawcett, 1965; Bunney, Fawcett, Davis & Gifford 1969; Levy & Hansen, 1969). However, this type of research is continuing and such work may succeed in identifying an important causal relationship between adrenal cortex functioning and acute stress.

Not only has research focused on endocrine functions, but it has also studied relationships between biochemical processes and the depressive syndromes that may undergird them in potential suicidal adolescents. Contemporary research strategies examine the neuropsychological correlates of suicidal behavior (Ostroff *et al.*, 1982).

Neuroscience is charting a new frontier in multidisciplinary research. One important joint discovery has been the identification of several neurotransmitters, molecules that either excite or inhibit nerve, muscle, or gland cells. *Serotonin* (5-hydroxytryptamine [5-HT]) is one of these neurotransmitters which is thought to be involved in the sleeping-waking cycle.

Neuroscientific research is studying the role serotonin may play in the etiology of behavioral syndromes, including suicide. Many of the drugs utilized to treat depression alter serotonin levels. Although it is not certain how these drugs interfere with serotonergic activities, neuroscientists suspect that these synthetic drugs may block receptor sites and decrease electrical activity within the cells. It is thought that the success of certain *tricyclic antidepressants* (i.e., imipramine) in elevating the mood of depressed persons is precisely linked to the structure-function relationship of serotonin.

This group of antidepressant drugs blocks the re-uptake of catecholamines into the synaptic terminal; the result is that the effects of these *catecholamines* (i.e., dopamine, norepinephrine, and epinephrine) are potentiated. Simply put, this means that the combined action of the synthetic drug with the catecholamines has a greater effect than the sum of the effects of each alone.

Serotonin systems may play a prominent role in the mood-elevating action of the tricyclic antidepessants. There is clinical evidence of reduced levels of 5-hydroxyindolacetic acid (5-HIAA), the metabolite of serotonin, in the cerebrospinal fluid of some depressed individuals and of reduced levels of both serotonin and 5-HIAA in the autopsied brains of persons who committed suicide (Coppen, 1972). One conclusion such evidence suggests is that some forms of depression, suicidal ideation, and suicidal behavior may be caused by a reduction in central serotonergic activity (Cotman & McGaugh, 1980). At this time it is difficult to establish direct relationships between drug interactions with serotonergic neurons and suicidal behavior. However, these avenues of research are being actively pursued.

Another interesting area of research is studying brain activity. Electroencephalographic studies of adolescents who have been hospitalized for suicidal behavior have revealed positive correlations between paroxysmal electroencephalograph (EEG) dysrhythmias and suicidal ideation. Acknowledging that correlations can only imply causation without confirming it, it is nonetheless interesting to note that such dysrhythmias may be associated with the inability to control ordinary functioning, particularly when a person is under significant physical or emotional stress (Struve, Klein, & Saraf, 1972).

A more complete discussion of epidemiological and biological aspects of adolescent suicide may be found in a comprehensive review article by Petzel and Cline (1978). They conclude that the biological aspects of suicide for youths has been insufficiently investigated. Too frequently, researchers are prone to interpret biochemical and medical aspects of adolescent suicide from the psychological perspective, without sufficient attention to the principal role the biological data may play in etiology.

Emotional Disorders

The three emotional disorders linked with suicide, not only among adolescents, but in all age groups, are depression, schizophrenia, and impulsive character disorders. These will be discussed in some detail, particularly in their relation to the incidence of adolescent suicide.

Depression

For a long time, the psychiatric community has been resistant to the diagnosis of depression in young persons. In the most recent revision of the *Diagnostic and statistical manual of mental diseases* (DSM-III) of the American Psychiatric Association (1980), a listing of depressive disorders in children and adolescents appears for the first time. Similarly, the diagnosis of childhood schizophrenia, now generally accepted in the psychiatric community, was also resisted.

Toolan (1962a, b) was regarded as a renegade in the medical community for his early thesis about childhood depression. He has consistently maintained his position that disorders like depression and schizophrenia have different symptoms at various stages of human development. Failure to recognize and classify these age-specific symptoms can contribute to the inability to diagnose accurately depression or schizophrenia in a child or adolescent.

There are a variety of approaches to tracing the etiology of depression in the adolescent population. It is important from the outset of this discussion to state that depression most probably has multiple causes, physical as well as psychological (Catryn, McKnew, & Bunney, 1980; Carlson, 1981; Pfeffer, 1981b). Which of these causes affects the others is still uncertain. What we do know is that there is an interaction between the physiologic and psychologic elements of depressive reactions (Lesse, 1981).

One theory which places strong emphasis on the psychodynamic aspect of depression, considers its cause as rooted in a lost love object that is loved ambivalently (Freud, 1957; Abraham, 1968). In this classic psychoanalytic formulation, the rage felt toward the lost object is turned destructively against the self. In the case of a child or adolescent, this loss of a love object most frequently would occur as a result of the death of a parent or sibling or because of a significant separation. Examples of the latter could be divorce in the family, foster home placements, or relocations that entail the loss of close peer relationships. A frequent adolescent loss involves the breakup of a romantic relationship. A suicide attempt may be understood as a concerted effort to regain contact with the lost love (Suter, 1976; Rosenthal, 1981).

Kathy, an attractive 16-year-old, was admitted unconscious to a hospital emergency room. She was discovered by her younger sister, who returned home in the late afternoon and found her curled up on the floor next to her bed. Patricia thought her sister was dead and she became hysterical. Her shrieking cry attracted the attention of neighbors, who came to her aid and summoned police; they provided emergency medical care and transfer to the hospital.

Kathy's mother had died suddenly in a tragic head-on collision three years previously. While this event was a shock to the whole family, Kathy seemed particularly affected by her mother's death. The persons she relied on most strongly included a close girl friend, Amy, whose family recently relocated to another state and a boyfriend, Carl, who was a student at the high school Kathy attended. Carl was having a difficult time handling all of Kathy's demands, particularly since Amy had moved.

He had suggested to Kathy that he and she might begin to see other people but still remain "friends."

Kathy became more despondent and withdrawn. Her father called the high school guidance counselor, who said that she would arrange to see Kathy immediately. They had talked, and Kathy seemed responsive to the initiative of the counselor; she cried profusely during their meeting. The counselor suggested another meeting the following day. After school, Kathy took a number of narcotic drugs that she had found in her father's bathroom cabinet.

Kathy's losses, both real and threatened, are evident. Her particular response to the loss of her mother, a loss her father and siblings had also experienced, underlines the fact that each individual's needs must be considered separately. Toolan (1981) maintains that the loss that affects an individual at different developmental levels produces different effects. While this may seem quite logical, in practice such a factor is easily ignored in assessing potential sources of loss in children. Toolan asserts that all depressions in children should be taken seriously and that cavalier explanations for functional disruptions in the young person's behavior should not be accepted without question. Glaser (1978) likewise notes that there are qualitative differences in a child's reaction to loss, depending on (1) the nature of the loss (death, divorce, rejection); (2) the child's developmental stage at the time of loss; (3) the child's ego strength; (4) the degree of personal independence enjoyed by the child; (5) the quality of the affectional bonds; (6) the available support system.

In addition to psychoanalytically oriented theories, numerous other theoretical approaches attempt to explain childhood and adolescent depression. Among them are cognitive and learning-behavioral perspectives. Learning approaches view depression and suicide as dependent upon significant shifts in a person's reinforcement patterns. In behavioral terms, this means that a person who judges his or her actual life to be fundamentally lacking in rewards may grow depressed.

The loss of a mother who is a primary reinforcement may trigger depression. Suicide threats and acts result from the deprivation of positive reinforcers, whether these losses are actual, fantasized, or anticipated. In behavioral terms, depression is a response evoked by aversive stimuli over which the individual seems to have no conscious control. Fundamentally, these aversive stimuli represent losses of gratification, whether they be persons or objects.

Kovacs and Beck (1977) posit a cognitive structure in which an individual maintains a negative attitude toward the self, the surrounding environment in which he or she lives (home, school, neighborhood, etc.), and toward the future. This negative mind-set exercises a major influence on the repertory of affective responses and is at the base of depression. The world is viewed through very dark glasses, and this constant bleak perspective on life translates into depressive affect which, if prolonged, can lead to suicidal behavior.

Finally, depression in children can be understood from the perspective of interpersonal interaction. According to this view, a child's depression may have its foundation in the depression of a parent or parental surrogate. Because an adult may be fully involved in his or her own intrapsychic life, he or she may be unavailable and unable to attend to the physical and emotional needs of the child. The child can respond to this prolonged deprivation by becoming depressed as well. Thus the depression in the child is seen to stem directly from interaction with the depressed adult.

There are many other attempts to understand the roots of childhood depression, particularly as this emotional disorder relates to the incidence of suicide among children and adolescents. Excellent review articles treat this topic in greater depth (Herzog & Rathbun, 1982; DenHouter, 1981; Cohen-Sandler & Berman, 1980; Glaser, 1978; Carlson, 1981; Kovacs & Beck, 1977; Glaser, 1981; Pfeffer, 1981a). The specific relationship of depression to suicide, in terms of symptomatology and treatment, will be discussed later.

Schizophrenic Reactions

The second emotional disorder frequently linked to youthful suicide is schizophrenia. While depressive symptomatology may be more common, schizophrenic reactions account for a certain portion of suicidal behavior among adolescents. The most striking characteristic of this behavior is a tendency to be withdrawn and immersed in a rich fantasy world in which visual and auditory hallucinations seem real. This delusional lifestyle frequently removes these young persons from meaningful interactions with their peers, parents, and other significant adults.

Many of these psychotic individuals report that their hallucinations encourage them to commit suicide. Because the adolescent is frequently quite withdrawn and uncommunicative, it is assumed that the susceptibility to hallucinatory suggestions of self-destruction is great in these individuals. It is evident from many reports of hospitalized adolescent attempters that such is the case. The same pathological indications hold true for adolescent homicides in which auditory hallucinations are blamed for the aggressive and fatal act. However, the complexity of schizophrenic pathology makes it difficult to generalize its relationship to suicide.

The following case exemplifies how an adolescent—in this case with a history of untreated personality disorder—attempts suicide in response to what he judges to be an order from God. The case highlights the fact that in schizophrenia even the method of suicide is empowered with symbolic importance. All of these details flow from the hallucinatory experience.

Duane is a bright, verbal 17-year-old high school junior. His parents described him as being "different" but they never judged it necessary to seek counseling for him until he was hospitalized after he attempted suicide by means of ligature strangulation.

When his parents found him in his own bedroom, he was unconscious. He had wrapped a rope around his neck, tying a knot with each of the seven circumferences.

When the police were called, they summoned an ambulance, since Duane still had a discernible pulse. Later the doctors explained to Mr. and Mrs. Schneider that the rope had cut off venous circulation and Duane had become unconscious. As he had fallen back on his bed, the tension on the rope had relaxed.

When Duane regained consciousness, he was wrapped up in the fantasy that God had appeared to him and told him that he must atone for the sins of the world. Each knot he tied would be penance for 100 years of history. Duane was energized with the sense that he was a savior, that God had chosen him, like Moses, to set his people free.

Aggression and Impulsive Character Disorder

Observers of child and adolescent behavior often comment on the impulsive characteristics of many youthful acts. Disobedience, temper tantrums, running away from home, and truancy are just a few examples of these behaviors. Psychologists and psychiatrists have attempted to understand the significance of these essentially impulsive behaviors. Some have preferred to look at them in terms of symptoms of "masked depression," considering the behavior to be the result of anger engaged by real or perceived losses. Adults frequently internalize anger, or direct it inwardly. Children, however, frequently express their anger outwardly, either toward themselves in self-destructive ways, or in blatantly aggressive and antisocial actions directed toward others.

When Paul was interviewed he had been hospitalized for 4 months in a private psychiatric facility. At the time of his admission he had attempted to end his life by jumping from the sixth floor window of his family's apartment. He had succeeded in making the jump, but his fall had been broken by the opened awning of a merchant's shop on the ground level. Nevertheless, Paul, aged 17, sustained multiple fractures of the leg and arm as well as some internal injuries.

Prior to his jump, he had been involved in a violent argument with his father, who was alcoholic. The father had been physically abusive toward his wife and children. On this occasion, Paul had yelled, "I can't take any more of this shit," had run to the window and opened it. The father had screamed, "Go ahead, jump." With that Paul had leapt out.

This account of an adolescent's impulsive self-destructive behavior is dramatic. However, it underscores how the alcoholic father's continued abuse of his family not only contributed to the depressing environment of the home but also became the catalyst for an impulsive and violent act on the part of his adolescent son. The impulsive suicidal act not only symbolized a release from this tension but was a means for the son to inflict pain on the abusive father.

Another explanation resides in what might be called "impulsive character disorder," which describes an adolescent whose development has lagged on some significant frontiers. If a child has encountered important failures in academic and interpersonal tasks and is experiencing difficulties in family life, the additional physical and psychological burdens of adolescence may prove to be insurmountable. Behaviorally, the adolescent may use aggressive and destructive acts as vents for his or her anger or frustration.

Of particular importance is the message contained in sexual maturation; the adolescent senses quite acutely the cue that he or she must grow up. The mandate may seem overwhelming, given a history of questionable success in this arena. The impulsive, acting-out behavior must be seen as symbolic and the symptoms need to be understood appropriately. Given the incidence of episodic dyscontrol behaviors, not only is the adolescent capable of self-destructive behavior, but anger or frustration he or she impulsively directs at a parent or peer can lead to homicide. Some parents have felt that these acting-out behaviors are manipulative, and indeed they may be. However, a judgment that they are manipulative is no license to ignore the rest of the meaning contained in them.

Another aspect of the issue of impulsive behavior is not, strictly speaking, psychopathological but is nonetheless related to suicide among adolescents. One of the by-products of the physical and psychological development of the adolescent is a new sense of independence. Linked with this independence is a certain belief in one's own power and ability.

Sometimes, an adolescent misjudges the limits of his or her strength and skill and consequently may take excessive risks. This kind of daring is evident in driving at high speeds or with reckless abandon. These impulsive decisions, grounded more in developmental exploration of the limits of one's ability and not in some more pathological self-destructive intent, can end in the death of the adolescent and his or her companions. The high percentage of accidental deaths among adolescents may find intelligibility in this nonpathological explanation.

Familial and Sociocultural Determinants

Derek Miller (1981) has noted that recent societal trends make adolescence, as a specific developmental period, extremely complex. These trends include the widespread disintegration of the nuclear family owing to the prevalence of divorce and the weakening of involvement with extended family. Miller further cites the erosion of consistent social ties and the easy access to and abuse of regressive drugs as contributing to the malaise that many adolescents experience. In a period of their human development when they need support to form and maintain important interpersonal relationships and to learn effective strategies to resolve adult conflicts and problems, such help may not be easily available.

This depiction of the American family and the adolescent's role within it may be an unfair caricature. Yet it does indicate the serious liabilities with which many adolescents must contend. Exposure to certain familial and social stressors may render a given adolescent more vulnerable to suicide. Frequently such an individual has had a long exposure to such sources of stress, and problems have surfaced before the adolescent years. Adolescence may simply be the "summing-up" period, when the young person takes stock of his or her personal experience. If the individual concludes that he or she has been basically unhappy in family and social relationships and senses that life is empty existence, then suicide may become an attractive option.

In some instances, the adolescent's parent or sibling may have previously suicided. Such a familial history of suicide places the adolescent at a particular risk. Earlier we asserted that suicide is not genetically transmitted; however, psychological identification and imitative behavior can be strong motivations in considering suicide (Pfeffer, 1981a, b).

Children can relate to a previous familial suicidal act in a variety of ways. The behavior of the deceased parent or sibling can be viewed as "permission" to do likewise to oneself. The grieving for the lost parent, and whatever bonding or attachment that relationship may have represented, may not have been adequately processed so that suicide for the child may symbolize the possibility of reunion with the lost source of gratification. Finally, suicide for the adolescent may be a vehicle for punishing the surviving parent. The child has witnessed the destructive effect of the prior suicide on family life and decides to inflict the ultimate disintegrating blow to the chaotic family system by his or her own suicidal act.

Some children grow up in environments that do not place a high premium on human life. This may be explained in part by the deprivations these social groups experience in daily living. Whatever the explanation, children who are thus exposed may be more prone to suicide. On the other hand, certain cultures may communicate such high expectations of their youth in terms of educational achievement and productivity that the youth who does not measure up to these indices of expectation may find suicide the only feasible option. This may explain the high rate of suicide among the youth in such countries as Japan, Switzerland, Finland, and Germany (Davidson *et al.*, 1972; Ishii, 1981; Kaizuka, 1977; Marcelli, 1978; Mouren & Soulayrol, 1978).

Finally, some parents find it difficult to distance themselves emotionally as their children mature (Richman, 1978). They continue to be too involved in their offspring's life and fail to provide the child the psychological space essential to establishing autonomy and independence. The burden can become so difficult for the child that suicide is the only solution an adolescent may see. For these children, suicidal behavior may be an effective way to gain distance from the stressful life circumstances of family and home.

Cohen-Sandler, Berman, and King (1982b) followed up 73 children and adolescents, aged 6 to 16 years of age, who represented 96 percent of a previously reported sample of suicidal, depressed control groups discharged from an inpatient psychiatric unit (Cohen-Sandler, Berman & King, 1982a). What they noted is that for these children, suicidal behavior was a powerful, albeit pathological, coping strategy. Since the children sampled were all hospitalized as a result of their suicidal attempts, they were at least successful in getting themselves physically removed from the stressful environment of the home. The researchers noted that many were not returned home upon discharge, but placed in a more supportive foster home milieu or in residential treatment centers. Before discharge, special arrangements were made for ongoing family therapy and for supportive school services. The results of these intervention efforts seem to have been successful, since the follow-up studies noted a significant lowering of measured stress scores.

Occasionally, it is the parent who seeks a way to escape from emotional or physical involvement with the family. A parent who psychologically abandons the child, permitting the child freedom in every domain and showing little interest in what the child is doing, can be catastrophic for the emerging adolescent. This kind of parental rejection can be a catalyst to suicide. In each of these instances, the family and social context provides messages, incentives, and motives to an adolescent who may be considering suicide. These messages may unconsciously sanction suicide as a reasonable solution to what is considered an insurmountable problem of continued living.

Sharon was the younger of two children in an upwardly mobile, suburban family. The older child, a son, was 5 years older than his sister and was in his senior year in a prestigious New England Ivy League college. The father of this family was the vice-president of a major manufacturing conglomerate and did extensive international travelling. Sharon's mother was actively pursuing her own interests in corporate real estate development. The family lived in an exclusive suburb of metropolitan Boston. Sharon was a boarding student at a private coeducational secondary school.

Although she was a bright student, her grades were beginning to slip, though not so drastically as to attract her parents' attention. She was involved in smoking marijuana, which was readily available at school. Some of her friends invited her to experiment with cocaine, which she did.

Sharon confided to her roommate that she felt very much alone. She resented the fact that her parents had sent her to this private school. They expected that she would move from this excellent preparatory school to a college, just as her brother had done. Besides, school provided a release for the parents from being involved with their children. At least, this is how Sharon argued the case with her roommate.

This was the story that the startled roommate told school authorities when they investigated the attempt that Sharon made on her life. She was discovered by this same companion in the bathroom of their suite. Sharon was fully clothed, sitting in the shower. She was semiconscious, with her wrists slashed. The note she had written simply stated: "I won't be a burden to you anymore." It was not addressed to anyone in particular.

Suicidal Behaviors

Whatever its particular etiology, suicide serves some specific psychic purposes. These purposes have been generally classified under three categories: intentional acts, marginally intentional behaviors, and accidents that raise the suspicion of suicidal intent. We would like to consider each of these categories of suicidal behavior.

Intentional Suicidal Behaviors

Operationally defined, intentional suicide is deliberate and planned. The individual usually provides some evidence of intent through conversations with others about the subject of death, or by warning others that suicide is being considered. Frequently enough, these allusions to death or suicidal intention may be so subtly interwoven with other topics of conversation that they are either missed or disregarded. The communication structure in which an adolescent is engaged may be already so stressed that any important messages may be obscured.

It is only in ex post facto reconstructions of the final encounters with suicide victims that survivors recollect veiled messages concerning intent. For this reason, it is very important that the declarative statements of people be taken seriously. There is a potential for manipulation in suicidal threats, but one cannot risk an actual suicide simply in trying to avoid being manipulated.

Sharon's roommate recalled other conversations with her [Linda]. Sharon had asked her if she ever thought about what it would be like to be dead. Linda had told Sharon that she never thought about it and considered it a weird question. Why would anyone think about death? Sharon had replied that she often thought about it and did not find the thought to be so bad. In fact, being dead was not a bad thing. At least then you would not have any hassles. Linda recalls saying: "Hey, let's change the subject; this is freaking me out." Sharon agreed and the conversation on death ended. Later, Linda recalled this conversation and commented, "Lately, she seemed to be thinking about death a lot. She told me that she was going to do a paper on the subject for her English course in American fiction."

Not all potential suicidal adolescents will share their intent in an expressive form with others. There are illustrative cases of seemingly well-adjusted students, with no evident psychiatric problems and no significant developmental stressors, who committed suicide. Even in such cases, in retrospect it is evident to trained observers that the adolescent may have been more psychologically withdrawn than had been noted. Because the child was making no demands within the family nor causing any difficulty in school, the pervasive intrapsychic conflict was neither detected nor treated. The best evidence about these kinds of suicides comes from attempters who survive and who subsequently receive appropriate psychiatric care.

Some seemingly adjusted adolescents are in far greater interior turmoil than many would suspect. If suicide is attempted, it may be a way of escaping from this inner chaos or emptiness. Some researchers would maintain that such individuals may have been depressed or schizoid, even though these conditions were never clinically diagnosed. These conditions could be *endogenous*, that is, triggered by biochemical processes within a person. They could be the result of significant emotional deprivations or exclusions (*exogenous*). While the child survives and maintains the semblance of normal functioning, coping is not at all as effective as it would appear.

Miller (1981) reported that some adolescents under stress display a particular genetic vulnerabililty to depression. He further notes that their strategy for coping involves exceedingly compliant behavior in order to stave off psychic pain. This pattern of behavior would positively correlate with the clinical picture above, wherein the individual at risk appears relatively healthy and balanced. However, when this same individual is faced with the developmental demands of adolescence, particularly those involving autonomous and independent functioning, the reservoir of defensive protection may prove insufficient, and the young person succumbs to the attractive escape that suicide offers.

This vulnerability to the ravages of depression may be exacerbated by involvement with alcohol or drugs. These substances, if abused, may further weaken coping abilities and may trigger a significant loss of ability to control function. As noted earlier, there is fairly consistent evidence that certain drugs exert their clinical effects through some interaction with brain catecholamines. An abnormality in brain catecholamines may be responsible for drug-induced depression, which might potentiate suicide. Not only might this be possible in individuals being treated for depression with certain tricyclic antidepressant medications, but it can also be true for youth who experiment with a wide variety of drugs so readily available today.

The most frequent type of intentional suicidal behavior among adolescents involves retaliation. Because the young person has experienced rejection—familial, parental, peer—he or she conceptualizes suicide as the ultimate form of punishment to the rejecting persons. A particular rejection may trigger this behavior, although it may in fact be only a symbol of many experiences of disapproval and emotional distancing. When adolescents choose to leave notes detailing their reasoning, it is not uncommon to find expressions of rage directed toward their parents, siblings, or a former boyfriend or girlfriend. Suicide punishes the survivor for the rejection the suicide victim perceived.

Sometimes the expression of this rage reflects the ambivalent feelings the adolescent may feel toward a parent. One such note, left by a 20-year-old young woman, graphically makes this point.

Dear Mom and Dad,

You have succeeded in making my life miserable. No matter what I did, it was never good enough for you. Everything I ever loved you destroyed. The best thing for me is to be rid of this burden. I simply cannot take it anymore. Take care of Bernie [a pet dog].

Love,
Elizabeth

In summary, the etiology of intentional suicidal behavior can be found in any of the factors discussed above, but is most frequently related to emotional disorders that are masked so that they do not attract attention. There is a distinct possibility that a certain neuroendocrine vulnerability may be involved in triggering certain suicidal behavior, but this is not easily verifiable.

Marginally Intentional Suicidal Behaviors

Marginally intentional suicidal behaviors are extremely difficult to distinguish. Adolescence is almost by definition a period in life where experimentation and certain risk taking are sanctioned. Adolescents do in fact test many limits of their abilities in efforts to gain a better appreciation of their potential. Body image becomes increasingly more important to the adolescent, and much energy can be invested in exploring the ways in which the body can be manipulated.

Among the most common causes of death in the adolescent age group are those associated with automobile fatalities. Driving at excessively high speeds, abusing drugs and alcohol, and demonstrating mastery and skill may combine to produce a tragic accident involving several youths. These scenarios are all too common in the local newspapers and other news reports.

Some of these incidents are genuinely accidental and are directly attributable to lack of experience and judgment on the part of the adolescent. However, some adolescents are involved in a number of distinct but related "accidents," enough to raise the question whether marginally suicidal intent may be behind them. A repetition of these acts should alert parents and school personnel, as well as primary care physicians, to the possibility of suicidal intent. Whereas an intentionally suicidal youth may provide a verbal message to others, the marginally intentional youth may be acting out the conflict in potentially self-destructive and homicidal ways, with the unconscious intent of attracting attention in order that someone will rescue him or her.

Experimentation with and abuse of alcohol and other drugs by adolescents present distinct problems for parents and adolescent counselors. On the one hand, adolescents have been raised in a society that has become quite comfortable with the use of drugs. On the other hand, the statistics on drug-related deaths among adolescents are alarmingly high. It is obviously not enough to simply advise youth about the dangers of these substances; greater attention must be focused on the reasons undergirding such frequent use and abuse. The very abuse of these drugs may be a manifestation of marginally suicidal intent. If such abuse were understood in this way, efforts to intervene might be more aggressive.

Finally, the death of Karen Carpenter and recent media discussions have focused public interest on certain eating disorders, particularly *anorexia nervosa* and *bulimia*, and the risks inherent in radical weight reduction programs. Anorexia is a psychophysiological condition, most commonly diagnosed in girls and young women. It is characterized by severe and prolonged inability or refusal to eat, sometimes accompanied by spontaneous or induced vomiting, extreme emaciation, and other serious biochemical changes. Bulimia is an abnormal increase in the sensation of hunger. A bulimic craves food and becomes involved in food binges. As in the case of anorexia, it is not uncommon that self-induced vomiting follow a period of inordinate eating.

Deaths related to these causes are not uncommon. The actual cause of death may not be identified as an eating disorder but will be masked under the physiological consequence, such as cardiac arrest or acute congestive heart failure. There can be a certain furtiveness in the symptomatology of these eating disorders, and it may be difficult to detect the seriousness of the problem. Because adolescents are so vulnerable to the way they perceive their bodies, they can be particularly sensitive to being overweight. This is a greater problem for women, although young men are not excluded from this danger. In some adolescent eating disturbances there is the possibility of suicidal intent.

Accidents Raising the Suspicion of Suicidal Intent

"Accident raising the suspicion of suicidal intent" may, at first sight, appear to be a questionable classification of behaviors. It describes those acts that end in one's own death but in which suicidal intent is reasonably assumed to be absent. A simple example of this is the case of an adolescent who dies in an attempt to climb a mountain. Although a novice, the adolescent judges his or her physical stamina and athletic abilities to be sufficient to the task. The adolescent's inexperience, and not any intentional or marginally intentional decision to die, is ultimately determined to be the cause of the lethal fall.

In addition to the implicit risks in exploring the parameters of their abilities, the environments in which many young people are nurtured must also be considered. Cultural protections for children—for instance, from the "facts of life"—and reinforcements of omnipotence—for example, on TV—lead children to conclude that they are virtually invulnerable. Within a frame of reference that does not sufficiently set limits, some adolescents move far beyond the boundaries of safety and discretion in the feats they attempt.

Occasionally, an adolescent will express rage in an explosive and destructive act. The young person may put a fist through a window or door. The person might storm out of a room and accidently fall down a staircase. These accidental acts, with their roots in anger and impulsive response, occasionally prove fatal. Any behaviors of this sort require attention, since ignoring them entirely may lead the young person who continues to succumb to anger and impulse to marginally intentional or intentional suicide.

Diagnostic and Treatment Issues

Previous discussion has identified some salient etiologic issues that contribute to an understanding of adolescent suicidal behavior. Different modes of suicide have been discussed with emphasis on the role of intentionality and motive. This body of knowledge assists in the identification of adolescents at risk and can be beneficial to parents, teachers, and primary care physicians who are in the best positions to make appropriate interventions. However, it is all too frequent that potentially suicidal teenagers come from homes with disturbed familial relationships, which may be actually contributing to the perceived difficulty. Parents may not be tuned in to the signals the adolescent is transmitting. Likewise, school personnel may not accurately interpret certain conflictual behaviors in the classroom, truancy, or other symptomatic acts as potentially self-destructive "cries for help." Finally, should the child actually be seen by a family practice physician, some of these same behaviors may be assigned a low weighting in an overall diagnosis.

Recognition and Identification of Symptoms

Cohen-Sandler and Berman (1980) reported on a study of primary care physicians in the District of Columbia. From their analysis they concluded that it was likely that respondent physicians (27 percent of the 375 contacted) were only aware of a fraction of their depressed and self-destructive patients. The researchers pinpointed areas where physicians might err in making an accurate differential diagnosis of childhood depression and suicidal vulnerability. Principal among these is the possible relationship between frequency of accidents and suicidal intent.

Toolan (1981) would seem to concur, questioning as he does whether there are many genuine accidents in life. In the terms of this discussion, Toolan would maintain that most accidents are marginally intentional. Cohen-Sandler and Berman (1980) reported that accidents are the major cause of death of children ages 5 to 14 years, confirming the statistics discussed previously on adolescent accidental deaths. Physicians need to be alert to the possibility that some of these accidents may be masked attempts at suicide by the young persons they are treating.

Unrecognized and therefore untreated, these children become prime candidates for suicide completion. The most important need is for greater sophistication in recognizing and correctly diagnosing possible suicidal behavior and then implementing effective treatment strategies to address the problem. As noted before, the psychiatric community has shown itself ambivalent toward the notion of childhood and adolescent depression, and has only recently begun to establish diagnostic criteria that can aid in identifying certain young persons at risk. Herzog and Rathbun (1982) assert that the final challenge in the arena of childhood depression is the basic reluctance of many adults, both professionals and nonprofessionals, to admit the possibility that a child has a depressive illness. The high incidence of adolescent suicides may be related to the fact that clinical depression is not accurately diagnosed in children, whose fragile equilibrium is significantly disrupted by the normal developmental stresses of the adolescent period.

Hospitalization

Treatment frequently is not begun until a serious attempt on one's life has been made. The most frequent therapeutic response is hospitalization, which in many respects can be beneficial. For an adolescent, hospitalization can be a reassuring gesture since it affirms that someone has finally understood the seriousness of the problem. It likewise communicates this same message to the other significant persons in the adolescent's family. If the attempt represents the adolescent's last effort to cope with or escape from a stressful situation at home or in school or with interpersonal relationships, the hospitalization provides a safe haven and respite from those negatively perceived engagements.

The hospital environment is a protective one, structured to keep the adolescent safe while he or she begins to deal with the anxious and negative feelings that may have triggered the suicidal attempt. To the adolescent who has attempted suicide, the world seems to have fallen apart; the hospital recognizes and accepts this perception and tries to supply a milieu in which the young person's internal disorganization might begin to regain some order.

Hospitalization also provides a point of transition in which the adolescent can engage in building a relationship with a therapist. Because many adolescents share in common a problem of social isolation and withdrawal, it is not easy to engage in helping relationships with them. Frequently these young persons have had previous difficulties in establishing relationships, and adolescence may have only intensified these problems. In fact, the adolescent's suicide attempt may have represented the culmination of perceived failures in these interpersonal tasks. Some adolescents acknowledge that they feel that no one cares about them, that there is no one on whom they can depend for support. The period of hospitalization can begin to build the foundation of relationship that is essential to any effective psychotherapeutic process.

The most significant contribution the hospital makes to the adolescent suicide attempter is to prepare the young person for re-engagement with family and social life. This is a complex and often difficult task, placing the hospital in a variety of roles. As an advocate for the adolescent, the hospital serves a liaison function with the family and the school to ensure that, to the degree possible, unnecessary stresses are avoided.

However, there are some contraindications to hospitalization. Some psychologists and psychiatrists are uncomfortable working with suicidal patients. Toolan (personal communication, July 30, 1983) commented that such therapists might prematurely or unnecessarily refer suicide patients to a hospital simply because he or she is too uncomfortable with the level of anxiety present. Occasionally, a hospital admission might be effected at the insistence of the adolescent's parents; the therapist's cooperation in this decision might be seen by the adolescent to be collusion with parents against himself or herself.

Hospitalization, particularly in situations where seclusion or round-the-clock observation are deemed necessary, may be a terrifying experience for the adolescent. This kind of intensive supervision is depressing and dehumanizing. Ordinary activities like urination and defecation are observed. The patient who has been unsuccessful in the attempted suicide may experience these precautionary measures as completely demoralizing. There are numerous cases where patients have succeeded in completing a suicide even while they have been monitored by staff in these intensive supervisory capacities (Hendrin, 1982).

Whether hospitalization is deemed necessary and useful to further treatment goals, it is important to keep effective channels of communication open with both the patient and the family. The hospital can provide a protective environment in which relationships with patient and family can be established —and valuable therapy begun.

Psychotherapy

Depending on the theoretical position, the goal of psychotherapy with suicidal adolescents is variously expressed. The psychodynamic formulation speaks in terms of replacing satisfying object relationships, particularly lost love objects. Or therapy might involve helping the adolescent to identify and regain control over the stresses that have triggered anxiety. A behavioral objective might be to teach better methods of control over impulsive reactions, particularly those that are self-destructive. This goal aims at reordering thinking and reasoning and modifying behavior. A family system approach might focus on the network of the family, trying to situate the locus of intervention in improving the interactions within this primary group.

Glaser (1978) correctly comments that the modality of therapeutic approach necessarily must be tailored to the specific needs of the individual adolescent. He further observes that this might entail switching from one method to another. For example, early on in treatment the conflict with parents or family may be so intense that family therapy sessions may not be beneficial. Perhaps after some individual sessions with psychodynamic and behavioral objectives, and some peer group therapy, the adolescent may be prepared and willing to invest in productive family work. Glaser concludes that a flexible, eclectic approach without rigid bias to one mode of treatment or another seems to be the best strategy for approaching psychotherapy with an adolescent suicide attempter.

Numbers of researchers who have studied the various modalities of psychotherapeutic care for suicidal adolescents share the view that parents should be involved in treatment plans (Pfeffer, 1981a, b; Tishler, McKenry, & Morgan, 1981; Toolan, personal communication, July 30, 1983). Family therapy is not always easily mounted nor sustained, but it is a therapy of choice (Richman, 1978). Parents are sometimes resistant to acknowledge that the youngster has attempted suicide. In his extensive therapeutic experience, Toolan has noted that children and adolescents are far more able to acknowledge suicidal ideation and behavior than are their parents (personal communication, July 30, 1983). In fact, Toolan has found that the greatest obstacle to the treatment of a suicidal youngster lies not so much with the child or adolescent, who is often responsive to the offer of help, but with the parents, who wish to maintain the facade that everything is fine. For these and many other reasons, every effort should be made to engage parents and other family members effectively in the therapeutic process, despite the resistances often encountered.

Psychopharmacological Treatment

Whatever the theoretical approach, some psychotherapy seems essential in helping the adolescent to understand and cope with the issues that have contributed to or precipitated a suicidal attempt. In some isolated cases, antidepressant medication has been effective (Puig-Antich, 1979), but drug treatment is not the treatment of choice for most adolescents. In the Cohen-Sandler and Berman (1980) study, pharmacologic treatments for depressed and suicidal adolescents were the least preferred modality. Where drugs were used in the therapy plans, the antidepressants were the most frequently prescribed, although anxiolytics, neuroleptics, and antihistamine-sedatives were also utilized.

Drugs often communicate a confusing message to the adolescent. They reinforce a feeling that things are completely out of control and someone else has taken over control of his or her life. While this in fact may adequately translate the reality, the symbolic value of the drug program may be countertherapeutic. The adolescent, who may be acutely sensitive to the chaos in his or her personal life, may conclude that he or she is not capable of assuming control. The psychotropic drugs may appear to the adolescent as an attempt on the part of others to control thought and behavior and may trigger paranoid reactions in the patient.

If the adolescent has been energized by the suicide attempt to deal with personal problems, it would seem counterproductive to tranquilize him or her and thus blunt the constructive affect. Apart from an initial effort to quiet the anxieties of the recent attempter, many physicians prefer to wean the adolescent from any chemical dependence and provide sedative assistance should the young person specifically request some aid in sleeping.

Drug involvement and abuse is not infrequently one of the precipitating factors in the self-destructive behavior. Detoxification and withdrawal may be a more relevant therapeutic concern. In cases where physiological addiction may not be at issue, the adolescent may have developed a psychological dependence on certain drugs. Therapy would necessarily have to contend with this compelling need before it could more successfully address itself to the developmental and environmental problems of which the drug abuse may be symptomatic.

Questions concerning the use of psychotropic medications in the treatment of depressed and suicidal adolescents remain issues of debate. Regardless of the strength of personal opinion on this matter, the consensus among all professionals is that psychotherapy is an essential ingredient to any successful intervention program. The majority of practitioners seem to favor an approach wherein drug involvement is kept to the absolute minimum.

Prevention of Suicide

Primary Prevention

One of the most common expressions voiced by the survivors of a suicide is "if only I had paid attention to that sign, I might have been able to prevent his or her death." So much guilt among survivors is linked to nonrecognition of signs of suicidal ideation in adolescents. The presuicidal person, as previously noted, frequently displays numerous clues of intention. The goal of a *primary prevention* effort is to recognize and interpret correctly these behavioral clues in order to prevent the person from carrying out the self-destructive act.

Numerous illuminative reports have attempted to provide a resumé of the specific behaviors that can signal suicidal intent. Some of these behaviors are linked to depression; it is for this reason that the proper diagnosis of depression in children and adolescents is so critical to the prevention of possible suicidal acts.

Among children and adolescents the behavioral shifts that are most noteworthy include the following. The child's eating and sleeping patterns may shift. The young person may become agitated and resistant to any efforts to control him or her. This rebelliousness is sometimes ignored because it is thought to be a normal manifestation of adolescent development. Adolescent revolt can mask depression. For this reason, it is difficult to isolate what is normative behavior in the process of adolescent differentiation, and what may be more appropriately considered depressed affect.

It is not unusual that these behaviors cluster together. The portrait of numbers of suicidal adolescents verify this assertion. Not only is the individual withdrawn and agitated at home, but the same kinds of behaviors are noted at school and in peer relationships. The presuicidal adolescent may act out in school, become delinquent in assignments and show erratic attendance patterns. Friends note similar belligerence and withdrawal of investment in group activities. When confronted with these dramatic changes, the adolescent may be prone to dismiss the observations as exaggerated or unimportant or may refuse to become engaged in a reciprocal effort to communicate. This makes intervention an exceedingly difficult project and explains in part why some parents, teachers, and peers retreat from initial efforts, assuming that in time the troubled adolescent will emerge from this "temporary" gloom. When disengagement is reinforced in this way, the trajectory to further deterioration is prepared.

In addition to specific behavioral shifts, other personality characteristics should be noted. Hostile behaviors or agitation can mask anger and rage that may have been present for a considerable time in the young person's history. Some of this affect may be linked to deprivation or abuse, some may be attributable to negative self-imaging and self-depreciation. A young person may be extremely sensitive to external sources of evaluation and therefore may be prone to overreact to academic failure, defeat in competitive sports, or critical judgments made by parents or peers. This vulnerability to criticism, whether its genesis is found in the self or in other persons, can expose an individual to depression and self-destructive thoughts.

The environmental factors discussed earlier in the section on etiology play an important role in prevention. If it is accepted that certain factors disturb the stability that is very important in a child's development, then attention should be paid to them. Principal among these factors are the following. In a mobile society, families are constrained by the pressures of parental employment and career development to make frequent relocations. These geographical shifts can have negative impact on children who must change schools and leave behind important childhood relationships. Other cultural phenomena, including increased divorce and remarriage and single-parent families, can also be more traumatic to a child than may initially be evident (Maris, 1981). Some children are skilled in covering up their reactions to these changes in family relationships.

Any traumatic loss for a child can dispose the individual to depression; undiagnosed and untreated, such depression can lead to suicidal thoughts and acts. The isolated or withdrawn young person may be responding to an inner experience of having been abandoned. This abandonment is most often related to parental loss, whether through death, family separation or divorce, or desertion.

Finally, catastrophic or chronic illness, disabling accidents, and serious physical disfigurement can render the adolescent extremely vulnerable to suicidal ruminations. These events in a young person's experience can make the prospect of adult life seem quite tenuous and bleak. At the time when bodily development and body imaging become factors of particular concern, the handicapped adolescent may see suicide as an effective escape from the dilemma of debilitating illness and its sequelae.

In all of these issues, what distinguishes one young person from another who may have similar experiences is the learned ability to cope. Some psychologists believe that children can be taught strategies for conflict and stress management, just as adults can learn to appropriate these skills. In addition, active efforts need to be made to keep children engaged, and not allow them to regress into dangerously prolonged and isolated withdrawal. Children need to experience success; occasionally parents and teachers have to plan activities in which such success can be achieved. In situations where emotional continuity and stability is not provided within the family, the other adult figures in the young person's life may be able to provide the closeness and warmth that can act as an antidote to the familial deprivations. For this reason relationships with teachers, guidance counselors, and coaches in interscholastic sports activities can be important agents of positive mental health in the life of a presuicidal adolescent.

All of this is predicated on the awareness of certain *prodromal signs* and making timely intervention. Prodromes in medicine are warning symptoms that indicate the onset of a particular disease. The challenges of effective primary preventive interventions are great. Since many adults are conditioned to deny the real possibilities of suicide among adolescents and are too willing to dismiss the importance of certain indicative behaviors and affect, many of these signs go unnoticed and without effective response.

Secondary Prevention

It is not until a person actually attempts suicide that effective reponse is engaged. **Secondary prevention** addresses the issue of treatment of the attempter. The defense of denial is so pervasive that some adults—parents and teachers—will still not accept the presence of suicidal intent in an adolescent, even when some actual attempt has been made. When these adults are helped to acknowledge the fact of an attempted suicide, these same persons feel impotent. They do not know what to do.

Mental health professionals have directed efforts to educate parents and school personnel about adolescent suicide and strategies for assisting the young person at risk. Suicide prevention centers and crisis hotlines are providing important information and assistance to families and teachers as well as to individuals who are on the verge of committing suicide. Some physicians are reluctant to become involved with needy adolescent patients and may unconsciously deny the seriousness of some of the symptomatology presented to them in routine physical examinations.

The value of educating those constituencies who might be of some assistance to the adolescent who actually attempts suicide cannot be underestimated. The skills used in early intervention efforts can make the difference between success and failure in saving the victim's life. Training programs for appropriate crisis intervention with suicidal individuals are available in many community health centers. Through such didactic and experiential learning activities, effective intervention skills are developed and enhanced.

Tertiary Prevention

At the beginning of this chapter it was noted that suicide is grossly underreported, particularly its incidence among the youthful population. Not only is it problematic to assess the actual epidemiology of suicide, but it is difficult to provide effective support to those noncompleters. Over the short-term, it may seem that masking of the suicide is in the best interest of the family, but the short-term gain does not offset the long-term liabilities. This is the objective of **tertiary prevention**, namely, to minimize the negative physical and mental health consequences of a suicide for survivors.

Parents internalize much of the blame for the death of a child, even though they may attempt to rationalize and excuse their culpability. They may feel certain resentments and blame others who did not recognize the signs and do something to prevent the young person's death. Much of their negative affect can be projected onto others. None of this, of course, can be expressed openly because the suicide has been relegated to the level of secrecy.

The normal social supports that could be very beneficial to the parent and family are unavailable. The internal feelings do not have an appropriate channel for ventilation with friends and relatives. Some people are reluctant to accept help from professionals or clergymen.

In these circumstances, skill in gaining the survivors' trust is essential. It must be assumed that such individuals not only need assistance but find themselves blocked from both the recognition of this need and the knowledge of how to receive such help. As in all crisis intervention efforts, the earlier the contact with the survivors, the more effective such intervention can be. Early understanding and support can dispose the survivors to accepting subsequent offers of help. The frank and comfortable acceptance of the reality, without judgment or blame, establishes an important foundation for effective work with survivors. Physicians, clergy, and funeral directors have a privileged opportunity for effective intervention because of their proximity to the family in the early moments of the crisis. They are privy to more information than may ultimately become public knowledge. With this entrusted information, they are in particularly advantaged positions to facilitate the process of grief resolution.

Not all health care providers are ready to assume responsibility for the difficult follow-up work with the families of survivors. Whenever survivors are able to share their feelings and experiences in support groups, the results are often quite productive. The more comfortable professional health providers are in dealing with the families of adolescents who commit suicide, the more effective will be their efforts to assist these families in the process of their recovery from and integration of their traumatic loss.

Summary

Suicide among adolescents and young adults has become an increasingly pressing societal problem. Not only is this one of the leading causes of death in this age cohort, but the incidence of suicide among younger children (aged 6–12 years) is also escalating (Pfeffer, 1981a, b). From all sectors of the society the call is raised for better criteria with which to assess a young person's potential for suicide. Implicit in this demand is a greater willingness on the part of society to acknowledge that suicide among youth is a genuine mental health problem. This recognition has not been the case historically. Suicide has been shrouded in secrecy, as both a social and familial taboo. This attitude of denial has camouflaged the available statistical and demographic data. The number of actual suicides is underreported. For this reason, the published statistics on suicidal death in this age group are quite sobering, for we must assume that the actual numbers are significantly higher.

The first question people generally ask when they hear a report of a suicide, particularly that of a young person, is: "Why?" Is there some logical explanation as to why a person chooses to terminate his or her life? A number of sources of explanation have been reviewed in this chapter. Is there a genetic predisposition to suicidal ideation and suicidal behavior? There is no credible evidence to support a genetic hypothesis, although it is likely that environmental variables and family history may place some children at greater risk for suicide.

Biochemical and neurophysiological research offers a fertile field for inquiry. One branch of neuroscience studies the biological bases of behavior, and specifically the ways in which the nervous system controls people's responses to situations. Since the 1960s, this relatively young field of study has been interested in relationships that might exist between cortical functioning and stress. For a long time, it has been a popular thesis that individuals decide to take their lives when they feel stressed. A word that concretizes this state of extreme stress is *depression*.

The expanding wealth of knowledge about neurotransmitters and the functions they serve in behavioral syndromes is potentially the most significant new frontier in biochemical research. One of these neurotransmitters, serotonin, has been attracting considerable attention. Depression is routinely treated with a classification of drugs called tricyclic antidepressants. It is thought that these agents block receptor sites and interrupt serotonergic activity within the cells. Behaviorally, these antidepressants act to elevate mood.

Some postmortem studies of suicide victims have revealed lower than normal levels of serotonin and a metabolite of serotonin (5-HIAA). This has led some researchers to hypothesize that a reduction in serotonergic activity may be causally linked to suicidal ideation and behavior.

Finally, the monitoring of brain wave activity of persons hospitalized for attempted suicide or threat of suicide has produced some interesting data. Dysrhythmic EEGs may be linked to intense suicidal ideation in these patients. One might reasonably ask whether the behavioral crisis has contributed to the abnormal brain activity or whether the behavior is being triggered by the changes in brain wave functions.

Although none of this research offers conclusive answers to the question posed: "Why does a person commit suicide?", it does open some stimulating new avenues of study.

Three behavioral syndromes have been traditionally associated with suicide: depression, schizophrenia, and character disorders. Biochemical research has studied the role that these behavioral patterns are thought to play in the etiology of suicide.

For a long time, depression was considered an adult syndrome; children did not get depressed. After years of debate among clinicians, the American Psychiatric Association has included the diagnostic criteria for childhood depression in its most recent revision of the *Diagnostic and statistical manual of mental diseases* (1980). Depression is a life-cycle concern and by its very definition, involves many variables, physiological, functional, and social. Depression can entail psychomotor retardation as well as significant changes in mood. All of this suggests that depression implies an interaction among many variables of psychobiosocial functioning.

Numbers of researchers and theorists have attempted to describe these interactions. For a long time, the formulations of Freud and his associates in the psychoanalytic tradition have dominated the discussion. Psychoanalytic theory hypothesizes that depression is rooted in a lost love object that is loved ambivalently; the wounded ego redirects the rage it feels toward itself.

Other theoretical approaches in contemporary psychology include those of the behaviorists, according to whom depression is thought to result from changes in the reward/punishment reinforcement pattern. Any significant loss of a person or thing that was positively gratifying to the person is experienced as an aversive stimulus. Depression is defined as a behavioral response to these negative stimuli. How these theories of depression relate to adolescence has been explored.

Schizophrenia commonly describes a variety of serious mental disorders, characterized by misinterpretation and retreat from reality, delusions, auditory and visual hallucinations, ambivalence, and inappropriate affect. A schizophrenic is frequently withdrawn and may display bizarre or regressive behavior. The seriousness of the disorder frequently requires hospitalization, although a person may only occasionally experience episodes of schizoid behavior, sometimes violent. While otherwise appearing normal, this individual may suddenly commit aggressive, antisocial acts or display violent motor activity.

Adolescents who display schizophrenic symptoms may be more disposed to attempt and commit suicide. Hallucinations may be translated by a schizophrenic youth as a mandate to take his or her own life. The detachment from reality and the retreat into an elaborate world of fantasy—characteristics of schizophrenia—are an invitation to some people to self-destruction.

The state of ego functioning has been judged as a significant variable in adolescent suicide (Pfeffer, 1981a, b). Impulsive behavior, an irresistible imperative to act in a particular (frequently destructive) way, is linked to weak ego control. Some clinicians have suggested that adolescent impulsive acting-out behavior may mask depression. Our discussion considered suicidal potential in adolescents who are prone to aggressive and impulsive behaviors.

Family dynamics, particularly communication patterns within families, have consistently been associated with the incidence of suicide in adolescence. Previous suicides within the nuclear family may be a predisposing factor in the subsequent suicide of an adolescent member. The inability of some parents to achieve a psychological separation from their adolescent children is thought to be a factor in the suicidal behavior of some young people. Suicide, for some adolescents, describes a pathological attempt to cope with stressful aspects of one's family of origin.

The search for the answer "Why does a person attempt or commit suicide?" is complex. It appears that the answer does not lie in one field of inquiry, but in the interaction of biochemical, emotional, familial, and socio-cultural variables.

Suicidal acts have been reviewed under three broad headings: intentional, marginally intentional, and accidental behaviors. The most clear category is the first: a person systematically prepares for his or her death, considering details of time, place, and method. In this process, the person intending suicide ordinarily provides some clues to the intention to commit suicide, although frequently these hints are not correctly perceived or understood, or they are ignored. Some of the more common reasons for which adolescents might intentionally plan and attempt suicide have been reviewed, including the frequently cited issue of retaliation—against parents, friends, lovers.

The classification of "marginally intentional suicidal behavior" is ambiguous. With respect to adolescence and young adulthood it describes activities that are potentially self-destructive and/or homicidal. The personality expansion tasks of the adolescent years imply testing of the parameters of one's life. Use and abuse of alcohol and other drugs are part of youthful experimentation. However, it has been suggested that some of these behavioral abuses may be symptoms of dissatisfaction with life and constitute pleas for help.

The eating disorders of anorexia nervosa and bulimia, common problems among young persons, may be related to the issue of suicide. Although neither could strictly be termed "suicidal," there is evidence to suggest that they are marginally intentional suicidal behaviors.

An obscure and challenging issue concerns fatal accidents of adolescents and the intent, suicidal and otherwise, that may lie behind them. Cultural factors may explain why many adolescents fail to accurately judge the realistic limits of their abilities. Some of these youth may lose their lives because they consider their strengths and abilities to be limitless.

Effective and timely treatment of those prone to suicide depends upon recognition and accurate interpretation of symptomatic suicidal behaviors. A number of common behaviors suggestive of suicidal ideation have been reviewed. Hospitalization of an adolescent who has attempted suicide is not always advisable. A number of psychotherapeutic approaches to the treatment of suicidal youth have been developed. Glaser (1978) has concluded that a variety of approaches may be needed, and a switching from one method to another may be the most beneficial to the adolescent and his or her family.

The use of psychotropic medications in the treatment of adolescent depression and suicidal response is an important issue. Many clinicians feel that antidepressant drug treatment is not the treatment of choice for most adolescents. Not only does the use of drugs give a mixed message to the adolescent, but the physiological effects may compound the individual's vulnerability to suicidal ideation (Cotman & McGaugh, 1980).

Suicide prevention is society's responsibility. The task involves three distinct strategies. The first, primary prevention, means doing whatever possible to recognize, interpret, and respond to the physical and behavioral cues in pre-suicidal youth. Secondary prevention addresses the issue of the responsibility of appropriately intervening with an attemptor, as well as that of educating family and society to be aware and responsive to the prodromal signs of suicide. Tertiary prevention is concerned with the care of the survivors of a completed suicide. It attempts to mitigate the negative psychological effects of this crisis.

The rate of adolescent suicides has been increasing over the past decade. This chapter has attempted to look at this phenomenon from a variety of perspectives, considering the underlying pathology of this problem for young people, etiologic issues, and behaviors that may mask suicidal intent. The role of the family, both in the precipitation of adolescent suicide and in its effective treatment, has been underscored. Together, new biological and psychological insights have enlarged scientific and humanistic perspectives on the problem of suicide in the transitional years into adulthood.

6
Catastrophic Life-threatening Events in Adulthood

Myocardial Infarction and Sudden Death, Burns and Lethal Thermal Injuries, Multiple-trauma Accidents

Coronary Heart Disease
- Psychological Prodromata of Myocardial Infarction
- Physical Activity and Coronary Heart Mortality
- Richter's Paradigmatic Research on Hopelessness and Sudden Death
- Human Physiology and Sudden Death
- Psychological Problems of Hospitalization and Convalescence
- The Coital Coronary
- Intervention with the Family Survivors of Cardiac Death

Life-threatening Thermal Injuries
- Life-death choices
- Prediction of Burn Mortality
- Postburn Adjustment and Adaptation
- Disfigurement and "Social Death"
- Effective Coping Strategies
- Special Needs of Burned Children, Adolescents, and Their Parents
- Geriatric Thermal Injury
- Burn Death

Multiple-trauma Injuries
- The Nature of "Critical Care"
- Anxieties Concerning Survival and Recovery
- Psychological Dynamics of Coping

Summary

Myocardial Infarction and Sudden Death, Burns and Lethal Thermal Injuries, Multiple-trauma Accidents

Throughout the human life cycle, individuals and families are subjected to numerous life-threatening experiences. Although advances in emergency medical care and technology have significantly reduced the mortality statistics for many life-threatening events, accidents and acute illnesses continue to suddenly confront people with the possibility of imminent death and with the thoughts and feelings associated with death. This chapter will consider three such critical events: coronary heart disease, burns, and multiple-trauma accidents.

Coronary heart disease is a major cause of death in the United States. Sudden cardiac death due to *ventricular fibrillation*, an arrhythmic contraction of the heart muscle, is perhaps the leading cause of death in the industrially developed world. *Myocardial infarction*, commonly called "heart attack," is another. Individuals are often not prepared for a myocardial infarction. Often they delay in seeking medical assistance, putting themselves at greater risk of dying from the infarction (Hackett & Cassem, 1979).

More than 80 percent of persons hospitalized with major burns survive. *Burn mortality* is influenced by numerous factors, including the age of the patient, the total burn area, third-degree burn area, prior bronchopulmonary disease, abnormal PaO_2 (arterial oxygen tension), and inhalation injury (Roi et al., 1981; Roi et al., 1983; Tobiason, Hiebert & Edlich, 1982; Zawacki, Azen, Imbus, & Chang, 1979). While an assessment of these and other factors upon admission are useful prognostic indices in treatment programs, they tell us little about how the burned individual and his or her family will respond to the trauma.

Motor vehicle and work-related accidents can plunge families into sudden crises. The proliferation of critical care centers in large metropolitan areas reflects the kind of intensive, specialized, comprehensive care that multiple-trauma victims require (Zschoche, 1981). Since accidents are the principal cause of death in the cohort of persons under age 40 and the third leading cause of death in the general population in the United States, this chapter will consider the special needs and concerns of multiply injured accident victims and their families.

In each of these three acute traumatic events, individuals and families are brought close to an encounter with death. In some cases, an afflicted individual, his or her family, or both may face decisions about the use of heroic, life-sustaining treatments. The highly specialized care required to treat successfully these various traumas may not fully meet the needs of patient and family, however. The chapter will discuss appropriate hospital care as it relates to these issues.

Coronary Heart Disease

Psychological Prodromata of Myocardial Infarction

Numerous efforts have been made in the medical and psychological literature to document the warning signs of an imminent infarction (Gentry & Williams, 1979). A *myocardial infarction* (MI) is gross necrosis, or death, of the myocardium, the middle and thickest layer of the heart wall, which is composed of the cardiac muscle. Necrosis of the heart tissue results from oxygen insufficiency over a significant period of time. An infarction can also result from an interruption of the blood supply to the area due to an obstruction of circulation, most commonly by a thrombus (a clot that obstructs a blood vessel) or an embolus (undissolved material carried by the blood current and affecting some part of the vascular system). The obstruction blocks a coronary artery and diminishes blood supply to some portion of the left heart ventricle, which then dies.

After reviewing much of the behavioral science data about coronary heart disease (CHD), Appels (1980) suggests a dynamic model to describe the process that may lead to a heart attack. This process begins with exorbitant efforts to receive recognition and response from the environment. Requiring significant energy, this striving can disrupt the body's chemistry by, for example, raising blood pressure and elevating the levels of cholesterol and glucose in the blood. When this type of self-induced stress becomes chronic, it may not only entail emotional disturbances but it may trigger a snowballing mechanism whereby alleviation of symptoms is sought in the very conditions that produced them—overexertion and alteration of body chemistry.

Clinically, a person prone to the onset of MI is characterized by vital exhaustion and depression. Any research that attempts to identify factors that have predictive validity for CHD must reconcile the debate concerning the origin of these conditions. The *Type A Personality* construct (Friedman & Rosenman, 1974) has garnered enormous popularity because it presents a cogent psychogenic explanation of the prodromata of MI. In fact, Friedman asserted that the cluster of psychological factors including tiredness, loss of vitality, helplessness, hopelessness, depression, exhaustion, sleep disturbances, and hypochondriacal concerns should not be construed as simple personality traits, but as symptoms of CHD. In research like Friedman's, however, it is difficult to determine whether such traits reflect physical symptoms present in the infarction-prone person or whether the self-induced stress is cardiotoxic due to neurohormonal correlates (Appels, 1980; Glass, 1977).

Physical Activity and Coronary Heart Mortality

In trying to identify those who might be more vulnerable to cardiac death, researchers have isolated physical activity as a possible indicator. A regular regimen of physical exercise is thought to be a beneficial prophylactic against the life-threatening medley of clinical conditions related to coronary heart disease.

The results of a 22-year study (1951–1972) of some 6,351 longshoremen working in the San Francisco Bay area were reported by Paffenbarger and Hale (1975). The goal of the study was to evaluate the relationship that might exist between physical exertion and the risk of fatal heart attack. The men participating in this study were between the ages of 34 and 74 at its inception in 1951; they were followed until age 75 or their death. Care was taken to compute their total work experience in terms of high, medium, or low caloric output. Other variables that could influence outcome, particularly psychologic and other selective influences, were not considered.

The findings seem to support the position that physical output is associated with reduced risk of coronary mortality. Within this group for whom objective, detailed, and reliable information was gathered, those who were in the physically most demanding jobs did better in avoiding CHD than did their associates who gradually assumed less taxing jobs on the docks. The study noted that the workers in the high-caloric output positions were required to expend energy in repeated bursts of peak efforts, while those in situations of medium or low-caloric output might perform at constant, but less intense, energy levels.

In analyzing their data, the researchers indicate that the intense, peak efforts of the high output group, may have had a beneficial effect on the cardiovascular system. The steady, lower-level output did not seem to provide the same conditioning. The logic informing this conclusion is that high-intensity energy outbursts may prevent or diminish the lethal chain of events involved in MI, beginning with ventricular ectopic activity, fibrillation, and sudden death. The high energy expended in strenuous physical activity increases the efficiency of cardiac action and cardiac output and may slow the heart and regularize its rhythm. As such, it may serve a protective function in reducing the risks of infarction.

What this study reports from a particular population of longshoremen has some application to the general population, and many physicians encourage preventive cardiovascular conditioning as a way of reducing or delaying the risk of death due to coronary artery disease. In fact regular physical exercise is thought to temper the negative effects of other factors possibly related to coronary heart disease, including *hypertension* (persistently high arterial blood pressure), *tachycardia* (excessive rapidity in the action of the heart), *obesity* (increase in body weight beyond the limitation of skeletal and physical requirement), *hyperlipoproteinemia* (excess of lipoproteins in the blood) and *hypercholesterolemia* (excess of cholesterol in the blood).

The following case study illustrates the complex interplay of factors that often leads to myocardial infarction.

Neil Clark is a 52-year-old sales executive with a major computer manufacturing company. He has been with this company for the past 18 years. During that time his career has progressed according to his own timetable. At the time of his heart attack he was a regional vice-president of the company's microprocessing division.

During his recent routine company physical examination Neil was advised of his elevated blood pressure and his increasing weight. He was counseled to monitor both of these factors. In addition, some of his associates noticed an increase in his consumption of alcohol. While none was prepared to boldly label him an "alcoholic," certain symptomatic behaviors indicated that this might be a more serious problem than Neil was prepared to acknowledge.

Neil's family life was also stressful. His three late adolescent and young adult children were concerns to Neil and his wife. The oldest was finishing college, living with a girl friend, and attempting to start a small landscape design business. He did not get along well with his father, and clearly desired not to be involved with him.

A college-aged daughter had resumed her studies after a period of psychiatric hospitalization for attempted suicide. She had overdosed on barbiturates while at school. She continues to see a psychiatrist for psychotherapy.

The youngest child is in her junior year in high school. Being the only child living at home, she feels enormous tension, particularly with her mother who is a tense, compulsive person, who tends to be smothering and overprotective.

Neil and his wife do not experience major difficulties in their marital relationship, although they seldom share significant communication with one another. Their marriage has developed on parallel tracks; Neil occupied himself with his career while Joan assumed almost total responsibility for the home and children.

Joan was very concerned about her husband's drinking, his overeating, and the stress under which he generally placed himself. She was constantly nagging him to follow the doctor's advice and make some changes. Neil became hostile when Joan brought up these concerns and responded by walking away from her or by telling her to get her own act together.

It is not easy to draw a clear distinction between the physiological and psychological factors in Neil's medical history and the psychosocial environmental factors that may have disposed him to CHD and a fatal infarction (Jenkins, 1979). Engel (1971) noted certain stress-related factors in the 170 case histories he reviewed of individuals who died of a heart attack. Although the circumstances were different in each of these cases, the deceased shared some common features. The stressful stimuli could not be disregarded, and the stressors appeared to engage strong emotional responses that transcended volitional control.

The sum of these factors may dispose a person to feel not only helpless, but hopeless. Several investigators have described this as "the giving up—given up response" (Saul, 1966; Schmale, 1968; Engel, 1968). The psychological constructs of helplessness and hopelessness have contributed significantly to hypotheses that explain death as the organism's ultimate response to stress. Much of the foundational research in this area was conducted with infrahuman animals. The conclusions of these early studies have contributed significantly to theories about the psychophysiological relationships in acute coronary deaths.

Neil confided to a close friend with whom he regularly golfed that he was feeling somewhat overwhelmed by the pressures both at work and at home. He had great concerns about his children, especially his daughter who had attempted to kill herself. Although she seemed to be doing much better, he still confessed that he was afraid that she might attempt suicide again, and succeed. He did not feel that he could talk openly with Joan about these concerns because she gets too upset. The job was also beginning to get to him. He admitted that he was spending longer hours at the office but that he didn't seem to be as productive as he once was. Besides, he was a bit heavier and credited this for his feelings of fatigue.

Neil's situation was not desperate, but he did sense a certain inability to control aspects of his family life, his marital relationship, and his job. When he recounted these facts to his golf partner, he concluded: "There are times when I feel pretty helpless, and wonder, what's the use. . ." (Williams, 1979).

Richter's Paradigmatic Research on Hopelessness and Sudden Death

In 1957 Richter published the data and conclusions of the first animal studies that established a relationship between hopelessness and sudden death. Later Seligman (1975) would adopt the term "helplessness." Engel (1971) and others use the term "giving up." All of these terms are interchangeable; each seeks to establish a relationship between psychological surrender and physical death.

Richter constructed swimming cylinders in which he placed various hybrid, laboratory-bred rats and recently captured wild rats. Experimental procedures isolated two factors as significant in the drowning deaths of rats. The rats' vibrissae, or whiskers, were shaved, thus severing an important perceptual contact the rat had with the outside world. Restraint of the rats by experimenters was also observed to be sufficient to trigger death.

Monitored by underwater electrocardiographic recordings, the dying rats displayed *bradycardiac rhythms*, that is, heart beat slowed to a pulse rate lower than 60. The rats' hearts stopped in diastole, during the period of dilatation of the heart. This observation was confirmed upon autopsy, where the heart was noted to be suffused with blood. It is interesting that these experimental conditions did not catalyze adrenergic activity in the animals' heart function. Richter, in reporting on the reverse reaction, namely, slowing of heart rate, concluded that the rats died a vagal death. This, he speculated, resulted from overstimulation of the parasympathetic nervous system rather than the sympathicoadrenal system.

Discussing these findings, Richter concluded that hopelessness is the best explanation for the sudden death of rats exposed to these experimental conditions. His early studies have inspired numerous similar studies (Griffiths, 1960; Lynch & Katcher, 1974; Rosellini *et al.*, 1976; Binik, Theriault & Shustack, 1977). In a careful review of the scope of psychological research of sudden death in infrahuman animals, Hughes and Lynch (1978) concluded that both the research design of the original Richter studies and the modifications introduced in subsequent research are useful for monitoring the physiologic parameters that mediate stress-induced death. They are not willing, however, to make the leap from these data to the conclusion that death resulted from "hopelessness."

Hughes and Lynch do not deny that the concepts of hopelessness, helplessness, or giving up may be a valid explanation of the animal's response to the experimental stressors. However, they note that it is not easy to assess the subjective feeling states of animals. It is one thing to track the behavior of a rat who passively drowns in an unfamiliar, overtaxing situation. It is quite another thing to conclude that the animal responds in this way because the situation is perceived as "hopeless."

In considering the leaps that some clinicians might be ready to make in extrapolating from research with infrahuman animals, Hughes and Lynch caution against conclusions that are too facile. They correctly note that the data they are reviewing report on physiological variables from which certain psychological conclusions have been drawn. Granting that the inferences may be correct, Hughes and Lynch conclude their discussion by observing that there may be certain psychological variables in human research that either have no counterparts in infrahuman species, or if they do exist, cannot be adequately tested.

Hughes and Preskorn (1980) state that it is hard to conceive of animal research that could successfully quantify the psychological states of infrahuman animals in verifying causal relationships to sudden death. It is not justified to assume that there are some nontestable psychological mechanisms at work when the only verifiable data are physiological. They feel that the physiological data, apart from the psychological inferences some scientists might draw from these data, are quite useful in themselves.

Human Physiology and Sudden Death

As stated earlier a clear division between physiological and psychological variables is not useful to the discussion of sudden death. This applies as well to cardiac arrhythmias. These variations in the normal rhythm of the heart beat may have a clear physiologic origin—*heart block*—but they can also be attributed to psychological factors as well—e.g., *paroxysmal tachycardia* (attacks of rapid action of the heart having sudden onset and cessation) or *atrial tachycardia* (rapid cardiac rate, usually between 160 and 190 per minute). Today it is generally recognized that the autonomic nervous system is not without higher cortical influence. Therefore, it is very important to consider the ways in which psychological factors may influence cardiovascular activity.

Lynch and his associates (Lynch *et al.*, 1974; Lynch, 1977) studied the effects of human contact on cardiac arrhythmia in coronary care patients. In ordinary routine procedures such as pulse taking, they documented heart rate changes of more than 30 beats per minute, a frequency double that of abnormal heart beats. Human contact can be stressful for the cardiac patient (Thomas & Lynch, 1979). However, even certain transient, low-level stresses in non-coronary-prone persons can precipitate cardiac abnormalities. Driving in adverse weather conditions or in heavy traffic, public speaking or performance, or other common potentially stressful situations may induce ectopic beats, occasional premature ventricular contractions, and tachycardia.

The popularity today of *biofeedback* is due to its successful management of these potentially stressful events. Biofeedback demonstrates that, to a certain degree, heart rate and arrhythmias can be responsive to learning (Olton & Noonberg, 1980). For example, patients subject to chronic *premature ventricular contractions* (PVC) can learn through biofeedback techniques to control heart rate and reduce the life-threatening risks this chronic condition represents. A PVC is a contraction of the ventricle that occurs prematurely in the heart beat sequence: increased heart rate reduces the rate of PVCs.

Acknowledging that coronary artery disease may be the underlying pathologic condition in heart disease, many cardiologists admit that certain neural activities may trigger arrhythmias in one patient and not in another. Today greater credence is placed in the relationship between central nervous system (CNS) functions and potentially lethal cardiokinetic activity. Sudden death, therefore, may not simply be cardiogenic but may have its triggering mechanism in CNS responses to external stimuli.

In their 1978 report on ventricular premature beats, stress, and sudden death, DeSilva and Lown support the position that stimulation of higher *sympathetic nervous centers* are involved in the incidence of arrhythmic activity and ventricular fibrillation. In fact, the regular use by many cardiologists today of *beta-adrenergic blockers*, which successfully inhibit response to sympathetic impulses and to catecholamines and other adrenergic amines at beta receptor sites, seems to check or at least reduce life-threatening arrhythmias. The apparent success of this attempt to regulate an otherwise electrically unstable myocardium vulnerable to erratic ventricular arrhythmias, has lent additional support to the hypothesis that the sympathetic nervous system may have an etiologic role in the incidence of fatal heart attacks.

Adopting the working hypothesis that higher cortical activity triggered by psychological factors can significantly affect cardiac electrophysiologic properties that may result in both ventricular premature beats and in lowering the threshold for ventricular fibrillation, Lown, DeSilva, Reich, and Murawski (1980) further studied this psychophysiologic relationship. The researchers designed animal studies in which an experimental group of dogs were placed in cages where they were restrained in Pavlovian-type slings. These animals received mild electric shocks during three successive days. The control dogs were placed in similar cages but were neither immobilized nor shocked. All of the animals were electrocardiographically monitored. When the experimental animal was removed from the cage and its heart rate had returned to normal, the mere return of the animal to the sling triggered ventricular tachycardia. The placement of the animal in the stressful environment elevated blood levels of catecholamines.

This research likewise established a direct relationship between increased stress and vulnerability to ventricular fibrillation. When the instrumentally aversively conditioned animals were given Tolamolol, this beta-adrenergic blockade sufficiently inhibited sympathetic autonomic discharge and changes in cardiac vulnerability were obviated.

When Lown and his associates (1980) translate to humans the significant findings of their extensive animal research and the models that derive from them, similar phenomena are seen. While many scientists are prepared to support a putative relationship between ventricular fibrillation and some psychologically induced triggering mechanism in the brain, the precise factors have yet to be determined. Lown and his associates conclude that considerable evidence supports the possible influence of CNS inputs on fatal heart attacks.

Despite the little human data to support related findings from animal studies, what is available tends to support these hypotheses. As useful as the beta blockers have been in stalling fatal rhythm disorders, they have not been universally successful, from which it can be inferred that numerous CNS mechanisms may be involved in arrhythmic activities.

Neil had alluded to the difficulties he was having at work in his conversation with his golf partner. Things were actually far worse than he described. The monthly sales reports indicated a significant slippage in his division. The morale among his managers was low. Neil seemed to be more and more reliant on alcohol and this was beginning to seriously affect not only his performance, but his mood.

The senior executive from the company's headquarters to whom Neil directly reported was aware of this situation and requested a meeting with him. In that meeting, Neil was confronted with his excessive drinking—a fact which he attempted to deny. He was informed that the company was prepared to support him in a rehabilitation program if he were willing to accept this offer. If he were unwilling, the senior officer told him that the company would have no other option than to accept his resignation.

This was a serious blow to Neil. He neither expected nor welcomed this ultimatum. He had thought that the meeting was requested because of the slump in sales, something that was happening in some other regional divisions as well. He did not consider that the company had a different agenda with him.

That afternoon he felt very tired and returned home early. Joan was not there when he arrived. He stretched out on the sofa in the family room, staring at the ceiling. He felt chills and began to perspire. There were radiating pains through his arms. He thought he might be getting the flu.

When Joan returned in an hour, Neil was in the same position. She became quite alarmed when she saw how ashen-colored his complexion was and how profuse the perspiration. She called the doctor and described Neil's symptoms. The doctor asked if it was possible to speak to Neil. When Neil confirmed to the doctor what Joan had described, the physician immediately ordered that an ambulance be summoned to take Neil to the hospital.

Neil had suffered a myocardial infarction. Could this heart attack have been precipitated by the stressful conversations he had had earlier in the day with the senior executive? Even though his physical condition and general lifestyle made him vulnerable to MI, did this additional source of stress catalyze the attack? It is difficult to make such a determination, but it is likely that certain psychophysiologic mechanisms could have triggered the attack.

Dimsdale (1977) would support this conclusion. He notes that neither the psychological or the physiological explanations of the causes of MI and sudden death are firmly established. Despite this fact, it is unquestionable that there is a connection between somatic and psychologic factors. He believes that interdisciplinary psychophysiological research involving both psychiatric and cardiac professionals will continue to shed greater light on what combination of factors disposes a person to a fatal heart attack.

The Psychological Problems of Hospitalization and Convalescence

Cardiac care is specialized and a potential source of stress to the patient. Not only can the environment of the coronary care unit be overwhelming to the person being treated, but it can create difficulties for the families as well. Other aspects of the treatment program may be similarly disturbing (Kiely & Procci, 1981; Hackett & Cassem, 1979).

Neil was somewhat relieved when he was transferred from the coronary care unit. He viewed the transfer as a positive sign that he would survive this heart attack. He actually appeared to be somewhat upbeat in his new hospital surroundings. He joked with the nurses and actually became a bit bawdy in the kinds of stories he related.

Joan was very nervous and became overly cautious when she was with him. She attempted to avoid any subjects that might be upsetting to him. Neil was anxious to get back to his work and asked his secretary to begin to send reports and correspondence to him. He ordered a dictating machine be brought from the office so that he could begin to catch up on a backlog of memoranda. Both Joan and his physician cautioned him about resuming this sort of activity prematurely, but Neil argued that he was feeling fine.

On one occasion when Joan tried to suggest that he not take on too many company burdens, he retorted, "If you don't stop pampering me, I'll sign myself out of this place."

Much of Neil's optimistic behavior masks a certain amount of denial and depression. He does not want to face the realistic consequences of his heart attack. His difficulties with alcohol and his work situation and his family problems have not evaporated as a result of his infarction. Hospitalization has provided a temporary relief from these tensions, but he is preparing to return to many of these same sources of stress. The heart attack has alerted him to the dangers these stresses represent for him, but he is not receptive to the advice the hospital is trying to provide in preparing its discharge plan. (See Gulledge, 1979.)

When Neil returned home, Joan was oversolicitous. While Neil understood and appreciated her efforts to monitor his diet and medication, he admitted that he felt like he was one of the children. She became nervous when he attempted to do some ordinary things, like taking out the garbage.

The illness brought them closer together. For the first time in many years, they actually began to talk about themselves. Neil said he was going to lay off the alcohol and try to get his work situation under control. The company was extremely supportive to him in this illness. Joan was somewhat relieved to hear him talk this way, but she later admitted that he had said these same things so many times before.

Neil was feeling better and wanted to resume sexual relations with his wife. She was quite anxious about his choice, fearing that he was not physically strong enough to be involved in intercourse. Neil protested that he was perfectly fine. Joan reluctantly consented, but she was not at all comfortable with this decision.

The Coital Coronary

The 1969 review by Hellerstein and Friedman on sexuality and the CHD patient reports that two variables—sexual activity and coronary heart disease—have not received much attention in the medical-psychiatric community. In a survey of the major cardiology textbooks, the authors found fewer than 1,000 words written on this subject. During the past 15 years, that silence has been broken and issues related to the sexual life of the cardiac patient have been explored.

While attention has been given to the entire psychosocial needs of the cardiac patient, including his or her sexuality, there has been virtually no research on the issue of the role sexual intercourse plays in the death of such an individual. The epidemiological data on sex-related deaths is simply not available. Derogatis and King (1981) claim that most of what is currently being reported in the field can be described as "hypotheses supported by logic and minimal data."

Engaging in a bit of speculation themselves, Derogatis and King attempt to describe the incidence of sexually related fatal heart attacks. They use the statistics reported in the often cited 1963 study by the Japanese pathologist, M. Ueno, that .6 percent of the 5,559 cases reviewed in a 4-year period were sex-related. Since these cases were almost exclusively extramarital and Derogatis and King conservatively estimate that sex between spouses is at least three times as frequent, they estimate that the risk of sudden death directly related to sexual activity is close to 2.5 percent.

Since there are approximately 450,000 fatal heart attacks each year in the

United States, it is possible that 11,250 of these may be sexually related. The actual incidence may be greater or less. Until serious research addresses this issue, the precise role that sexual activity plays in fatal heart attack will remain a mystery.

The physiological demands of sexual intercourse have been studied by Masters and Johnson, who have documented increase in heart rate, blood pressure, and respiration during the peak period of coitus. Responding to the concerns cardiac patients have about resuming ordinary sexual activity, Hellerstein and Friedman (1969, 1970) state that, except for individuals in congestive heart failure, intercourse presents no particular risk. The little research that has been done on physiological output in sexual relations by individuals with CHD concludes that the extent and duration of physical demands do not appear to be extensive and do not place the individual in life-threatening circumstances (Nemec, Mansfield, & Kennedy, 1976; McNaughton, 1978; Gulledge, 1979). However, it is possible that the intense sympathetic nervous system activity associated with sexual intercourse and the elevation of blood levels of norepinephrine and total catecholamines may destabilize the electrical activity of the myocardium and leave the person vulnerable to fatal arrhythmias.

Six weeks after Neil's admission to the hospital he was back to work. The doctors had recommended a restricted work schedule and a weight reduction program. He had been successful in regaining some control over his drinking difficulties—an achievement which was encouraging to both his wife and his company.

Neil quickly found himself overengaging in business activities. His colleagues tried to encourage him to slow down, but he was insistent that he was feeling perfectly fine. It was apparent to everyone that he was trying to prove to himself that he was capable of the kind of work that had contributed to his promotion to a managerial position.

Old habits began to replace the routines that had been suggested to reduce his risk of subsequent coronary problems. The vicious circle of stress entangled him, and he began to resort to old methods of coping, including the use of alcohol.

Ten months after his initial infarction, while attending a meeting of division heads at corporate headquarters, he suffered another infarction and arrested. Efforts to resuscitate him failed.

When Joan was notified by telephone of his sudden death, she stoically replied: "He would not listen to anyone; he insisted that he was perfectly fine."

Intervention with the Family Survivors of Cardiac Death

Death resulting from a fatal heart attack, stroke, or some other cardiac-related difficulty places a family in a crisis situation. For the past 20 years or more, mental health intervention with families in such crises has been guided by numerous theories about optimal care. Primary among these is the work of Gerald Caplan (1964), who reasoned that people in crisis are the most receptive to the assistance that is offered to them. Caplan asserted that even minimal help offered during the early period of the crisis can be parlayed to maximum gains. These principles of *preventive psychiatry* have influenced the strategies of many practical efforts to aid people in need, although some researchers would maintain that people in crisis are not as open to therapeutic intervention as Caplan might suggest (Bernstein, personal communication, January, 1984).

Williams, Lee, and Polak (1976) undertook a controlled study to examine the effects of a short-term crisis service that was provided to a group of families who were recently bereaved through a sudden death. They were interested to test the reliability of the principles on which so many community mental health programs and clinical practices are based. It has been assumed that preventive crisis intervention following soon upon the onset of the crisis of sudden death can alter the potentially negative physical and psychiatric sequelae among survivors.

In mounting their research they hypothesized that family members provided with competent crisis services would display better coping behavior, lower indices of physical and/or psychiatric problems, and less social disruption than similarly bereaved families who did not benefit from such services. The design of their study involved three distinct groups: an experimental group, composed of bereaved surviving family members who received crisis intervention assistance; a similarly bereaved control group who received no intervention help; and a nonbereaved control group who did not receive any preventive crisis services.

The results of this carefully monitored study confirmed the fact that sudden death indeed has a significant impact on bereaved families in terms of increased risk of ill health, coping behavior, and disturbed social functioning when they are compared with nonbereaved families. Surprising, however, were the indications that short-term crisis services did not appear to influence the post-bereavement adjustment.

The treatment that the experimental group of families received focused on strengthening their adaptation to sudden death. A member of the clinical team would accompany the medical examiner to the location of the death and contact the surviving family members within an hour or two after the death. This early session generally lasted for about two hours. Families were then followed for one to 10 weeks, with an average of 5 sessions per family.

When the bereaved families in the experimental and control groups were assessed in terms of their health, the health indices were similar. Ironically, those in the experimental group who received supportive services reported greater difficulties in coping with the ordinary problems of familial and social reintegration and adjustment. The one positively beneficial result of the clinical intervention efforts was that families receiving treatment reported better decision-making abilities than families not receiving postbereavement assistance.

Following up on this research in primary prevention, Williams and Polak (1979) reported that sudden death may have a two-stage impact upon the surviving family members. In focusing on the long-term adjustment patterns of families exposed to sudden, unexpected death, they paid particular attention to the environmental stresses at the time of death. They hypothesized that intervention strategies that concentrated upon person-centered characteristics may not be as effective as those that take into account the network of the entire family as well as the specific environmental factors surrounding the death. Their research took into account the complex determinants of both family functioning and problem-solving capabilities in the course of adjustment and showed how these individual/familial variables are compounded by the stresses and environmental conditions that attend the sudden death experience.

Williams and Polak (1979) confirmed the findings of Parkes and Brown (1972), which had established an increased risk of ill health among family survivors and close bereaved relatives. This research had noted early increases in subjective psychological and somatic-anxiety-type symptoms. Coping had proved least effective in both familial problem solving and individual decision making. These inadequacies seemed to contribute to a feeling that the quality of life had diminished, both within the family system and in the arena of personal functioning. Williams and Polak described this as "first-phase" reactions. After the first year of bereavement, as Parkes and Brown (1972) had also observed, families exhibit "second-phase" problems focused around more concrete issues of finances and the quality of their familial life.

Considering the kind of cathartic, person-centered, supportive services provided to the families in the experimental group and the seemingly contradictory results, Williams and Polak (1979) questioned the benefit of such structured interventions. In fact, the data gleaned from multiple regression analyses hint that such interventions may have actually had a negative effect on the course of bereavement. This purely statistical observation was shared by the members of the clinical teams who actually provided the services and monitored the period of adjustment. These clinicians felt as though they were intruders in the families, even though the families were open to their offers of help and generally appreciative of their efforts. The researchers suggest that such efforts might be more beneficial if the family actively seeks such assistance, rather than being passively made the recipients of such services. It may be, too, that the clinical strategies and modalities of intervention may not be as effective as initially assumed. More serious is the possibility that such efforts may compound the problems of bereaved families and delay their normal course of adjustment.

Research of this sort, which attempts to test assumptions that have remained virtually unchallenged in more than two decades of community mental health practice, is extremely important. It will necessarily force clinicians in the medical and psychological specialties to define more precisely the role and function they play in the care of families who are suddenly bereaved by an unexpected death.

Life-threatening Thermal Injuries

The experience and technology currently available in critical care burn units explain the fact that more than 80 percent of those hospitalized with major burns survive. Mortality statistics present only a partial picture. In critical burn situations, patients and their families are often faced with difficult options concerning treatment. The procedures and technologies of intensive burn care units are intended to rescue and sustain life against often doubtful odds.

The success of these interventions is impressive. However, that success is not without physical and emotional costs to both the burn patient and his or her family. People survive burns today that would have proven fatal 25 years ago. The heroics involved in many of these rescue efforts—to treat, for example, extensive *full thickness* (third degree) *burns* over a major portion of the body, lead numerous medical and psychiatric personnel to muse about the ethics of these attempts. Those who ultimately survive the trauma of the burns and the intensive, prolonged medico-surgical treatments may find themselves ill-equipped to deal with the psychosocial dimensions of their handicap.

Life-death Choices

Medical science is not immune to the moral and ethical issues that are inextricably related to its highly successful efforts to rescue extensively burned patients. Imbus and Zawacki (1977) have discussed their philosophy in rescuing severely burned patients whose survival is judged to be without precedent. They strongly believe that patients should be informed of this judgment and be encouraged to participate in strategic decisions about whether they should receive heroic life-sustaining treatment. Imbus and Zawacki maintain that patients can be active partners in these decisions and that such involvement preserves a burned patient's autonomy.

The choice between life and death is an ultimate one. Philosophically many physicians would tend to agree at least in principle with the Imbus and Zawacki approach. Others question whether a severely burned patient is capable of making a free and reasoned decision. McCrady and Kahn (1980) believe that persons in the extreme critical situations following major thermal injury are incapable of making life-death choices. They question whether a patient admitted to a burn unit in the first few postburn hours is sufficiently lucid to understand the medical assessment and the life-death options available.

McCrady and Kahn, challenging the assumptions which seem to inform the Imbus and Zawacki approach, state that patients who might be evaluated upon admission to be without precedent for survival may actually recover. Cases continually extend the parameters by which the chances of survival are predicted. Even though certain objective norms are available to guide predictions of burn mortality, it is questionable whether critically burned patients can sufficiently grasp and assimilate the facts to make an informed and reasoned decision concerning care.

It is difficult for a physician to outline options to a patient without introducing subjective biases that might weight the choice in a particular direction. In presenting treatment choices to a person whose survival is judged to be without precedent, it is unlikely that the physician can sufficiently maintain neutrality. Because burn patients are generally receptive to medical judgment, it is questionable whether they are free to make crucial decisions about heroic interventions to save their lives.

Prediction of Burn Mortality

Zawacki, Azen, Imbus, and Chang (1979) studied 1,535 burn patients during a 4-year period in an attempt to better understand what distinguishes survivors from nonsurvivors. Utilizing multifactorial probit analysis, they calculated the contribution of numerous factors that could contribute to the probability of fatal outcome.

When a patient is admitted to a hospital burn unit, routine initial treatment ordinarily includes cleansing of the burned surface, debridement of loose tissue, and topical treatment of the burned area with silver sulfadiazine cream or aqueous silver nitrate. Subsequent protocols include hemodynamic and fluid resuscitation, antibiotics, inhalation therapy, early removal of third-degree burns, and skin grafting (Allyn & Bartlett, 1981).

Traditionally, the *Baux rule* is used to assess burn mortality. This evaluative judgment is based on two essential factors: age and the total body surface area (BSA) burned. By adding the patient's age to the percentage of BSA burned, a quick determination can be made. The basic assumption is that a score higher than 75 presents a poor prognosis and almost certain death. Zawacki and his colleagues (1979) attempted to introduce greater discrimination into this assessment by considering other factors they judged to be important. These include third degree burn area, prior bronchopulmonary disease (bronchitis, pneumonia, asthma, emphysema, chronic obstructive lung disease, and so on), abnormal arterial oxygen tension (PaO$_2$ [less than 70 mm Hg]) and airway edema. Using this 6-factor mathematical model, Zawacki and his associates concluded that this enriched schema enhanced their ability to estimate the probability of fatal outcome in burn patients.

Roi, Flora, Davis, Cornell, and Feller (1981) developed a biostatistical method for estimating mortality risk for the burned patient, using the two normative variables noted above, but adding the factor of the presence or absence of perineal burns. Perineal burns involve the area between the thighs, bounded in the male by the scrotum and anus and in the female by the vulva and anus. The severity grading chart they constructed is intended to provide a graphical method for quick computation of admission severity for the burned patient. The biostatisticians utilized data from 11,200 patients at 12 burn treatment centers in the United States. Their intention in providing such a chart is to aid assessment of the level of care needed and to aid in determining the priority of need and proper place of treatment.

Tobiasen, Hiebert, and Edlich (1982) have developed an Abbreviated Burn Severity Index (ABSI) that is based on age, sex, presence of full-thickness (third-degree) burn, presence of inhalation injury, and percentage of BSA burned. For the purpose of their analyses, the researchers studied 590 patients treated at two Virginia burn centers. They compared the standard Baux and modified Baux scores (Stern & Waisbren, 1980) with the ABSI. Reporting superior results with the ABSI in estimating whether or not a burned person will die, the authors feel that the ABSI is the most accurate and comprehensive simple assessment tool currently available. They feel that it provides a useful objective measure to complement clinical observations and judgments.

In 1983, Roi, Flora, Davis, and Wolfe published two new burn severity indices under that title (Roi *et al.*, 1983). As in their earlier research cited above, they make use of the same data gathered from the dozen U.S. burn centers. Each of these new indices estimates the risk of death utilizing 5 variables: (1) patient's age, (2) gender, (3) size of burned area, (4) perineum involvement and, (5) the elapsed time from the event of the burn to hospital admission. The two indices differ in the specificity of the burn size information used. The first index uses only the percentage of total body surface burned. The second additionally considers the amount of full-thickness burn. The more detailed index enhances the accuracy of the estimate in determining a patient's prognosis and could aid in assessing the benefits of new treatment modalities.

Such severity grading scales use many of the same variables, with slightly different emphases. Each of them is useful to medical professionals engaged in providing emergency care to burned individuals. Each of these statistically derived assessment tools potentially adds greater accuracy and specificity to the task of estimating outcomes for persons sustaining major burns.

Despite the enormous odds against survival, persons with more than 80 percent BSA burns do in fact manage to hold on to life. Bernstein (1976a,b) has incisively described these individuals as "triumphs of medical care but tragedies of human life." For some surviving burn patients, the reward for their accomplishment is the sentence of a living death. It is this form of "death" that will now be discussed.

Postburn Adjustment and Adaptation

Serious, life-threatening burns present adjustment problems not only for the victim, but for his or her family (Davidson *et al.*, 1981). If a patient survives the initial trauma, progressive treatment involves extended care that places burdens on the entire family network. In addition, the degree of disfigurement, even with the best cosmetic and reconstructive surgery, can present psychosocial problems for patient and family alike. Serious thermal injuries are an acute problem requiring emergency assessment and treatment. However, for the victim who survives and his or her family, they become chronic problems.

For many persons who face the crisis of serious burns, there is little knowledge or experience on which to rely. The world of the burn unit is foreign and can intensify the patient's perception of loss of control. Because serious burns may not be part of one's personal experience, many people do not grasp the implications of extensive thermal injuries. It is not unusual that people entertain unreasonable and somewhat magical expectations about what medicine and surgery can accomplish. When applying these to serious burns, parents and family members not only expect that their burned child or relative will survive but that he or she will be restored to normal function and bodily integrity. Despite efforts to establish reasonable expectations about survival and cosmetic possibilities, parents and families may not be emotionally prepared to hear what is being communicated.

Mark is a 19-year-old college freshman who survived a collision with a tanker trailer carrying flammable chemicals. He was pulled from the car in which he was riding by another motorist at the scene of the accident. Although he was still conscious, his clothing was on fire, but with quick action by the man who rescued him, the flames were extinguished.

When emergency medical help arrived at the accident scene, they were able to *triage* (sort out and classify the injuries and determine priority of treatment needs and best place for this treatment) the patient and determine that he required specialized care for his thermal injuries. This judgment was made on an initial assessment of third-degree burns of the face and neck, arms and hands, chest and legs. With the assistance of a medical helicopter, he was airlifted to a primary burn care facility in a nearby major city.

When he arrived at the hospital a nasotracheal tube was inserted because Mark was experiencing difficulties oxygenating and ventilating. Intravenous infusion had already been initiated by the EMT [emergency medical team]. Since his condition was unstable, Mark was not able to be moved to the hydrotherapy room for routine bathing. These initial procedures were carried out in the treatment area, where intensive monitoring and therapies were in progress.

Mark's parents were notified by telephone of the serious accident and the initial assessment of the extent of their son's injuries by the police. They made immediate plans to depart for the hospital, which was about a three-hour automobile drive from their home.

When they arrived at the hospital, they were deeply disturbed by the sight of Mark. He was in a semisitting position in the bed in the burn unit. Tubes were extending from many parts of his body. An intra-arterial catheter had been inserted through his left arm, where a peripheral IV had also been attached, and a pulmonary artery catheter had been floated into him, as well as a urinary catheter. Fluid replacement therapy had begun, and he was receiving blood and plasma transfusions. His hands were elevated and pinned to splints. Significant surface eschar excisions, or removal of burned tissue, had been accomplished.

Mrs. Sorrentino cried uncontrollably at the sight of her son. Her husband tried to calm her, and when she had regained some composure, they were able to tell Mark that they were close to him, that they loved him, and that they were praying for him.

Mr. and Mrs. Sorrentino were anxious to speak with the doctors. A resident who had participated in the initial treatment of Mark was available to talk with them. He was very sensitive to them and tried to be as responsive as he could be to their random and repeated questions about Mark's burns, his chances, his general health, the extent of his disfigurement. While the physician tried to be as hopeful as he could be in answering these questions, it was clear to him that neither of the parents was prepared to hear about the extent and seriousnessness of Mark's injuries, and the present and future dangers that threatened his life. Whenever they asked the question (which they did several times in this initial interview) whether Mark was going to live, the resident responded that there were no guarantees and that his chances were fair. Mr. Sorrentino, in what became a repetitive refrain, said: "Mark's tough; he'll pull through."

Once the imminent danger of death has passed and survival seems likely, the burned person and family begin to assimilate the full significance of the injury. If successful adjustment is to be made, an effective liaison must be forged between the patient and those important individuals who can support him or her during the long and arduous treatments that follow. Social adaptation is not easy, particularly if the face and external limbs are severely scarred and disfigured, as was true in Mark's case. This is not a simple matter for families, or for the wider social community. Such disfigurement can seriously interrupt the communication between the burned person and his or her social network (Bernstein, 1976a; Davidson *et al.*, 1981).

Disfigurement and "Social Death"

Our society places a high premium on physical appearance. This ideal is internalized by many individuals in the course of personality development. People harbor a picture of their ideal body image and often struggle to achieve this ideal even when certain dimensions are not possible. Serious disfiguring burns present special challenges to the survivor's sense of body image.

Initially, surgical interventions have the goal of managing trauma and retaining maximum function. When the person's condition has been sufficiently stabilized, then attention may shift to reconstructive and cosmetic surgical objectives. Although they attempt to restore whatever normalcy is achievable through plastic surgery, surgeons are careful not to raise the patient's or the family's expectations that everything will be as it was before. Despite the impressive accomplishments in reconstructive surgery, there are still limits to what can be done.

Bodily deformity, particularly facial disfigurement, affects the burned person's relationship to self, to family, and to others in the wide social community. Bernstein (1976b) observes that the ability to cope with burn disfigurement cannot be defined by some neat personality profile that is tied to anticipated adjustment. Some individuals approach the challenge of personal and social adaptation in an active mode. They marshal their physical and emotional resources and seek ways of reinvesting these assets. The opposite reaction may be more common. Some people respond to their thermal injuries and disfigurement by withdrawing from familial and social involvement, retreating into a self-imposed isolation. This coping strategy is not productive and can lead to apathy and depression. For some individuals it seems as if the isolation unit in which they were or might have been placed during hospitalization becomes a symbol of what the rest of their life is destined to be.

Social disengagement may be rooted in the person's acute awareness of scarring or disfigurement. Self-esteem is often related to body image and appearance. A person who is anxious and ashamed of his or her physical appearance may seek refuge in privacy and obscurity. While this social detachment may mitigate some of the suffering associated with the stigma attached to physical handicap and deformity, it does not erase the problems that result from debasement and lowered self-esteem.

Heightened sensitivity to other people's reactions contributes to the problems associated with social reintegration. The disfigurement resulting from serious burns elicits a variety of reactions within the family and from others. Some younger children are reluctant to approach disfigured parents; in some instances they perceive them to be "monsters." Spouses may find it difficult to approach a mate sexually (Garts & Garland, 1983). They may avoid touching the scarred areas of the spouse's body. Parents may feel renewed guilt each time they see a burned child (Bernstein, 1983; Kavanagh, 1983a,b). Burn victims can become preoccupied with the ways in which people take notice of them in public and with the expressions of horror, pity, and revulsion that they perceive in their reactions (Murray, 1983; Weinberg & Miller, 1983). All of these varied subjective experiences can diminish a person's sense of self-worth, and contribute to a feeling of being socially dead. In the extreme, these perceptions and feelings can subtly force an individual into a form of psychosocial exile.

Effective Coping Strategies

Others seem to integrate their deformities into a comprehensive picture of self (Blades, Jones, & Munster, 1979). Their defenses, particularly denial, may be sufficiently strong to offset the negative reactions they encounter in familial, school, work, and other social milieux. Certain features of the disability may be repressed, and emphasis is shifted to constructive potentials. This positive attitude on the part of the burned individual can influence environmental acceptance and adaptation. This approach asserts the ascendancy of "mind over matter." While excessive denial associated with suppression and repression may not be in the long-term interest of the severely disfigured or disabled person, the defense may be both necessary and useful in helping the person regain some control over his or her personal and social functioning.

In this whole process of psychological adjustment, people will rely on a varied repertory of responses. Some find solace in humor (Bernstein, 1976a). They may find that self-initiated humorous comments about their disfigurement or disability may diffuse the tension they would otherwise encounter and make social exchange easier for themselves and others. Humor can subtly mask conflict and may actually be a reaction to it. For some individuals this may be a useful way to manage the conflictual feelings they have in social settings.

Others may derive satisfaction by sublimating the negative feelings and reactions they have about their disabilities into socially beneficial efforts. By investing himself or herself in worthwhile endeavors that offer some degree of personal gratification and social recognition, a person is able to minimize somewhat the importance of his or her disfigurement.

Much of the success of these efforts to cope with burn disfigurement depend upon the understanding and acceptance the burn victims find in their marital and familial relationships. If the environment is healthy and loving, and communication open and effective, then a disfigured person has a good opportunity to make the necessary psychological adjustments to resume a productive human life. A healthy family will be able to weather the negative aspects of that adjustment, including the bitterness, rage, and blame that are part of the vascillation many people experience. Strains within families are inevitable consequences of efforts to understand, to adjust, and to respond. To manage these stresses and strains successfully, a family may need some outside support and reinforcement. The extended human services of the hospital and health care community may be best able to respond to these families' needs (Cahners, 1978; Cahners & Bernstein, 1979, Weinberg & Miller, 1983; Marvin, 1983).

Special Needs of Burned Children, Adolescents, and Their Parents

A family in which a child survives a major thermal injury often experiences a form of death. For some families, the long hospitalization and painful treatments place severe stress on relationships between spouses and with other children. Marriages that experienced difficulties prior to the burn trauma may not be able to withstand the pressures of this crisis.

Parents sense the need to mourn. This is obvious in the case of a family whose child may have succumbed to some bacterial infection or metabolic breakdown after weeks of heroic efforts by the burn team to save his or her life. But parents also need to mourn when their child is out of danger and when the prospect of full recovery is promising. They must come to terms with the loss of function and the disfigurement that are consequences of the burns. They need to deal with feelings of guilt, self-reproach, and blame. One spouse may harbor resentment toward the other spouse, who is judged to have been neglectful of the child, or rage toward an individual who in some way is responsible for the accident that resulted in the child's catastrophic burns. All of these feelings are as much "mourning" issues as those directly related to physical death.

It has long been recognized in the psychiatric community (Cope & Long, 1961) that the family constellations of some burned children are emotionally disturbed and disorganized. It is important that this observation not be over-generalized. However staff need to be able to differentiate normal stress and grief from psychopathology. Whatever its circumstances, the family may be able to benefit from appropriate psychiatric consultation.

The presence of psychopathology in the family and the consequent neglect of children may be a contributing factor in the serious burns sustained by children. Not only is staff faced with the practical issues of physical care and rehabilitation, but more importantly with strategic decisions concerning protection of the child and prevention of further harm.

The injuries and scarring sustained by the child certainly aggravate and compound the feelings of the parents. The child's serious injuries may be the first occasion the family has had to receive support and counsel. While their needs place additional burdens on the psychiatric and social service departments, the long-term rehabilitation of the burned child depends on the success of these interventions (Mendelsohn, 1983; Weinberg & Miller, 1983).

Clarke (1980) points out that parents may need to mourn their lost unblemished child who seems to have changed so much in facial and bodily image, as well as in attitude. To minimize the estrangement, parents should be encouraged to resume responsibility for the ordinary care of their burned children as soon as it is feasible. Being thus involved enables them to understand and accept the realities of the thermal injuries and disfigurement in the context of a renewed relationship.

The fear of death haunts some children even when their medical condition is stable and the prognosis of recovery is good. Staff and parents need to be sensitive to the clues of these death-related concerns and not simply dismiss them because they cause discomfort. Such clues indicate a need on the part of the child to process these fears; to help requires sitting, listening, understanding, and supporting.

Solomon (1981) remarks that most burned children undergo some emotional disturbance, whether it is due to a fear of death or some other apprehension or anxiety about their injuries. His extensive experience in pediatric surgery confirms his judgment that patience and gentleness, coupled with careful explanations of procedures and responses to a child's persistent questioning, do alleviate many of a child's fears and anxieties.

Returning home and gradually resuming normal play and school activities is traumatic, not only for the child and family, but for others who will encounter the seriously disfigured child. School personnel, classroom teachers, and fellow students may need some advance preparation so that reintegration is as smooth as possible. Hospital staff often will participate in this preparatory, educative process (Cahners, 1979). All of these factors contribute to the child's emotional well-being and minimize the degree of psychological disturbance he or she may experience in the adjustment process.

The approach of adolescence can be a crisis for a burned child, whose disfigurement may present new difficulties in social, recreational, vocational, and sexual activities (Bernstein, 1976b). Ideally, some issues would have been anticipated and supportive preparation begun prior to the onset of puberty and menarche. Adolescents are realistically concerned about their sexual desirability and intimate realtionships. Some may become depressed and actually experience a form of social death. Bernstein (1976b) appropriately labeled this as "life in a minor chord."

A dejected and socially withdrawn adolescent, despairing of the possibility of a satisfying life, can entertain thoughts of suicide. While it is difficult to estimate the incidence of suicides among burn patients, burn team personnel all acknowledge personal experiences of individuals who succeeded in killing themselves.

Summarizing what he considers to be the most important features of optimal care of the burned child, Clarke (1980) lists the following points:

1. The burn accident is a **family** event.
2. Parents need to maintain their parenting role.
3. It is important to recognize and deal with the child's anxieties.
4. Children need assistance to learn how to deal with others about their burns and disfigurement.
5. It is important to assist the child in maintaining his or her place in the peer group.
6. Parents need support and help to process their own feelings.
7. Parents and children need constant information in the long course of rehabilitation.
8. Health care professionals need to interpret to parents, siblings, and school personnel the patient's changed physical and emotional capacity.

These points summarize well the major therapeutic needs of the child who survives major thermal injury. They underscore the importance of a trusting and dependable long-term relationship between the hospital team and the family.

Geriatric Thermal Injury

Persons over 65 years of age who endure major burns present different challenges to medical management and rehabilitation. As a group, their mortality rate may be considerably higher than younger adults and children with comparable BSA burns. The possibility of coexisting chronic diseases complicates the treatment strategies and may negatively influence the prognosis of survival.

Slater and Gaisford (1981) reviewed 108 elderly patients treated in the Western Pennsylvania Hospital and Burn Care Center over a period of 6 years. Of these patients, 68 died and 40 survived, yielding a mortality rate of 63 percent. Those who died had a mean age of 76.4 years and mean BSA burns of 44.8 percent whereas survivors were on the average 73.5 years old and had mean BSA burns of 16.7 percent.

In many of the elderly patients in this survey, significant medical histories were noted. In the case of those who did not survive their thermal injuries, complications were noted in their treatment records. The most common indications included renal and pulmonary failures. Preexisting heart and lung disease were also considered to be related to survival.

Recognizing the particular problems presented by an older person with major thermal burns, new approaches promise increased survival among older persons. Resuscitation techniques specifically tailored to the medical requirements of older persons may decrease the mortality rate reported in the Slater and Gaisford (1981) review.

The ethical questions, however, loom high in deciding whether or not to attempt resuscitation of a seriously burned older person. Decisions of this sort are not easy, regardless of the age of the patient. As noted earlier, the recuperative powers of persons can defy even conservative medical judgments about mortality risk. However, with an older person, questions about quality of life must be balanced against the demands of extensive treatment. Staff will experience great anguish as they attempt to resolve these issues in consultation with the elderly patient and his or her surviving relatives. Whenever extreme measures of resuscitation and life support are demanded, the medical community must wrestle with the ethical implications of such actions.

Burn Death

Severe thermal burn injury is a complex disease process. This was evident in the brief case summary presented earlier of Mark Sorrentino. While tremendous medical advances have been made in understanding and treating the various aspects of burn wound pathology, management efforts are not always successful.

Mark, whose burns were assessed to extend to 80 percent of his body, survived the initial resuscitative period. During these initial few days he showed signs of clinical improvement and his doctors and parents were guardedly optimistic. Mrs. Sorrentino continued to weep whenever Mark's condition was discussed. Mr. Sorrentino, on the other hand, was decidedly overcontrolled, unwilling to entertain any suggestion that Mark might not survive these massive injuries. The "he's tough, he'll pull through" refrain was his strongest defense.

On the fifth postburn day, Mark's condition began to deteriorate. Although Mark had certain circulatory and metabolic dysfunction from the time of admission to the burns unit, these problems intensified and the complications proved to be fatal.

His parents were not present with him when he died; they had returned to their hotel at the suggestion of a staff nurse. When the resident physician called them, he asked them to return as soon as possible to the hospital. He did not tell them on the phone that their son had already expired.

When they arrived at the burns unit, they were met by the staff nurses and doctors who were on duty. They were quietly informed that Mark had died forty minutes earlier. Since they wished to do an immediate autopsy, they had to make this request at once. The parents were in shock at the news and Mr. Sorrentino signed the permission form without any discussion.

The couple were invited to see their son's body, which had been removed to a private examination room. The supporting apparatus had been removed and the body was draped, ready for the anticipated autopsy. Mrs. Sorrentino kissed her son's forehead and then turned away, with heavy sobbing. Supported by one of the nurses, they left the room and were brought to a nearby lounge where they were met by the hospital chaplain and one of the doctors.

Although parents may not have been even remotely responsible for the accident that caused the thermal injuries to their children, they are all too often ready to accept the blame. One of the themes Mr. and Mrs. Sorrentino continued to introduce during Mark's hospitalization and in the conversation after his death was: "We should never have bought him that car." The fact that Mark had been drinking, that he had been exceeding the speed limit when he crashed into the tanker trailer truck that had stopped for a traffic light did not enter into his parents' thinking. All they could do was assess their own culpability.

Everything medicine could have done for Mark had been attempted. His prognosis from the outset of the treatment had been marginal, yet he was showing some improvement. The parents clung to these positive signs and were not prepared for the cardiopulmonary and metabolic complications that caused Mark's death. They were angry with the doctors for not being able to check these imbalances. Their feelings were extremely ambivalent: they felt gratitude toward the entire medical staff for the care and attention both Mark and they had received, yet they felt anger toward them for allowing him to die. "Why did you let him die?" was the unanswerable question that Mrs. Sorrentino kept sobbing throughout the final hospital meeting.

A follow-up meeting was arranged with the Sorrentinos to communicate the data derived from the autopsy. On the day of the scheduled interview, Mr. Sorrentino called and said that he and his wife would be unable to make the meeting. He requested a written report of the autopsy. He thanked the hospital and staff for the help they had provided to them and for the sensitivity to them after Mark's death. He reluctantly confessed that his wife simply would not go back to the hospital because the memories were too painful. Mr. Sorrentino was told that the staff was always ready to assist whenever this might be useful and appropriate, and the conversation concluded.

Multiple-trauma Injuries

The Nature of "Critical Care"

Since the 1950s, critical care centers have increased in number throughout the United States, particularly in the more densely populated metroplitan areas. These emergency medical centers are specifically staffed and equipped to treat comprehensively the multiple trauma resulting from work or recreation mishaps, motor vehicle accidents, or some acts of criminal violence and assault. The knowledge and skills that have been gained over the past thirty or more years, coupled with technological advances, offer a better chance of survival to multiple-trauma victims (Meislin, 1980).

The nature and circumstances of multiple-trauma injuries challenge the competencies and skills of the medical team, not only in the direct physical care of the injured patient but in the management of the stressed family (Moonilal, 1982). Acute, catastrophic injuries interrupt the homeostasis of the family system. Although the mortality rate in critical and intensive care settings may be as low as 20 percent of all intakes, each family of a multiple-trauma victim must seriously confront the possibility of death. Should the patient be stabilized, the family may confront other forms of "death" caused by amputation, permanent functional loss, permanent brain damage, or irreversible coma.

For most families, a life-threatening injury to one of its members is perceived as a crisis. The goal of any intervention with families in acute critical situations is the same: the reestablishment of physical and emotional equilibrium. Too often traditional medical practice has been so absorbed in its life-rescuing mission with the injured patient that attention to the needs of the vigilant family members has been relegated to a diminished position in the hierarchy of concerns. It is understandable that the critical care emergency medical team might be so fully absorbed in the direct care of patients that interaction with the patients' families would be reduced to periodic medical conferences and bulletins. Without compromising the priority of care required by the patient, however, the concept of critical care no longer relegates the simultaneous care of the patient's family to a peripheral position. Comprehensive care now includes effective work with family members (Mann & Oakes, 1980).

It was midday when 25-year-old Patricia was brought unconscious to the emergency room. She and her husband and their 15-month-old son had just returned from a summer vacation. Larry, her husband, was an officer at the nearby Air Force base.

When they returned to their apartment, Patricia decided to go to the store to get some groceries, especially some milk for the baby. She went alone in the family car. In order to get to the local store she had to enter the highway and travel two exits. As she was entering the highway, her car was struck on the left side by an oil delivery truck, which was travelling at least 50 mph in the extreme right lane into which Patricia was entering when the accident occurred.

When emergency medical help arrived, the fire department was already on the scene. Neither the oil truck nor the automobile exploded on impact; however, it was impossible to manually extricate Patricia from her vehicle. The fire department was using mechanical "jaws of life" to rip away the twisted car frame.

Upon initial examination, Patricia was not conscious and was unresponsive to verbal or painful stimuli. Pupillary response was also abnormal. There were no fractures and no external bleeding. Precautions were taken to prevent any additional spinal cord injury, and she was moved by ambulance to the hospital.

By the time her husband was located and was able to get to the hospital, x-ray studies and a CT scan (computerized axial tomography) had been done of Patricia's head; the neurosurgeon was anxious to have Larry's permission to take Patricia to the operating room to do an angiogram and to relieve the intracranial pressure to her brain. This pressure was creating cerebral edema. Larry nervously signed the request and the neurosurgeon departed. The dazed young husband was left alone in the emergency room waiting area.

Margaret Epperson (1977) has described the dynamics often encountered in caring for families confronted with a life-threatening injury to one or more of its members. The emotions most frequently displayed by affected families include heightened anxiety, denial, anger, remorse, and grief. It is important to consider, if only briefly, the issue of family dynamics and the ways in which competent management can assist families in their adaptive efforts.

Anxieties Concerning Survival and Recovery

Anxiety is generally defined in terms of external symptoms. Somatic responses to apprehension and uncertainty include tachycardia, sweating, tremor, agitated movements, strictures of neck and shoulder muscles, syncope (fainting), and diarrhea. The death or catastrophic injury to a loved one, particularly sudden death, can set in motion a number of these anxiety-related reactions. Physicians who identify these normal reactions may be hasty to prescribe *anxiolytic drugs* like *diazepam* (Valium), *chlordiazepoxide* (Librium), or some other minor tranquilizer of the benzodiazepine family to reduce or dispel the anxiety. However, although the symptoms of anxiety may be greatly relieved by the prescription of a sedative, and its prescription may be appropriate, the causes of anxiety can only be adequately confronted by effective psychological attention.

Effective management of an anxious person can often be accomplished without resorting to the prescription of benzodiazepines. Anxiety frequently stems from having to confront something that is unfamiliar and that appears to be beyond one's control. Hospital emergency waiting rooms are peopled with many anxious individuals reaching for whatever information they can about their injured loved ones. People in these circumstances are greatly helped if they are given simple but accurate information about the patient. To the degree possible, techniques and procedures need to be explained to the family. Because it is generally not possible for the family to be readily admitted to the treatment area, a mental picture of what procedures are being taken should be painted for the family. Some professionals argue that this type of communication with family members can only intensify their apprehension. Others reason that honest, accurate periodic reporting helps family members to maintain some sense of control, establishes effective communication between them and the treatment team, and gradually prepares family members for eventual contact with the injured person or for the possible unsuccessful outcome of emergency efforts.

One of the medics who was at the accident scene sought out Larry in the waiting area. He introduced himself and asked Larry if he would like to talk about the accident. Larry was very ready to learn whatever he could about his wife's condition. The EMT related the circumstances of the accident as well as he could reconstruct the facts. He told Larry that Patricia had been scarcely conscious when the fire department had arrived, and was unconscious when they began to work on her at the accident scene. She was provided supplemental oxygen and was immobilized to avoid any spinal complications. Once she arrived at the hospital, extensive cardiovascular, respiratory and metabolic assessments were made and a neurological consultation was requested. It was the neurological evaluation that identified the intracranial hematomas that were now being treated by emergency surgery.

Although the technician did not have any other specific information to communicate, Larry appeared to be a bit more relieved to have some first-hand details. He thanked the technician for what he had done "to save my wife's life." He also thanked him for taking the time to talk with him.

The goal of such communication is not one-sided reporting. While certain information needs to be transmitted to the family and may need to be repeated and explained in several different ways, this is only one aspect of the communication. Family members' anxiety is dissipated to the degree that they can express their subjective feelings. Many different thoughts, ideas, and fantasies fuel anxiety. With little encouragement, most individuals welcome the opportunity to ventilate some of these inner experiences and feel relieved to be able to verbalize these concerns to another understanding person. To the extent that this type of communication pattern is established early between the injured patient's family and the critical care team, the family is given a headstart in weathering the crisis.

Psychological Dynamics of Coping
Denial

Unconscious denial commonly serves to protect a person in the face of facts and consequences that one is unwilling or not prepared to entertain. Denial is a complex mental mechanism that has important relationship to healthy adjustment. As a defense it has its legitimate place in a person's psychological armory. It takes time to assimilate facts about a loved one's condition, especially when the information communicated is tentative or not promising. Equally stressful is the news of possibly irreversible breakdowns in mental and physical functions.

Denial is misunderstood by too many clinical practitioners, who fail to appreciate its beneficial functions. The information and prognosis communicated by the medical professional may be incontrovertible; families may appear to dismiss these assessments and prefer to entertain unreasonable expectations of recovery. Initially, the family is best left secure in its denial. Often this is a transitional state, denial serving as a bridge between the wished-for world and the real world. Paradoxically, the unrealistic hopes and expectations attached to denial can emotionally prepare a person to deal with things as they are. Of course, denial can assume pathological proportions; this presents a different challenge to effective management.

As the family dynamic processes denial, gradually the family finds effective ways to absorb realities concerning the condition of the injured member. Little by little the family relinquishes its corporate and individual denial.

From the accident site Patricia had been taken to the nearest hospital that had a multiple-trauma emergency team. It happened to be a church-affiliated hospital. The Catholic chaplain [author] met Larry while he was still in the emergency room reception area. Larry had been raised as a Baptist in rural Texas but had not been involved in religious practice since his youth. He was open to the chaplain's interest in him and his wife and was very talkative.

Since the chaplain had been alerted at the time of Patricia's admission, he had been present in the treatment area when her condition was being assessed. This information was very consoling to Larry and this helped to establish a relationship between him and the chaplain. "I'm sure everything's going to be all right with Patricia, Reverend, 'cause you were there to say some prayers for her. God is going to listen to you."

The chaplain was comfortable enough with Larry's attempts to deny the seriousness of the initial assessments of his wife's injuries. This position became fixed throughout the next several days. During that time the chaplain became the most important link between Larry, the medical staff, and Patricia, who lay unconscious in the intensive care unit. Each day Larry would say: "Keep up those prayers, Father; maybe today she will open her eyes and say hello to us."

Anger and Hostility

The suddenness and seriousness of the injury to a loved one generate feelings of uncertainty and powerlessness that can, in turn, provoke anger and hostility. These feelings can take many varied forms. Some individuals may mask their feelings under a cloak of self-blame. "If only I had . . ." statements are common. When attempts are made to relieve the person of this self-imposed blame, these may be met with a hostile rebuff. Other individuals will look for someone or something to scapegoat. Unsafe automobiles, defective heat and smoke detectors, faulty safety equipment at work, or lack of proper police support or protection can become the object of angry protest. Because the hospital is the immediate context in which these angry feelings can be processed, it is not unusual that many conflicts are projected onto the hospital and its staff.

During his daily rounds the neurosurgeon met Larry. By temperament, the physician was not very communicative. It was clear that he did not respond well to Larry's insistent questions. His responses were always guarded, and it was clear that his most conservative judgments about Patricia's condition were not optimistic. Should she ever regain consciousness, it would be impossible to predict the extent of her brain damage. She was being supported on a ventilator; in the surgeon's judgment, without this life support she would not survive.

Larry had extremely hostile feelings toward the neurosurgeon and was quick to ventilate them to his trusted confidant. The chaplain listened to the young husband as he described frustrations with the hospital staff. The young man was virtually alone. Both his family and Patricia's were in Texas; Patricia's mother and Larry's sister were due to arrive the following day. Larry was trying to provide care for his small son and keep a continual vigil outside the intensive care unit. It was evident that the physical and psychological stress of this routine was taking its toll on him. It was not unusual that he had the chaplain paged once or twice a day, just to have someone to talk to. "She's going to get better, Father, despite what that doctor keeps saying."

For some staff, the expression of these feelings by the patient's family can excite negative reactions. Although the hostile accusations may be unmerited, it is important that there should be no response in kind. The anger may be situationally related to the current crisis, or it may be more deeply rooted in a whole series of other relationships with the patient and family that transcend the present crisis. Because the ventilation of angry feelings on the part of one family member can engage other members of the family and unite them in a common expression, it is understandable why some medical personnel will avoid such a family or will abruptly abandon them once this dynamic is set in motion.

It is important, however, that families express their feelings. If the family is allowed to work through angry thoughts and feelings, some of which are legitimate and insightful, the power and rage that fuels them gradually diminishes. The distillate from this process can be helpful in the family's reorganization. Epperson (1977) has found in her work with families in crisis situations that they often come to see that they are angry at the patient himself or herself, whose injury has seriously disrupted the family's homeostasis and burdened its members.

A family or family member may act out anger in socially unacceptable ways, causing a certain embarrassment. Such individuals soon regret the verbal and physical assaults they make on members of the critical care team who try to work with them. It is very helpful to assure families that what they say and do is understandable, given the difficult circumstances in which they find themselves. This empathic and forgiving attitude on the part of the medical support team members can help a family come to terms with its ambivalent angry feelings. A family that is able to work through these feelings will be more effective collaborators in the important work of rehabilitation for the injured family member. If the patient does not survive his or her injuries, then the family will have already begun, in the course of its vigil, to reconcile the potentially destructive feelings generated by the crisis. For these reasons, despite the discomfort involved, staff should encourage families to ventilate their anger.

Replaying the Events

The waiting period throws a family into a state of suspended animation. Life continues to go on around them, but they are grouped together, uncertain whether the next minutes or hours will bring hopeful or fearful news. Emotionally, they make preparations for either outcome. Unlike the situation of certain death, wherein a family may become involved in anticipatory grieving, a multiple-trauma crisis creates an emotional limbo. Identification with the injured patient may be intense, and the family may judge itself to have been an accomplice in the circumstances leading up to the catastrophic event. A family may need to rehearse detail upon detail, recreating the scenario in which the accident occurred. However obsessive, this family dynamic is therapeutic. The family alone has the power to absolve itself and reconcile itself to the unfortunate circumstances. Families should be encouraged to talk it out together, inviting each person to share whatever he or she feels may have been his or her own part in the event.

"Patricia and I got married despite our families' opposition. She got pregnant and we decided to get married although we both had decided to get married even before we knew about the baby. Her parents did not come to the ceremony, except one of her sisters. This really hurt both of us. We haven't been very religious, though we both believe in God. Do you think God is punishing us for our lives?"

On many occasions, Larry was involved in this kind of remorseful and soul-searching rumination. He kept rehearsing the circumstances of their return from vacation and her decision to go to the store. He had volunteered to go to the store himself, but she had insisted. Larry frequently said: "She wasn't used to the highways here; she panics in those kinds of situations." He wondered whether she even saw the oil truck approaching, or whether she applied the breaks instead of accelerating.

The driver of the truck came to the hospital; he was greatly shaken by the accident and needed to express his sorrow to Larry. This meant very much to Larry. The driver told him that he saw the car accelerating on the ramp and making its approach. The distances seemed safe and he presumed the car would continue its speed. For some unexplained reason, Patricia must have applied her breaks just as she entered the travel lane. It was too late to avoid hitting her; the driver admitted that he had attempted to swerve, but he could not avoid impact.

Grieving

Waiting for news of the multiple-trauma victim can engage grief reactions among family members who may begin to ruminate about certain aspects of their relationship with the injured person. A spouse informed that her husband is completely paralyzed may be drawn to grieve the loss of a sexual partner and the physical aspects of their relationship. A father informed that his son's leg has been amputated may grieve the loss of the pleasure he derived from watching his son play competitive sports. These reactions may be accompanied by emotional outbursts, sobbing, and crying. Some family members become very withdrawn and mildly catatonic. Grief of this sort is a necessary condition of adjustment. It is the emotional counterpart of acceptance and integration. If a person is to resume a working relationship with the injured person, the realities that govern the patient's condition must be understood not only intellectually but affectively. As family members begin to come to terms with these realities in their own personal ways, they very much appreciate the understanding and encouragement, albeit tacit, of staff. This kind of support, offered and accepted during this early phase of adjustment, is extremely important.

Patricia's condition did not significantly change for the better part of two weeks. The neurosurgeon effectively concluded that there was little chance of her recovery. He anticipated that at some point she would experience convulsion, arrhythmias would develop, and she would die. Orders not to resuscitate were noted on her chart.

Larry kept his hopes alive, frequently entering her cubicle in the ICU, holding her hand and through his tears telling her how much he loved her, needed her, and wanted her to wake up and get better. Through these futile pep talks he was beginning to reconcile the possibility that she would never be able to accomplish these things. Larry hoped for a "miracle."

At eleven o'clock on the sixteenth day of her hospitalization, Patricia died. Larry was not at the hospital, but he was telephoned and asked to return. The chaplain was with Patricia when she died and remained at her bedside until Larry arrived. When he entered the cubicle, he bent down and embraced his wife, kissing her and sobbing deeply. After a few moments of silent embrace, he looked up at the chaplain who was next to him and threw his arms around his neck and wept. When he regained his composure, he said, "Father, could we go down to the chapel and pray?"

After about ten minutes together in the darkened chapel, Larry got up and said, "I can never thank you enough for all you've done for me during these past two weeks. I could never have gotten through this without your help. I feel sure that Patricia is with God and that she's going to help me and Rick [the 15-month-old son] to make it. We'll always be a family and we'll never forget you."

Summary

There are numerous developmental challenges that adults must negotiate. In addition to the normal, maturational *crises* associated with choosing an occupation, choosing a mate, and deciding for or against parenthood, other events require that the adult confront his or her own mortality. The death of a parent or sibling may be the occasion for this encounter with death. This chapter has focused on three catastrophic life-threatening events: myocardial infarction and sudden death, major burns and thermal injuries, and multiple-trauma accidents.

Coronary Heart Disease

Heart disease is the leading cause of death among adults in the United States. The incidence of fatal heart attacks and other coronary-related deaths begins to become significant in the cohort of ages 35–44 and increases steadily thereafter. Americans are beginning to seriously consider how certain aspects of culture, lifestyle, and diet may be contributing to heart-related diseases.

Some of the prodromata or events that may induce heart attacks have been reviewed. Primary among the psychological variables is self-induced stress. The Type A personality (Friedman & Rosenman, 1974) has been identified by cardiologists to be a principal behavioral precursor of a life-threatening heart attack. As described by Friedman and Rosenman, Type A behavior involves an habitually stressed lifestyle.

The value of regular physical activity has been recognized. It is believed that the high energy expended in strenuous physical activity increases cardiac action and output, slows the heart, and regularizes its rhythm. A consistent regimen of physical activity may decrease the risk of a fatal heart attack.

An important interaction may exist between physiological and psychological factors in the incidence of myocardial infarctions. The major psychophysiological formulations that influence contemporary theorizing about heart attacks have their roots in studies on hopelessness and helplessness performed with infrahuman animals. For example, Richter's (1957) celebrated research on rats exposed to swimming experiments studied the physiological parameters that mediate stress-induced death.

Scientists have been tempted to extrapolate from animal research and apply its conclusions to human subjects. However, it is likely that the psychological variables applicable in human research have no counterparts in animal behavior and that even if they do, these variables cannot be properly tested.

Numerous efforts have been made to document the ways in which psychological factors in human subjects influence cardiovascular activity. One area of research studies the effects of human touch on cardiac arrhythmia (Lynch, et al., 1974). Another approach explores the potential for controlling heart rate and arrhythmic activity using biofeedback methods. A fascinating field of inquiry involves the specific ways in which external stimuli trigger central nervous system reactions (DeSilva & Lown, 1978). This latter research investigates the possibility that some psychologically induced mechanism in the brain may trigger life-threatening instability in the myocardium, characterized by arrhythmic activity or ventricular fibrillation. Although the research effort in this area of psychophysiological investigation is well established, its conclusions are still tentative and often contradictory. The various researchers agree that there appear to be important causal relationships between psychological and physiological factors in the incidence of heart attacks.

The care of a cardiac patient involves these same factors. It has been observed that the environment of the coronary care unit in many hospitals is perceived by patients as stressful. Posthospital adjustment is likewise stressful for the patient and family. The fact of a myocardial infarction may significantly alter sexual relationships. Some heart patients fear that the physical effort involved in sexual intercourse may precipitate what has been termed a "coital coronary."

Since cardiac death is a frequent occurrence in medical practice, intervention strategies with the surviving family members are of utmost importance. The chapter explored the benefit of structured intervention programs. The research of Williams, Lee, and Polak (1976) concluded that the clinical strategies and modalities of intervention that have been virtually unchallenged for years may not be as effective as once assumed.

Burns and Thermal Injuries

Clinical experience in treating burns and ever-improving technologies to assist in their treatment explain the high survival rate of burn patients. This progress, however, has created a new set of physical and emotional problems that survivors and their respective families must deal with.

Patients admitted to a specialized burn treatment unit are routinely assessed with respect to survival prognosis. In the case in which survival is judged to be without precedent, some physicians maintain that the patient and family should be informed of this judgment and should participate in decisions about extraordinary life-sustaining interventions. Others question whether a severely burned patient is capable of making informed choices about heroic interventions.

Numbers of new burn severity scales have been developed to aid in making informed determinations about survival. These scales assess a number of variables, including age, sex, size of burned body surface area, presence of full-thickness (third-degree) burns, presence of inhalation injury, perineal involvement, and elapsed time from burn to hospital admission. A number of these burn severity indices are discussed.

Seriously burned persons who survive have been described by one psychiatrist as "triumphs of medical care but tragedies of human life" (Bernstein, 1976). The crisis into which the patient and his or her family has been thrown may last for many years. Successful coping and adjustment depend to a great extent on the strength of the relationships formed between patient and family and the health support team.

One of the most crucial adjustments is to disfigurement, particularly facial disfigurement. Society highly values physical appearance. Although advances in plastic and reconstructive surgery have been impressive, there are limits to what can be done to restore burned patients to normal appearance. Bodily deformity and disfigurement can bring about *social death*, a withdrawal from interpersonal involvement with family and others. This social detachment is rooted in the weakening of self-esteem and related to the perception that people do not want to see a deformed individual. Self-banishment or withdrawal is not a solution: many patients who socially withdraw continue to be victimized by their own negative self-judgments. Rehabilitation involves work not only with the patient but with his or her family.

Individuals use a variety of strategies to cope with the long-term consequences of their thermal injuries. Denial, though not in the long-term interest of a severely disfigured or disabled person, may be necessary and useful in initial efforts to regain personal control over many aspects of social functioning, including relations with family and in the world of work. Humor can often help to ease tensions that both patient and others sense. It can also be a way to manage conflictual feelings in a social setting. Some persons deal with disfigurement by becoming involved in productive endeavors that yield a high degree of personal gratification and social recognition. The success of efforts to cope with disfigurement depends to a great extent on the support the burned patient finds in marital and familial relationships.

Although the focus of the chapter has been on adults, it has briefly considered the special needs of burned children. Since adult parents shoulder the most serious responsibilities for a child's rehabilitation—a burden that often places enormous stress on marital and familial relationships—their needs must be considered as well. Parents frequently are burdened with a sense of guilt, self-reproach, and blame for their children's injuries. In a real sense, they need to mourn lost dimensions of their child's bodily appearance and function.

Parental adjustments require support and counsel from psychiatric and social work professionals as well as from those more directly involved in the continued physical care of the burned child. Parents need direction as they begin to assume normal resonsibilities for the child's care. They need assistance to deal effectively with their child's fear of death and other psychological concerns.

Hospital personnel can be instrumental in providing consultation to school administrators and teachers to facilitate the reintegration of a burned child into the school environment. Since the school plays a major role in a child's social and developmental life, it is imperative that school personnel be helped to support effectively the child and family.

Finally, older persons with serious burns encounter specific problems. Preexisting chronic health problems affect the assessment and treatment of thermal injuries of the elderly. Quality of life must be balanced against the demands of extensive treatment when decisions about the care of older persons are made.

Multiple-trauma Injuries

Critical-care medicine has helped to reduce the number of deaths caused by multiple trauma. However, the circumstances that surround medical emergencies and the intensive care required to manage a critically injured patient, place great stress on families. Comprehensive critical care includes intervening with families in crisis to help them regain physical and emotional equilibrium.

The final section of this chapter looked at some of the psychological dynamics frequently seen in families involved in a multiple-trauma crisis. Families are anxious about the life-death outcome of their injured member. Much of their anxiety stems from the lack of information provided to them. Communication between medical staff and family members not only supplies needed data to aid understanding, but it provides important opportunities to anxious families to express and ventilate their feelings.

Families cope with the reality of traumatic injuries by seeking comfort in denial. Denial provides a safe haven in which to gradually assimilate the facts physically heard, but emotionally rejected. As such, denial serves a beneficial function in bridging the gap between wish and reality. Denial buys important psychological time that is often crucial to acceptance and coping.

The path from denial to acceptance may run through a maze of psychological feelings and responses. Some families display angry and hostile feelings toward each other, the injured patient, the person or circumstances responsible for the injury, or toward the medical staff who are providing care. Families must be encouraged to express these feelings and not to repress them.

Processing of feelings makes the replaying of events a necessity. Families tend to rehearse repeatedly the events leading up to the injury. This repetition assists in the process of adjustment and acceptance.

Finally, grieving is a common emotional experience in the dynamics of families faced with multiple trauma. As in the other reactions discussed, this form of response enables families to accept the various outcomes of serious injuries.

In each of the three situations considered in this chapter, families are confronted with the distinct possibility that one of their members may die as a result of a life-threatening event. Despite low mortality statistics as a result of advances made in early assessment and effective treatment of patients, the very crisis engages strong emotional conflicts within the family system. Effective medical management extends to the families of the patient, and comprehensive care includes attention to a multiplicity of death-related concerns.

This chapter has examined the issues surrounding three catastrophic, life-threatening events. The discussion has not only focused on medical and psychiatric management of the patient but has considered the impact of these events on the patient's family. Medicine has long debated how far the boundaries of its responsibility for the patient reach. It is clear that these boundaries must reach out to include the emotional care and guidance of families faced with what can be extended crises.

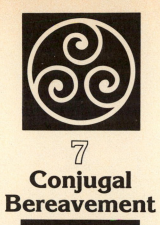

7
Conjugal Bereavement

Introduction

Psychodynamics of Grief and Mourning

- Pathological Grief
- Early Analytic Formulations

Contemporary Approaches to the Process of Normal Grieving

Anticipatory Grief

- Freudian Thought on Anticipatory Grief
- Neoanalytic Formulations of Anticipatory Grief
- Sociopsychological and Sociocultural Aspects of Anticipatory Grieving
- Assessment of the Preventive Value of Anticipatory Grief

Sequelae of Conjugal Bereavement

- Physical and Psychological Morbidity During Bereavement
- Psychiatric Morbidity During Bereavement
- Vulnerability to Suicide
- Mortality Patterns Among the Bereaved
- Epidemiological Conclusions

Clinical Management of the Bereaved

- Age as a Factor of Adjustment
- Health Care Management of the Bereaved

Summary

Introduction

One of Freud's earliest and most celebrated case studies involved the treatment of grief of a certain Anna O. (Freud, 1957a). Nevertheless, conjugal grief and bereavement have received relatively little attention until recently. This neglect may be partially explained by the fact that many spouses complete the process of bereavement without developing major psychiatric problems. Mental health practitioners have not considered grief to be pathological in nature, although many would readily acknowledge that certain deviations from the normal resolution of grief are occasionally observed. In the United States alone it is estimated that there are approximately 10 million widowed persons. Most of these individuals have not required special medical or psychiatric attention in their efforts to cope and adjust to their losses.

In their social readjustment scale Holmes and Rahe (1967) attempted to weight variably a number of stressful human events and found that loss of a spouse is rated as the most stressful life experience. Similarly, Paykel, Prusoff, and Uhlenhuth (1971) rated conjugal bereavement as high among losses on the human life crisis continuum. While conjugal bereavement may entail normal grieving processes, the fact remains that conjugal loss is a major stressor and can affect both the physical and psychological health of the widowed survivor.

This new awareness explains the significant efforts in contemporary research to understand the dynamics and function of grief in the recovery and readjustment of bereaved persons. This chapter will consider the principal conclusions of these efforts and will relate these findings to intervention strategies with conjugally bereaved persons.

Psychodynamics of Grief and Mourning

The terms *grief* and *mourning* are frequently used interchangeably to describe behavioral responses to loss. While this synonymous usage may be acceptable, it is important for the present discussion that these two concepts be differentiated. *Grief* refers to those very personal, subjective feelings and behaviors that attend the conscious recognition of loss. Grieving refers essentially to a personal experience and to the particular constellation of feelings and behavioral responses that characterize an individual.

Mourning, on the other hand, refers to the "social face of grief" (Parkes, personal communication, 12 October 1983). It involves social and cultural expressions of grief and specific mourning practices. These are viewed as ways of demonstrating love for and devotion to the deceased and in many respects are felt by the bereaved person to be a duty. For example, in some cultures, a widowed woman is expected to dress entirely in black, regardless of her age. To wear colorful clothing would be interpreted as a desecration of the memory of the deceased. In another culture, a widower might refrain from cutting his hair and shaving for a designated period of time. These mourning practices may help the person recognize and deal with the reality of the loss and negotiate the necessary steps to personal adjustment.

However, the performance of prescribed sociocultural rituals do not always resolve grief. In American society, there are no universally recognized 'mourning' rituals. Hence, there are few social and cultural supports for grieving persons. Apart from some limited religious practices that can facilitate grieving, the bereaved in many Western societies are left alone to process their grief. Grieving, therefore, is a complex human experience, involving both particular somatic and psychological feelings and behavioral reactions to loss and also various mourning practices that may encourage or discourage the processing of these feelings and behaviors.

Pathological Grief

A normal reaction to loss and therefore not inherently a psychiatric issue, grief can intensify to such a point that it virtually incapacitates an individual, affecting his or her processes of thinking, perceiving, reasoning, and judging. Grief can distort a person's ability to respond appropriately. When grief responses build to such intensity that they trigger maladaptive behaviors, they are considered to be pathological. One salient feature of *pathological grief* is the static quality of response sets. The individual appears to be locked into a particular feeling or behavior, unable to achieve any satisfactory resolution. This same characteristic identifies pathological mourning. The anticipated resolution of grief does not occur because the adaptive processes that should aid adjustment are dysfunctional.

The differences between the normal and pathological aspects of grief and mourning have been noted for a long time. The theoretical formulations concerning these differences are important inasmuch as they assist in identifying normal reactions and provide some insight into possible causes for pathological grief and mourning.

Early Analytic Formulations

The earliest and most important discussion of the issue of grief is found in Freud's *Mourning and melancholia* which was published in 1917 (Freud, 1957a). In this and in other related discussions, Freud attempted to detail the similarities and differences between the mental features of two principal grief reactions. Although some contemporary theorists and clinicians reject Freud's formulations, these provide important theoretical background to an understanding of grief.

Normal grief temporarily inhibits certain routine interests and activities and elicits feelings of emptiness and dejection. According to Freud, pathological grief includes additional features of panic, preoccupation with self, and lowered self-esteem. These maladaptive and regressive behaviors often result in self-hatred and, in some instances, self-destructive thoughts and acts (MacMahon & Pugh, 1965).

The common denominator in all grief reactions is the disappearance of something experienced as genuine loss. Freud coined the term "the work of mourning" to describe the process of resolving this loss. Several ingredients are essential to grief resolution. First, the loss must be recognized and accepted in conscious life, necessitating gradual withdrawal of the psychological attachments to the lost object. The "work of mourning" consists essentially in this process of psychic withdrawal whereby the ego becomes liberated and able to reinvest itself in other objects. Freud went no further in detailing this process.

Pathological grieving not only seems to abort this process, but in its place the bereaved person seems to experience remarkable self-devaluation. The loss for such a person is not something external to self but seems to coincide with the internal life of the bereaved individual. In contemporary terms, grief reaction might be termed a *reactive depression*. Freud, however, was of the opinion that *melancholia* (pathological grieving) was not simply a dysfunctional response to loss but that it reflected the actual psychological makeup of the bereaved individual. In other words, the loss may simply provide a theater for the more habitual, self-deprecating attitudes of a person to show himself or herself.

In attempting to explain how an external loss precipitates a sense of inner loss, Freud theorized that the lost object is internalized by the pathological mourner, whose original choice to incorporate the object was fundamentally narcissistic. While this is an important starting point in classical analytical theory, it is important to note that some contemporary clinicians do not find it helpful in understanding the dynamics of grief, feeling that the concept of narcissism does not sufficiently illuminate the reasons for which some bereaved people experience weakened self-esteem and self-hatred and become involved in self-destructive behaviors.

In his clinical work, Freud noted that self-accusations frequently described the lost object rather than the bereaved person. From this he concluded that while the bereaved appears to be attacking himself or herself, unconsciously the attack is directed toward the lost object. Essentially this means that pathological grief is an attempt to vent feelings of hatred and rage against the lost object whose loss has left a certain void in the loser; this hatred and rage gets directed toward the self.

To summarize simply, Freud viewed grieving as a normal process of internally saying goodby to a lost object and gradually withdrawing the psychological investments that once accounted for attachment to the lost object. As this process concludes, the ego is liberated to reinvest in other objects. Melancholia, or pathological grieving, results from an inability to accomplish this detachment because of a preexisting ambivalent relationship with the lost object. Because the object figured so importantly in the satisfaction of narcissistic needs, the lost object is punished for failing to continue to supply these gratifications. The punishment, though directed toward the lost object, is actually turned inward toward self and this accounts for expressions of lowered self-esteem, self-hatred, and self-destruction. In assessing the borderline between normal grief and pathological grief (melancholia), Freud looked to the meaning and quality of the previous relationship with the deceased and the ways in which the ambivalence that characterized that relationship expressed itself in the wake of the loss of that object.

Freud drew a clear distinction between normal and pathological grief, reasoning that a person who responds to loss with melancholia may possibly have a predisposition to psychopathology. His student and colleague Karl Abraham (1969) later suggested that some of the processes noted in melancholia might be normal components of grief and may not necessarily be reflective of an inclination to psychopathology. For Abraham, internalization of the lost object does not occur as an antecedent to grief but as an intrinsic part of the grieving process, allowing the bereaved to feel: "The loved object is not gone, for now I carry it within myself and can never lose it." According to Abraham, the work of grieving is not the ridding of the attachment to the deceased but the process of internalizing the deceased, allowing the dead person to become a part of one's inner self. Once this internalization has been achieved, the bereaved can reconcile the fact that external presence is no longer necessary; the inner union of memories and past experiences helps sustain the important dimensions of the lost relationship (Pincus, 1984).

This insight was further explored by Melanie Klein (1940), who viewed object loss in adult life in terms of infantile experiences. Just as a child gradually comes to learn that temporary or transitional losses do not seriously threaten or disturb basic safety, so this same lesson needs to be negotiated in the face of object loss in later life. Using the example of weaning from the breast in infancy, Klein noted that the child gradually recognizes that the breast is not the sole assurance of security and that it can be removed without essentially disturbing his or her fundamental equilibrium. Klein concluded that just as weaning can be a traumatic transitional loss for the child, so does object loss (death of a loved person) in later life, though devastating, offer similar opportunities for the redefinition of what constitutes safety and security.

The line between normal and pathological can be found in the ability or inability of the bereaved to allow others to assist in making the necessary psychological adjustments to restore inner balance. The child weaned from its mother's breast learns to identify and accept other symbols of its safety and security. Likewise, the bereaved needs to accept other relationships that can assist in the inner healing and promote the reestablishment of the equilibrium temporarily upset by the object lost.

Contemporary Approaches to the Process of Normal Grieving

The word *grief* can appear to be a static concept. Contemporary usage tends to favor the term *grieving*, which emphasizes the active and progressive dimensions of the process and which implies specific phases, steps, or stages.

In 1944, Lindemann published a report on his work with 13 survivors and families of victims of a tragic night club fire in Boston's Coconut Grove. As a staff psychiatrist at Massachusetts General Hospital where many of the burn victims were taken after the fire, Lindemann was in a unique position to monitor the grieving patterns of a number of individuals who had shared a common tragedy. He summarized his observations of these cases and others like them in what has become an archival treatise on the symptomatology and management of grief. The process of grieving, as Lindemann describes it, consists of five major features: somatic distress, preoccupation with the image of the deceased, guilt, hostile reactions, and interruption of usual behavioral patterns. As will be shown later, these components of grieving have significantly influenced the way in which other researchers have conceptualized the process.

In an important study of attachment and separation, the British psychiatrist John Bowlby, (1960, 1973) has attempted to identify certain phases of grieving. His formulations were based on clinical observations of children who had been separated from their parents in the course of routine hospitalization and who had been left in the care of other people. In collaboration with James Robertson, Bowlby identified three phases of grieving: protest, despair, and detachment.

By this classification Bowlby did not mean to imply some rigid stage theory but rather to suggest that a normative progression marks the process of separation. He readily acknowledged that there is a significant variation in the ways in which individuals will experience and express certain feelings and reactions. He noted that these phases seem to blend into each other, thus making precise definition extremely difficult.

Colin Murray Parkes (1972) enlarged upon Bowlby's formulations in his study of the processes of grief and bereavement in adult life. Parkes's earlier studies (Parkes, 1964; Parkes, Benjamin, & Fitzgerals, 1969; Parkes, 1970) and more recent studies of the reactions of widowed persons (Parkes, 1975; Parkes, 1981) brought the rigors of experimental design and statistical analysis to bear on what was largely a theoretical discussion. His work reflects careful clinical management and strict adherence to the conventions of scientific inquiry.

Like Bowlby, Parkes defined the grief process in terms of a phasic progression of psychological and social experiences. The phases roughly parallel the schema Bowlby had suggested and are similarly variable. They likewise tend to confirm the characteristics Lindemann (1944) had described as *pathognomonic of grief*—in other words, they sum up what is known about the normal process of grief.

The first phase in Parkes's approach is a period of **numbness**. This early reaction involves feeling stunned, paralyzed, dulled by the news of the death. In some ways, this initial reaction serves a protective, anesthetizing function, buffing the individual against the full effect of pain and suffering. This phase itself is not static. Parkes reported that some people vacillated between early periods of distressful emotional outbursts and this blunted state of disbelief.

When the telephone rang and it was Jack's boss, I felt a hollow feeling in the pit of my stomach. I braced myself for some bad news. Had Jack taken ill? Was he in an accident? What Mr. Pearson had to tell me was worse than even I had feared. Jack was dead.

He had left for work that morning at the normal time. He was looking and feeling fine. The house was chaotic with the children preparing for school. The kitchen was a beehive of activity. I quickly kissed him good-by; he said "I'll call you later this morning when I finish my sales meeting." With that he went to the garage and left.

I recall Mr. Pearson being very solicitous on the telephone, but I must admit that I did not hear much of what he said after he told me that Jack had died. I do remember that he said Jack had been taken to Columbia Presbyterian Hospital but that they were unable to revive him. I remember wanting to go to the hospital, perhaps so that I could verify the fact for myself. Mr. Pearson offered to send the company limousine to take me, but I quickly declined.

When I hung up the telephone I sank into the kitchen chair. I felt numb, almost like I had no sensation in my hands. It was as if I were in a daze; actually I felt faint. I don't actually know how long I sat there before I thought: "I better do something." I called my oldest daughter, who had been married three months earlier. She said, "Mother, stay right where you are; I'll be right over."

When she arrived, I was still in the kitchen. When she came in, we both began crying. This was like a watershed for me. When I was able to regain my composure, I felt able to begin to make the initial arrangements with the funeral director. . . .

In its normal course, numbness is measured in hours and days. It gradually yields to a second phase, which Parkes calls **searching**. Once the person comes face-to-face with the reality of the loss, a number of psychological processes are set in motion that have their root in the necessity to separate from the lost love object. Anxiety is one of the most characteristic expressions of this separation process. Without identifiable stimulus, the bereaved person feels drawn into preoccupied thinking about the deceased. Engaged in this way, the bereaved often experiences physiologic reactions. Sobbing and crying are not uncommon in this stage of grieving. Parkes indicated that this mental preoccupation with the deceased, coupled with this "pining" reaction, is the specific sign by which grieving can be identified.

Other researchers seem to concur that these symptomatic responses are indeed pathognomonic of grief. The term searching adequately describes the course of the behavior; it is as if the preoccupation with the deceased is an attempt to recover the lost object. In this vacillation between reality and fantasy, the bereaved may be subject to delusions. These delusions are *hypnagogic*, that is, they occur while a person is falling asleep. The delusion is a form of dreaming.

Widowed persons may report that they think they hear their spouses walking up a staircase and fully expect to see them enter a room. Another perceptual distortion might involve hearing a deceased spouse's voice in another room and actually going to that room anticipating the person will be there. These are normal components of this phase of grieving, although many widowed persons can be exceedingly troubled by these experiences and may be reluctant to acknowledge them to another for fear they might be interpreted as clear manifestations of mental illness.

The children were very comforting during the whole time of the wake and funeral. Jack and I had always been so proud of our large family. The three that are still at home are my greatest concern, particularly the youngest, who seems to have adjusted poorly to her father's death. The other four are on their own and are able to take care of themselves. I feel like I'm on my own to get these final three through school and adolescence. There are times when I wonder how I'll ever manage without him.

So many nights I've gone to our room and closed the door. There I find myself crying myself to sleep. Everything about that room reminds me of him. Robert cleared out his father's closet and dresser. Even the emptiness of that closet brings me to tears.

There have been many nights when I thought I heard Jack's car pulling into the garage. I thought, "How silly?" but still something in me expected that he would come up the stairs and say, "Hi Betty, Love." He always called me "Betty, Love" or "Mommy, Love."

One night I actually thought he was next to me in the bed. You can't believe the excitement I felt to think he was there; I must have been half asleep. I remember putting on the night lamp next to my bed, only to find Jack's place empty. I began to cry and recall saying to myself, "Betty, you must be losing your mind; he's dead and he's not coming back."

Normally this process peaks at 5 to 14 days after the spouse's death. Parkes and others have estimated that this phase gradually declines thereafter. It is not unusual that even a year after the death the widowed individual experiences feelings of pining and yearning. In some instances these feelings are still very pronounced. The emotional reactions of this phase can catalyze another set of responses.

As the bereaved searches for threads of the lost relationship, two principal emotional responses are common. The first is *anger*, as the bereaved begins to realize what the loss implies in practical and pragmatic terms. For some, this might mean the necessity of assuming economic and familial roles that the deceased spouse might have managed. In other cases, the death may have created significant financial or social alterations in lifestyle.

As the full import of these changes find their way into consciousness, the widowed person feels angry. Some widowed persons find it difficult to process their anger, judging it selfish and inappropriate to harbor negative feelings toward the deceased.

The repression of these feelings can give rise to the other dominant emotional response: *guilt.* Guilt is a normal consequence of repressed anger, whereby a person's affect is turned in on the self, and the self is subsequently punished. Guilt can also be the product of the searching process itself, which uncovers missed opportunities in relationships. Unresolved issues may also surface. The judgment that the surviving spouse could have done more for the deceased in the terminal process is not uncommon. Some may consider that they neglected doing something that may have contributed to the spouse's death. Any of these lines of reasoning can be a source for guilt feelings in the bereaved.

All my friends kept telling me how well I was doing and how they admired my ability to take over so many of the things Jack used to do. Little do they know how I actually feel inside. I'm embarrassed to admit that their comments infuriate me. To be honest, I feel robbed—and angry.

These are upsetting feelings, because I sometimes blame Jack for dying and leaving me with all these burdens and responsibilities. I relied on him so much that I really am struggling to take over the finances and all the other maintenance responsibilities for the house and kids. My son, Robert, and Linda [daughter] and Paul [son-in-law] have been very helpful, but they aren't Jack.

Kathy [youngest daughter] actually expresses some of what I feel inside. She feels cheated because Jack has died. She often says, "He didn't even say good-by." I'm worried about her more than any of the others. It was unfair that he should die and leave us with all these unfinished tasks. We needed him very much.

You must think this is a very selfish thing to feel about a man who worked hard to support a large family. He made good provisions for us financially and his company has been more than generous in helping me. But I still feel angry with him for leaving me alone with these burdens and God for taking him.

Anger and guilt require ventilation if they are to be appropriately resolved. To this end, widowed persons require an interpersonal environment that is accepting of what might otherwise be considered inappropriate emotional reactions. They need the support of other persons who are understanding of the ambivalence the bereaved individual feels and comfortable when this ambivalence expresses itself.

These supportive persons can become the object of the widowed person's anger, especially if they encourage the bereaved to accept the fact of the loss.

In some cases, a well-intentioned family member, a professional, or a friend of the bereaved can lack sensitivity to the particular dynamics of the person's grieving, or, misreading cues to readiness, can push prematurely for resolution of the loss. This subtle or direct pressure can trigger a very hostile reaction on the part of the bereaved that can unnecessarily complicate and intensify the whole process. A stance of careful listening is preferable to an intervention strategy that relies heavily on giving advice and urging to action. Effective counseling attempts to strike a balance between empathic listening and encouragement to action.

This constellation of feeling reactions can move the person into the third phase, which might be generally described as *reactive depression*, the characteristic features of which are sleep and eating interruptions, apathy and malaise, dysfunction in higher mental activities, and disorganization in certain other behaviors. A spouse's death, as noted before, is considered to be one of the most stressful life changes. This event for some persons temporarily throws everything into a state of chaos. The future is out of focus, and life is experienced as a day-by-day challenge. Depression is rooted in this inner experience of turmoil and disorganization; resolution depends on assuming gradual control over specific aspects of the disorganization.

Some widowed persons assume this control by taking over certain roles and functions of the deceased spouse. This may be a number of minor and symbolic roles, or it may involve major shifts. Occasionally, a spouse of an elected political official will seek to fill the term of office of the deceased or may stand for election to a full term. In the same way, a spouse may choose to manage the family business in place of the deceased. Some psychologists have understood this identification process as a means of resolving the confusion that attends a spouse's death.

Jack had always been encouraging me to go back to my career in nursing. Since Kathy is a sophomore in high school, I thought maybe the time is right. I enrolled in a refresher course at a nearby University School of Nursing. They were very kind and helpful to me. I have a peculiar interest in learning some of the specialized skills in cardiac intensive care nursing.

It has occurred to me, as it certainly must be evident to you, that there is probably some relationship between Jack's sudden death and my interest in the CCU [coronary care unit]. However, I'm pursuing that interest and I must say it has helped me quite a bit since I started the program. It's hard getting back into the routine of studying; I feel like one of my kids worrying about papers and tests. The kids have been helpful to old Mom, and I think Jack is saying in heaven: "Nice going, Betty, Love."

What is clear from this description is the fine line that does exist between phases of the grief process. As the bereaved person gradually assumes certain roles and functions of the deceased, or carves out new roles altogether, the depression begins to lift.

Tremendous variability marks the course of the resolution of grieving. Specific aspects of this variability will be considered in connection with the issues of clinical morbidity later in this chapter. Generally speaking, the majority of bereaved spouses complete the principal grief work within the first year of widowhood, although in some cases more time may be necessary or specific professional intervention required.

Anticipatory Grief

In studying the phenomenon of grief, researchers have focused on those factors that might attenuate the negative effects of loss. One process that has drawn considerable attention in this regard is that of *anticipatory grief*. This process might be described as a behavior pattern related to an awareness of an impending loss, to its psychological impact, and to the adaptive mechanisms through which emotional attachments to the dying person are gradually surrendered.

Freudian Thought on Anticipatory Grief

Although he did not use the precise term, Freud recognized the process of anticipatory grief. In two separate essays, "Premonitory dreams fulfilled" (1899) and "On transience" (1916) Freud asserted that the mourning process might possibly be unconscious and that certain premonitions of the impending loss of an object could begin to weaken emotional ties and prepare the person for separation (Freud, 1957b, c).

Freud conceptualized grief as the progressive loosening of psychic attachments. As these ties, or *cathexes*, initially established the psychological relationship, the bonding process is effectively reversed when death interrupts the interaction between love objects. In the topological scheme by which Freud explained intrapsychic functioning, the ego is charged with the important executive responsibility for maintaining the organism in equilibrium. In response to the imminent forced separation from a loved person because of death, the ego begins to mandate withdrawal of libidinal investment, even though this process may be resisted. Even a casual observation of human behavior shows that this process of withdrawing emotional investment (*decathexsis*) is neither easy nor welcome. Yet, according to Freud, this is the necessary emancipation toward which all grief work is targeted and without which a person will be hampered in making further reinvestments.

In suggesting that this process could be anticipated, Freud recognized that premonitory fantasies of impending separation could engage ego activity as a defense against the catastrophic effects of the loved one's death. In this way, the death of a loved person could be anticipated and certain aspects of grieving could be accomplished prior to the ultimate separation. Freud reasoned that this unconscious preparation for final separation could mitigate the psychological pain an individual might experience in the wake of the death of a significant person.

Neoanalytic Formulations of Anticipatory Grief

This concept was not further developed in Freud's writings and for a long time received little comment in the professional community. In 1944, Lindemann re-introduced the concept of anticipatory grief. His work with families of critically ill burn victims documented the existence of a grief process that anticipates the death of a loved one.

Lindemann reported evidence of certain dynamic features of grieving: depression, preoccupation with thoughts of the dying person, and fantasies of life without him or her. He judged that this process of anticipation of loss and the attendant grief responses served an adaptive purpose in lessening to some degree the impact of the prospective death of the loved one. In this sense, anticipatory grief could be a useful and effective coping mechanism.

Within an essentially psychoanalytic framework, what is proper to postmortem grieving can be applied to premortem grieving. If, as Lindemann believed, normal grief had a predictable and limited course, it followed that the longer a person had to process the prospective death of a loved one, the more advanced might be the grieving process. In cases where the terminal illness is of considerable duration, it is conceivable that some persons could complete the grief work prior to the loved one's actual death. In these circumstances, the bereaved would exhibit relatively few postmortem grief symptoms. Anticipatory grief work would serve an important adjustment function in cases.

Lindemann was sensitive to the potential danger in relationships in which anticipatory grief work is engaged but in which the mortally ill loved one regains health and function. Rather than limit his examples to the cases of terminal illness, he drew upon other clinical experiences. For example, he cited the case of a soldier who was absent for an extended time during the Second World War. During this prolonged separation, his wife "mourned" his absence to such a degree that she achieved apparent detachment and emotional decathexis. When he finally returned home, their former relationship was irretrievable. He had difficulty reconciling his wife's detached attitudes and in trying to understand her desire for a divorce. Dynamically it was evident that her anticipatory grieving had been so successful and complete that emotionally she was already divorced from him.

Since Lindemann rekindled discussion of this phenomenon, interest in it has been keen and debate heated. Fulton and Gottesman (1980) have prepared an excellent summary of the principal efforts to study anticipatory grief in a systematic way. They reviewed two major classifications of research: studies that explore the interactions between parents and their terminally ill children, and investigations of the effects of anticipatory grief on the primary survivors of terminally ill adult patients.

These diverse researches highlight the relationship that seems to exist between anticipatory grief and subsequent adjustment to loss. Although this relationship has been carefully studied, the results are often contradictory and inconclusive. Because the various investigators of this issue have set about researching it in different ways, utilizing somewhat diverse methodologies, it is virtually impossible to compare the conclusions they report.

Although the concept as introduced by Freud and later refined by Linde-mann and others appears relatively simple, it has not lent itself easily to defi-nition and measurement. Each researcher resorts to an operational definition of what anticipatory grief and adjustment to loss means and, in doing so, frequently focuses on the variable of the length of time available to the survivor in which preparatory work could be accomplished.

Anticipatory grief is not as conceptually neat as Lindemann's brief discus-sion of the topic might suggest. For example, it is difficult to establish con-sensus on what ensures that the processes of anticipatory grief have been engaged. Some have suggested that a definitive diagnosis of illness as termi-nal might satisfy that requirement. Clayton, Halikas, Maurice, and Robins (1973) have maintained that medical diagnosis alone does not ensure that prospective survivors will begin to prepare emotionally for anticipated death.

Classic symptomatic responses to depression have generally formed the basis of the conceptualization of anticipatory grief and have established the principal index of measurement. This is one useful way to conceptualize antic-ipatory grief since depressive responses may indicate that the message of the probability of a loved one's death has been received and is being processed. In some cases, however, even though he or she has been carefully informed about the likelihood of death, the spouse may ignore the data and effectively deny the prognosis. While depressive affect tends to confirm that the prospec-tive survivor has been engaged by the information communicated, the pres-ence of these symptomatic responses may not necessarily indicate anticipa-tory grief.

Most of the studies of anticipatory grief are retrospective investigations wherein adjustment is the dependent variable. This type of research relies on self-reporting with its obvious inherent methodological weaknesses. A survivor may be inclined to paint an unrealistically positive picture of a deceased spouse and likewise describe personal adjustment in more positive terms than do apply. People generally like to be perceived in a favorable light and may interpret experiences in ways that enhance this affirmative perception. Re-search that relies principally on interview protocols of present and retrospec-tive experiences may find it difficult to distinguish among the various infor-mations received, all of which may not be internally consistent or in accord with other clinical observations.

Sociopsychological and Sociocultural Aspects of Anticipatory Grieving

Fulton and Gottesman (1980) offer a psychosocial framework in which an-ticipatory grief might be refocused. Much research on anticipatory grief de-pends heavily upon the traditional psychoanalytic formulations discussed ear-lier, which place considerable emphasis on the process without paying sufficient attention to the sociopsychological and sociocultural factors that contextualize it. Fulton and Gottesman suggest three factors that might affect anticipatory grief.

First, they assume that the volume and intensity of grief is proportionate to the psychological value one person may have for another in a family system. Grief is determined to some degree by the particular social and cultural expectations of the index social group.

A second consideration concentrates on the knowledge a dying person has concerning his or her diagnosis and the attitudes that govern the way he or she prepares to die. Some individuals seem to prefer denial and pretense, while others may be open and direct. Dying is an interpersonal process. The knowledge the dying person has about his or her diagnosis and the expressed and unexpressed attitudes and choices that are known to family members affect the prospective survivors' ability to engage in anticipatory grieving.

In addition to the way a particular patient may control the environment, the leadership provided by health care professionals can influence the course of anticipatory grief. The ease and openness of communication among physicians, nurses, therapists and technicians, patient, and family members and the attitudes of the health care team toward disease, dying, and death can either promote or inhibit anticipatory grieving.

Finally, it is quite normal that some important family members may find it extremely difficult to digest the inevitability of a terminal diagnosis and may retreat into isolation as a way of coping. This is an important moment to consider effective intervention, since failure to do so may have serious consequences not only for the way the dying family member will face death but also for the future adjustment of the individual who has sought refuge in denial, separation, or abandonment.

A third issue that Fulton and Gottesman identify is society's attitudes toward bereavement. A cursory survey of certain Eastern and Middle Eastern cultures reveals elaborate and detailed traditional mourning rites. In almost every one of these ancient cultures, there seems to be an intact and respected ritual that not only legitimizes human grieving but accords it a privileged position in the hierarchy of social conventions. For whatever reasons, certain Western societies deemphasize mourning rites and rituals and accord little or no status to an institutionalized role for the widowed and bereaved.

This contrast between expressive Eastern practices and restrained or repressive Western attitudes is certainly indicative of the predominant mores of the American society. Americans tend to place minimal value on mourning rituals and generally offer little support to persons who grieve. If this is true of postmortem practices, it is even more true of anticipatory grieving, which in fact is often perceived as the "waiting vulture syndrome" (Davidson, 1975) and is socially discouraged and frowned upon.

Assessment of the Preventive Value of Anticipatory Grief

Whether or not anticipatory grief has a positive effect on a person's adjustment to the death of a loved one is clearly the most critical issue. Gerber,

Rusalem, Hannon, Battin, and Arkin (1975) correctly maintain that whatever theoretical position on anticipatory grief one holds, it is safe to assume that most individuals whose spouses face long, debilitating terminal illnesses will utilize that time in some way to prepare for the future. In addition to practical concerns about putting one's affairs in order (wills, estates, funeral arrangement details), this time is also important for ending important interpersonal relationships.

In November we learned that Paul had lung cancer. Then followed 28 cobalt treatments and what seemed to be temporary remission. Fortunately for Paul and for the family he was able to be at home during most of his illness. We had our annual Saint Patrick's Day party in March and it was bigger and better than ever and a great morale booster for all.

In June Paul returned to the hospital for 10 days and then went home again. Of course it was very sad to see him losing weight and feeling so bad and knowing the cancer was taking over.

On July 2 Kevin (the oldest son) arrived from Casper, Wyoming, with his son, Sean. We welcomed them and had a great family gathering. Then on July 7 we rushed Paul to the hospital and within 12 hours, with the whole family (five adult children) at his bedside, he passed away.

We all miss Paul terribly but I feel fortunate to have been his wife for 42 years and know the closeness we all enjoyed as a family. Those final months between November and July were important ones for me, and I think for each of our children. Even though we were initially quite hopeful that the cobalt treatments would stem the cancer, and were encouraged by the evidence of some remission, deep down in our hearts, Paul and I knew it would prove fatal. Gradually we were able to admit this to each other, and this was a great release. That admission, far from being hopeless, made it possible for us to prepare for that undesirable, but inevitable outcome. We lived those last months as fully as we could.

The family likewise benefitted from Paul's final months. Each in his or her own way was able to share something important with Dad, and I know that Paul derived enormous consolation from these encounters with the children. This was so evident at the funeral where the family became so involved. John gave a very moving eulogy in his father's memory. Later, in rereading his message, I came to appreciate even more how important those 9 months from the time of Paul's diagnosis to his death had been for all of us.

I can't say that I don't feel his loss terribly. I do. But, I must say that I did a lot of preparation before he died, and I was better able to face life without him because of what we shared before he died. The kids have all been just great to me, and I see them quite a bit, with the exception of Kevin and his family who live so far away. I thank God that we had that time with Paul; it has made his dying that much more bearable for me.

Clayton and her associates (Clayton *et al.*, 1973) did not find any significant difference in the indices of depression among elderly widows ($M = 61$ years) who displayed characteristics of anticipatory grieving from those who presumably did not do such grief work prior to a spouse's death. The same researchers found no important differences in the postmortem adjustment patterns of the elderly widows surveyed when they were compared as to the extent of their spouses' terminal illnesses. Those whose husbands had long-term illnesses seemed no better adjusted than widows whose husbands died after relatively short-term illnesses. The conclusion to be drawn from this and similar studies of older persons who survive a spouse is this: the extent of preparatory grieving in anticipation of an imminent death of a spouse does not prevent or reduce postmortem psychological adjustment.

These data report no positive effect of anticipatory grief work on the subsequent psychological adjustment of older widows. Other research considers the potentially negative impact of these same anticipatory processes. Gerber and associates (1975) collected data from 81 surviving widows and widowers 6 months after their spouses' deaths. Of the entire sample, 16 had spouses who died of short-term fatal illnesses while the remainder of the group experienced long periods of preparation with their terminally ill spouses. Comparing these two groups on the criteria of medical adjustment, the survivors bereaved after a long fatal illness adapted less well than those whose preparation was significantly shortened.

Not only did greater opportunity for anticipatory grief work not help the older survivors, but there is some evidence that the longer preparatory period may have actually contributed to a more difficult adjustment. In evaluating their findings, Gerber and associates concluded that an extended death vigil can be detrimental in a number of ways. Neglect of one's personal health in order to care for the terminally ill spouse is one common explanation. It may be only after the spouse's death that the consequences of this neglect become apparent. Not only may such extended care of a terminally ill spouse exact its cost in terms of physical health, but the emotional premium may be high. Long terminal illness can deplete the psychological resources upon which a survivor may need to draw in the postmortem period. Diminished reserves as a result of an extended death watch can place an elderly widowed person at added risk.

Gullo (1975) studied the psychological, psychophysiological, and somatic reactions in women who anticipated the death of a husband. This investigation was limited to the interval between discovery of the terminal diagnosis up to the time of the spouse's death. It did not consider the postmortem period. The study reported the types of life stress to which the wife was exposed as her husband's illness progressed. Among the conclusions, it was noted that the characteristic signs of grief appeared at the time of the spouse's terminal diagnosis: depression, anxiety, feelings of inadequacy, and changes in personal habits and role functions. The stresses clearly were tied to the major alterations in personal and family lifestyles as a result of the terminal illness of the husband.

Anticipatory grief reactions were highest at this early period in the course of the terminal illness, higher than at any subsequent period. Interestingly, the long phase of terminal decline did not serve the interests of the prospective widows. Gullo reported that these women became more fatigued as they appeared to put aside their own grief in an effort to attend to the physical and emotional needs of their dying spouses. Not only were they apparently not engaged in a grief resolution process, but their principal energies were heavily invested in the care of their dying husbands. In each case, this was judged to exact a high cost as the wife began to show deterioration in her own physical and psychological functions. Somatic complaints and symptoms of physical disorders became more numerous as the period of the terminal decline was extended. When compared to those of a control group, these behaviors were judged to be significantly different, leading to a conclusion that a long period of preparation for a spouse's death may not be as advantageous as once thought.

The data from the Gerber study and the Gullo exploratory investigations suggest that extended time to prepare for the death of a loved one is potentially hazardous for the survivor. The assumption that sudden death is more tragic than death after a long terminal illness is questionable, and it is not certain whether the forces that dictate the course of anticipatory grief are of positive or negative value to the survivor.

Sequelae of Conjugal Bereavement

The death of a spouse requires more adjustment and adaptation on the part of the bereaved widow or widower than almost any other stressful life crisis. This is true regardless of the age of the survivor. Some cultures may be more or less helpful to the widowed person than other cultures, but societal support does not change the fact that conjugal bereavement is a complex human experience. Contemporary research has yet to reach consensus on whether widowhood is more difficult for the young or the old, for men or for women, for one cultural or socioeconomic group or another. Despite the inconclusiveness of research on the effects of conjugal bereavement, various studies have contributed significantly to knowledge about grief and bereavement and about ways to assist widowed persons in their personal efforts to adapt and adjust.

Physical and Psychological Morbidity During Bereavement

While the number of carefully controlled studies of physical and psychiatric morbidity of the bereaved are few, there are far more retrospective reports than prospective ones. Many are anecdotal in nature. Present discussion will be limited to the major researchers and their conclusions.

Parkes stands out among these. His earliest efforts in the field of bereavement research involved retrospective analyses, but he has also contributed two noteworthy prospective studies. In 1970 he published the first report on a long-term study of 22 widows residing in London (Parkes, 1970). These women ranged in age from young to old, with an average age of 49 years. Under the National Health Service in Great Britain, all people are registered with general practitioners (their family doctors). The general practitioners who collaborated with Parkes in this research were asked to refer anybody of whose bereavement they had been notified and not to select people who required therapy. The participants, therefore, were not a completely random sample, but neither were they highly selected.

In one of his earlier retrospective studies, Parkes (1964) had noted that the consultation rates among widows under age 65 who presented with psychiatric symptoms appeared to triple during the first 6 months of widowhood. These figures were obtained from a study of the medical records of widows. Judgments were made on the amount of medication prescribed; Parkes observed that the ratio was 7 times greater during the first year and a half of widowhood than in the comparable control period.

When he tested out these observations in the London study, these data were confirmed. These women visited their physicians on the average of 4.7 times more during the first 6 months of bereavement. Parkes did not note any demonstrated deterioration in their physical health to warrant these more frequent consultations, and assumed that the increase in visits to physicians might reflect a developing dependency on the doctor resulting from the loss of conjugal support.

Parkes and Brown (1972) subsequently studied 49 widows and 19 widowers under the age of 45 years who had been bereaved for under 14 months. A well-matched married control group provided an excellent comparison over the course of the study. The conclusions of this investigation reveal that there was an increase in depressive symptoms among the bereaved sample, including eating and sleeping disorders, weight fluctuation, cognitive and affective dysfunction, and an increased dependency on drugs, including alcohol, tobacco, and sedatives. The bereaved were 4 times more likely to have been hospitalized for medical and psychiatric reasons than were the control subjects, despite the fact that no significant intergroup differences in general physical health were recorded. Differences were noted in the presentation of psychological complaints and somatic complaints related to stress, including classic descriptions of chest pains and palpitations, trembling and twitching, and generalized feelings of nervousness and anxiety. Of the 68 bereaved persons, 22 consulted a clergyman, social worker, psychologist, or psychiatrist during the first year because of some emotional problem related to bereavement. This statistic is compared with 5 individuals among the controls who sought consultation with a professional counselor.

These findings are consistent with those of a careful retrospective questionnaire study reported by Maddison and Viola (1968). This investigation included 132 Boston widows and 221 from Sydney, Australia. Similar symptoms were commonly reported and were not judged to be unusual among recently bereaved persons. Comparable patterns of autonomic nervous system arousal were noted, as well as increased consultations with counseling professionals.

During a 4-year follow-up of the bereaved subjects in the Parkes and Brown research, a progressive decline in these symptoms of depression was evident, so that by the third year the two groups were no longer different. Certain behavioral choices were evident, and widowers appeared less well adjusted than married men. Apart from these findings, time seemed to have had a restorative effect among the bereaved.

Clayton (1974) prospectively studied 109 widows and widowers seen one month after the deaths of their spouses. The average age of these widowed persons was 61 years. These people were matched for age and sex with married counterparts. Although psychological and somatic problems dominated the early weeks of bereavement, the bereaved group was not judged to be significantly different from the control group in the number of physician visits or in the need for medication to manage depressive symptoms. The small but significant increase (p less than .05) in the use of hypnotics may not be critical to the discussion since two-thirds of the bereaved used these drugs prior to their husbands' deaths.

Clayton introduced two definitions of clinical morbidity of bereavement. The first considers the person who seeks nonpsychiatric medical attention for symptoms occurring after the death. The second describes the widowed person who seeks psychiatric consultation in addition to or instead of medical attention. In both cases, the presenting symptoms may include specifically medical, psychological, or psychophysiological complaints that are considered to be directly related to the death of the spouse, or older conditions that have exacerbated as a result of the death. To accurately assess morbidity, these changes need to be recognized early in the bereavement, generally within the first 4 months after the death. Otherwise causal relationships can become obscured and other intervening factors may distort the clinical assessment process.

Utilizing Clayton's operational definitions of clinical morbidity of bereavement in reviewing the published studies, a few simple conclusions can be reached. First, there does seem to be an increase in the number of medical consultations during the first year of widowhood, and widowed persons increase their intake of prescriptive drugs. The comparative data seem to confirm that there is little difference between bereaved and nonbereaved subjects in the nonpsychiatric symptoms presented. Psychological symptoms and psychophysiological responses are frequently considered to be normal features of reactive depression. Assessments are ordinarily made in nonpsychiatric consultations and may be a part of routine medical treatment by internists and family practice physicians. Although the presentation of complaints ordinarily involves psychophysiological problems, these are not often referred for specific mental health consultation and treatment. This second classification of consultation is rare among bereaved persons.

Psychiatric Morbidity During Bereavement

The death of a spouse is a relatively rare cause of hospital admissions for depression, as opposed to other, more common types of loss. Significant numbers of people requiring hospitalization to treat depression have suffered major changes in their lives, usually losses, prior to the onset of a depression.

When Hudgens, Morrison, and Barchha (1967) reported on their study of 40 psychiatric patients hospitalized with affective disorders and compared this group with 40 carefully matched nonpsychiatric hospitalized control subjects, they found no significant differences with respect to remote or recent loss experiences. It is interesting, however, that in the 80 persons studied, not one had lost a spouse. Even when they expanded the group to include 100 persons, they still found not a single widowed person.

In a related investigation, which examined the relationships between life events and depression, Paykel, Myers, Dienelt, Klerman, Lindenthal, and Pepper (1969) sampled 220 inpatients and outpatients who had been diagnosed as depressed. These individuals were further screened and their depression was assessed on a scale from zero to 6. Only those rated 2 and above were included in the study. Finally, the subjects included in the final sample had depression as a primary diagnosis, not as one secondary to some other psychiatric illness. Of the 220 patients, 185 were carefully matched with non-hospitalized controls. For the purposes of our discussion, it is important to note that in the combined groups, only 16 of the depressed group and 4 of the control group reported a death within the family during the prior 6 months. While this number might be small, it is still interesting to note that 4 times as many bereavements had occurred in the depressed patients than in the controls. This coincides with the loss rate among depressed patients studied by Parkes (1972). In citing the study done by Paykel and his associates, Clayton (1973) noted that a personal communication with Paykel disclosed that only one of the 20 family deaths reported was that of a spouse.

Frost and Clayton (1977) studied some 344 psychiatric patients and matched hospitalized nonpsychiatric patients, looking for possible correlations with conjugal bereavement. In this large survey of hospitalized persons, they found less than 1 percent of the psychiatric patients and not a single one of the matched controls to have experienced the death of a spouse during the prior 6 months. When the definition of conjugal bereavement was extended to include the previous 12 months, no additional incidences of spousal death were recorded.

These various psychiatric surveys strongly suggest that conjugal bereavement does not usually precipitate psychiatric illnesses sufficiently severe as to require inpatient hospital care. The psychiatric sequelae may be intense for some persons, but many seem to respond to less drastic interventions than admission to a psychiatric hospital unit. All indications are that psychiatric consultations are rare occurrences in the period following the death of a spouse, and most adjustment reactions requiring medical intervention appear to be managed in routine family practice care (Clayton, 1982).

The fact that the significant majority of widowed persons neither seek psychiatric care nor require psychiatric hospitalization does not imply that these same people are without risk of mental illness. In fact, given the stressful nature of the loss and the multiple adjustments necessitated by such an event, it is understandable that the bereaved are considered a population at relatively high risk. This "high risk" label is applied to the widowed on the basis of a fundamental hypothesis of psychosomatic medicine that psychosocial stress affects health. It is therefore important to explore some of the ways in which the widowed may be at risk.

Vulnerability to Suicide

One of the earliest suggestions of the relationship between widowhood and suicide is attributable to Durkheim (1951), who conceptualized the loss of a spouse in terms of *anomie*. In a social vacuum, a widowed person may find himself or herself without the roles and functions that once provided structure and meaning to life. Loss of this structural support for some individuals can be so devastating that the future is perceived as holding little hope or promise. In this state of existential loneliness and hopelessness, suicide becomes an attractive solution and escape. Durkheim's studies reported that widowers were more vulnerable to suicidal ideation and were highly successful in their attempts.

MacMahon and Pugh (1965) undertook a very interesting retrospective study to test Durkheim's hypothesis. Reviewing the death certificates of 320 widowed persons who had suicided, they compared these records with those of a control group composed of a similar number of widowed persons who had died of other causes. When they checked the death certificates of the spouses of the deceased survivors in order to verify the length of the period of widowhood, they found 80 percent of the documents sought. Studying these records, they noted the following statistics.

Suicidal deaths seemed to cluster in the 4 years following the death of the spouse, with the highest incidence occurring during the first year of bereavement. MacMahon and Pugh estimate that the risk of suicide is 2.5 times higher during the first year of bereavement and 1.5 times higher in the subsequent 3 years. It appears that older widowers (aged 60 years and older) are the cohort at greatest risk during the first year. This trend remained constant throughout the 4 years surveyed.

Mortality Patterns Among the Bereaved

Other mortality studies (Young, Benjamin & Wallis, 1963; Cox & Ford, 1964; Rees & Lutkins, 1967; Parkes, Benjamin, & Fitzgerals, 1969; Stroebe *et al.*, 1982) used comparable methodologies and reported similar findings. Young and associates (1963) found that widowers were a higher mortality risk during the first 6 months of bereavement than were their married counterparts. After that critical period, no notable difference in mortality rate between the two groups was observed. A large sociological study (Rees & Lutkins, 1967) reported a significantly higher risk of mortality for the bereaved during the first three years of bereavement, with the highest incidence occurring during the first year. This study considered the mortality patterns of members of the extended family of the deceased; the most significant mortality statistics involved widows and widowers who were judged to be 10 times more vulnerable than bereaved parents, siblings, or children. As in other studies, the Rees and Lutkins research found widowers to be at greatest risk, particularly during the first 6 months of bereavement.

One of the few studies to challenge the direction established by these various investigations is the work done by Clayton (1974). In this research (*N* = 109 adult subjects), which was cited earlier in the section on physical and psychological morbidity during bereavement, Clayton reported a mortality rate of 4 percent for bereaved persons in the first year and a comparable rate of 5 percent among the married controls. Following up on these groups 4 years later, 16 percent of the 109 bereaved persons and 12 percent of the control group had died. The average age of the bereaved subjects, as noted earlier, was 61 years. Although the study was principally designed to consider psychiatric morbidity of the bereaved, it did not note any excess risk of mortality among the widowed persons in the study group compared with the married controls.

This issue of increased mortality among the widowed remains a controversial issue. Discrepancies mark the findings of the principal studies. The only evidence that seems consistent is that widows do not appear to be at particular risk during the early phase of bereavement, while widowers may be at somewhat greater risk. Clayton's sample (1974) and most of the others that have shown negative mortality results are too small to be generalizable. Mortality rates are counted in terms of deaths per thousand and cannot be studied in samples of less than a thousand. The Young, Benjamin, and Wallis study (1963), reported more than 20 years ago, is still the largest and best designed prospective study of mortality rates and no other publication has contradicted its findings.

Epidemiological Conclusions

Jacobs and Ostfeld (1977) have carefully reviewed the epidemiological literature on the mortality of conjugal bereavement. They suggest two alternate hypotheses that may help to explain the basic pattern of increased mortality among the bereaved. Both explanations assume that bereavement *per se* does not elevate the risk of mortality. Rather, conjugal loss spotlights a group that has an excessive risk of mortality for a number of *other* reasons.

The first explanation is based on the principle of attraction commonly referred to as **homogamy**; this assumes that like marries like. In the case of those who might be weak or ill, their partners might likewise be weak and ill, just as those who are attractive, athletic, and strong might choose partners who are similarly gifted. The second explanation considers the effect of **environmental stress**. This position considers the impact of living in an unfavorable environment that may be pathogenic not only for the deceased but ultimately for the surviving spouse.

These two hypotheses, which attempt to supply some theoretical support to the trend of increased mortality among bereaved spouses, remain unsupported by empirical evidence. It is unlikely that either of the two explanations will satisfy the epidemiological question concerning conjugal mortality. It may be that the reasons for increases in mortality lie in the complex psychological adjustment processes that directly affect health management and health maintenance practices of the surviving spouse. The mortality of the bereaved may likewise be connected to the intrapsychic processes more commonly known as the "will to live." Trends in mortality among the bereaved may hinge more on these psychological issues of adjustment and adaptation and their consequent impact on physical health and function than on extrapsychic, environmental variables.

Gallagher, Thompson, and Peterson (1982) suggest that a spouse's death requires more readjustment on the part of the bereaved than any other stressful life crisis. It is unclear, from various research studies reported in the world literature, whether this stress is greater for men or for women, although men seem to suffer more negative effects (Stroebe & Stroebe, 1983). From an epidemiological perspective, Gallagher, Thompson, and Peterson (1982) suggest that negative changes in physical health, mortality rate, and mental health status usually accompany widowhood. Arens (1983) in a similar report observes that many widowed persons experience "lower levels of well-being." She emphasizes that this phenomenon may only be incidentally related to widowhood and may be more a function of age, generally poorer health, and less active social life. Gallagher, Thompson, and Peterson (1982) summarize their investigations by stating that complex psychosocial variables, including a person's customary way of coping with stress and the quality of the familial-social network, may attenuate the potentially negative impact of widowhood.

Clinical Management of the Bereaved

Because the risk of mortality is judged to be relatively small and because major psychiatric illness is not ordinarily associated with bereavement, it is understandable that family members, friends, and health care providers may not recognize and respond to legitimate, albeit subtle, cries for help. Yet as has been shown earlier in the chapter, conjugal loss and bereavement is a genuine concern of preventive psychiatry, and the processes of grief and adaptation directly affect mental health. This final section will consider the clinical management and support that could be beneficial to widowed persons engaged in the recovery process following the death of a spouse (Arkin, 1981; Parkes, 1981).

Age as a Factor of Adjustment

The sparse empirical research that has been published on the adjustment patterns of widowed persons seems to indicate that age may be a significant factor. The early studies of Parkes (1964) and Maddison and Viola (1968) sampled mainly younger widows whose principal concerns may have been practical issues of financial and familial management. The existential world of the older widowed person may be considerably different from a younger counterpart.

Heyman and Gianturco (1973) specifically investigated the adaptation of widowed persons over the age of 60 years. They examined individuals who were already participants in longitudinal studies being conducted at the Duke University Center for the Study of Aging and Human Development. Widowers ($N = 14$) were an average 74.8 years of age and widows ($N = 27$) were an average 73.1 years of age. All of these individuals were living in relatively independent, noninstitutional settings. Participants in this study had been initially evaluated in 1955 while they were still married and living with their respective spouses. The mean interval between the death of spouse and subsequent assessment was 21 months. They were assessed again 3 years later.

The results reported by Heyman and Gianturco did not reveal any significant differences in the overall health level of men and women, nor was any significant difference in health status detected in pre- and postwidowhood assessments. The bereaved seemed able to maintain their previous levels of activity and continued to be engaged with family and friends. Of particular interest was the place church-related activities played in the hierarchy of involvements. This type of activity appears to be of major significance to older widowed persons.

The picture of the older widowed person that emerges from this study indicates that elderly persons adjust reasonably well to widowhood, maintaining relative stability in a lifestyle that may have characterized their lives prior to a spouse's death. As long as certain stabilizing elements can be maintained as constants (for example, the continuity of familiar relationships within neighborhood, home, church, and so on), adjustment to the loss of a spouse seems to be managed well. In fact, the data from the Duke studies seem to indicate that lifestyle changes and psychological sequelae are better explained by reference to the cumulative effects of chronic illness and restricted functioning rather than as the direct effects of conjugal bereavement. We noted this same conclusion in our discussion of epidemiological issues (Arens, 1983; Stroebe & Stroebe, 1983; Gallagher, Thompson, & Peterson, 1982; Valanis & Yeaworth, 1982).

It has been almost two years since Robert's death. After 58 years of marriage it is difficult being on one's own. However, I'd prefer to stay alone in this big old house than to become a burden on any of my children. I know that they worry about me and have many times offered to have me come to live with them, but I hope I'll never have to resort to that.

I thank God every day that I still have my health and am able to take care of myself. I am able to get out during the good weather and go to church regularly. The people in the parish are so thoughtful and kind to me. Everyone offers to drive me here and there; I feel very secure. On Wednesdays I have my Bible study group;

I get so much out of this meeting—only wished I had learned more about the Bible when I was younger. Then on Sundays, I continue to go to the Senior Citizens' Social. Robert and I used to go to this together; I enjoy the programs and the activities, but most of all the people I meet there.

Robert and I moved into our house soon after we were married, and we have lived in this town for—can you believe it?—sixty years." I know just about everyone; all of us "old ladies and gents" have a lot to reminisce about. We've shared a lot of common history.

All of these things have eased the pain of Robert's passing. If it weren't for my independence, my children, my friends, and my church, I don't know what I would do. As I said, I thank God every day that he has given me these gifts that make my life so rich.

This is not to deny the impact that a spouse's death may have on the way in which an older person maintains his or her health. Older survivors may neglect early evidence of disease. In some situations, the deceased spouse may have assumed the role of "guardian" in monitoring the health of the other. Without that surveillance, the widowed person might overlook significant dimensions of routine health maintenance. These practical aspects of loss in an older person may be far more significant in terms of health and adjustment than most of the other psychosocial issues of adaptation.

The relative ease of adjustment among older widowed persons may be explained as part of the natural course of human development whereby older married persons psychologically prepare for the prospective role of widowhood and gradually adapt themselves to this eventuality. In addition, as Gallagher, Thompson, and Peterson (1982) have hypothesized, adaptation may not be the same for young and old. Since personality is operationally defined according to the stable and enduring characteristics of cognitive and emotional functioning, the coping and adaptive abilities exhibited by some elderly bereaved individuals can be seen as the product of a full lifetime of crises met and adjustments made.

Religion may play an important role in this adjustment. Throughout adult life, the religious community serves as an important social resource in times of human need and offers a context in which the meaning of various life events can be considered. As an older person encounters the death of a spouse, the supports of traditional religious practice may be of paramount assistance in coping with the loss and making appropriate adjustments.

Younger widowed persons may not have the same developmental supports available to an older person. The majority of opinion supports the position that the severity of symptoms and reaction to spousal death is age-related, with younger persons significantly at greater risk than their older counterparts. Gorer (1965) reports an increased incidence of sleep disturbances among the younger bereaved. Maddison and Walker (1967) and Maddison and Viola (1968) found illness scores to correlate positively with the age of the widowed, with the younger showing higher indices of general health deterioration. These and other findings tend to confirm the position that widowhood for the younger survivor is frequently experienced as traumatic.

Ball (1977) concluded from a written survey and personal interview study of widows of various ages that age and mode of death were significantly related to the intensity of the grief reaction. Not only did younger widows (less than 45 years of age) display a greater number of the classic grief symptoms already discussed, but the severity of these symptoms was likewise judged to be more intense and prolonged. Lopata (1975) noted that family members and friends of the bereaved can prematurely encourage the bereaved person to surrender the newly acquired role of widow or widower. American society seems more comfortable allowing an older person to retain a certain degree of status and position in the role of widowhood than it is prepared to accord to a younger person. This tendency to encourage a younger widowed person to complete the work of grieving and put aside the role of widowhood may contribute to the difficulties in adjustment that some younger widows exhibit.

It was a shock when we learned of Tony's diagnosis. He did not want to admit how serious it really was; I honestly believe that he thought someday he would wake up and it would be all gone. This made it very difficult on me because he never seemed to want to discuss the possibility that he would not survive. In my own mind, I did not want to think about this possibility either.

He died seven weeks after his illness was discovered. Those seven weeks were difficult ones for all of us. We have two small children and Tony had his own successful advertising business in the city (New York). I tried to keep everything together during this time. My own father had died only four months earlier and my mother was taking his death very badly. I felt like I was going to have a breakdown myself; the pressures were just unreal.

Since his death I must say I have not been doing that well. I've decided to run the business. So far, things are working out OK in that area. I have a good day-care placement for the youngest child and a lovely woman is at home with the children until I return from the city around 6:00 P.M. each evening. She also starts the dinner for me.

But I'm afraid if I just stopped for a minute, the whole world would collapse. I know I have not come to grips with Tony's death. I'm not sleeping well; I find that I'm crying a lot. I am embarrassed to say this to you, but I'm angry at him (Tony) for leaving me with all of these burdens. It just doesn't seem fair.

I don't go out socially, although lots of people have invited me. I feel awkward. There are good-intentioned friends who would like to arrange dates for me. Even though Tony's been dead for almost a year, I don't feel right about it. Maybe, that's because I'm Italian and I was raised with a special respect for the memory of a deceased husband. My mother wears black all the time; she thinks I'm terrible because I never would wear black. Look at me now, a bright red dress! You must think I'm a real case of contradictions.

I never would have suspected that I would have found widowhood so terribly difficult. Of course, I never thought it would happen to me after only 12 years of marriage. Widowhood happens to people like my mother who was married for 48 years.

People think I'm doing so well; they admire the fact that I took over Tony's business and am making a go of it. Little do they realize that I feel put together with a thin layer of glue, which I feel is coming apart. The message I am constantly getting is this: get on with your life; think about yourself and your children. My life and my children were all tied up with Tony. Don't they understand that without him, a major part of my life is gone?

Lopata (1975), reporting on her extensive research with widows in the Chicago area, observed that some widows apparently remain deadlocked in their attempts to adjust to the loss of a spouse. She attributes this phenomenon to the fact that our society provides little assistance in helping a widowed person build a new identity. She uses the term "no where to go" to describe this experience of social and psychological immobilization. Since one of the most important aspects of the whole adaptive process is identity reconstruction, younger widows may need greater assistance in making the requisite modifications in terms of role and lifestyle. This not only includes issues of practical importance, such as being a single parent or source of financial support to a family, but it also involves the new conditions of being no longer married and being potentially available for dating and remarriage.

Health Care Management of the Bereaved

Jacobs and Ostfeld (1980) state that the physician, in caring for a bereaved person, performs humanistic, educative, and preventive tasks in addition to the normative task of curing illness. This perspective is well expressed and defines the scope of care that any health care provider should consider in ministering to a bereaved person.

The physician, clergyman or clergywoman, and the funeral director are commonly the professionals to whom the widowed will turn first for assistance. A helpful posture to assume is one that is receptive to communication and able to validate the bereaved person's experience of loss. To be maximally responsive, a caregiver needs to understand the dynamics of grief and be comfortable with expression of feeling. In some respects, a professional may be able to facilitate the process of validation of loss within the family and thereby positively affect the whole course of bereavement.

Because grief is not simply a psychological state but also affects biological functioning, a careful monitoring of physical health is often not only desirable but necessary. Research in neuropsychology is continually discovering significant correlations between adrenocortical hormones, epinephrine and norepinephrine ratios, testosterone, and multihormonal processes. Knowledge of these neuroendocrine relationships can be of major significance in monitoring the physiological course of grief resolution and may have predictive value in planning effective medical and psychiatric interventions.

One has to exercise prudence in monitoring the physical health of the bereaved. It is easy to increase the anxiety of bereaved people, who are likely to be overanxious about themselves at the best of times. In general, people need reassurance more than monitoring. A health care provider can provide this reassurance by offering information to the bereaved about the normal course of grief, its dynamics, and its objectives. This information can be extended in turn to the family of the widowed person and the broader social community. Physicians need to be knowledgeable about referral resources within the community that may be helpful to widowed individuals. Mutual help programs may be quite useful for some bereaved persons (Silverman, MacKenzie, Pettipas & Wilson, 1975). Clinical experience has led Parkes (personal communication, 12 October, 1983) to recommend a variety of mutual support groups backed by professionals who would be able to prevent some of the difficulties that arise when a group of bereaved people get together to help each other. One of the principal difficulties in such groups is containment of anger, which can erupt violently and lead to the disintegration of the group.

Primary care physicians are in a privileged position to assist bereaved persons. Although they share their responsibilities with other colleagues in the helping professions, theirs is a special position, concerned with balancing physical and psychological care as well as assisting in the tasks of social adjustment. Success in these therapeutic and humanistic goals depends to a great extent on the degree of understanding about the dynamics of human grief and the willingness to invest time and energy in accompanying the bereaved through often dark corridors toward resolution.

Summary

Widowhood is one of the most stressful of human crises. For this reason, the psychodynamics of grief and mourning have attracted the attention of numerous researchers.

Grief is a normal psychological response to loss. It includes those personal, subjective feelings and behaviors that accompany an individual's recognition and acceptance of a significant loss. The term *mourning* is often popularly used interchangeably with the term *grieving*, although, technically speaking, the two are distinct concepts. Mourning has been called the "social face of grief" (Parkes, personal communication, 12 October, 1983). It involves the social and cultural ways in which grief is expressed. Grieving is a complex behavior, involving somatic as well as psychological reactions. It is affected by various mourning practices, which may either encourage or discourage the processing of the thoughts, feelings, and behaviors associated with grief.

Although grieving is a normal response to loss, grief reactions can be so intense and prolonged that the bereaved ceases to function appropriately. This dysfunction may describe interruptions in thinking, perceiving, reasoning, and judging. Pathological grief places a bereaved person in a psychologically immobile state. It effectively prevents the person from making the necessary adaptations and adjustments necessary to resume normal functioning.

What causes pathological grief? Several theoretical approaches have been reviewed. Freud's discussion of normal and pathological grief in *Mourning and melancholia* (1917) sets forth an analytic hypothesis (Freud, 1957a). It assumes that the work of grief involves the process of withdrawing ego investments in the lost object and the reinvestment of those energies in other objects.

Freud did not believe that the death of a loved one *caused* the pathological reaction but that the loss may simply be the precipitant that uncovers habitual personality traits in the bereaved. He suggests that the bereaved may have had an ambivalent relationship with the deceased, a relationship that may have satisfied important narcissistic needs. For Freud, the previous relationship with the deceased person holds the key to understanding grief.

Other analytic authors have described grief in different ways. Abraham (1969) considered grieving as the process by which the deceased person becomes an internalized part of one's self. Klein (1940) saw grief work in terms of weaning; she identified the psychological task as one of letting go of a prime source of security and realizing that it is not the sole anchor of one's life.

Contemporary authors have addressed the same topic as these early clinicians and theoreticians. Lindemann (1944) published an archival monograph on the symptomatology and management of grief. In this treatise, he described a broad repertoire of physical and psychological behaviors commonly associated with grieving.

Bowlby (1960; 1973) later attempted to describe phases in the grief process. His work derived from extensive research into psychological reactions to attachment and separation. Parkes (1972) used the theoretical model suggested by Bowlby in elaborating his own description of grief and bereavement in adult life.

These researchers have each contributed to a better appreciation of the variables that together are pathognomonic of normal grief. Their descriptions of behavioral and emotional reactions have aided in understanding its dynamics and in considering ways to support and facilitate the grief of the bereaved.

Anticipatory grief describes behaviors associated with impending loss. It includes those adaptive mechanisms through which emotional attachments to a dying person are gradually surrendered. Although **anticipatory grief** is a contemporary term, it has its roots in the thought of Freud and other analytic authors. Freud noted that in the situation of forced separation from a loved person, the ego begins the process of withdrawing libidinal (emotional) investment, even though there may be strong resistances to doing so.

Lindemann documented this phenomenon in his work with critically ill burn victims and their families. He observed many of the dynamics associated with grieving in the responses of these families. He concluded that this preliminary grieving, antecedent to actual loss, was beneficial and helped in adaptation. He likewise underlined the implicit difficulties in such a process of withdrawal in those cases where the critical situation reverses and the patient recovers.

Fulton and Gottesman (1980) reviewed the numerous studies on anticipatory grief. Their extensive review leads them to conclude that the concept does not lend itself easily to definition and measurement. Their description is not as simple as that offered by Lindemann (1944). The chapter discussed some specific studies that illuminate some of the difficulties encountered in documenting the assets and liabilities of anticipatory grief.

In most efforts to study anticipatory grief, the psychoanalytic influence is pronounced. Fulton and Gottesman (1980) suggest that the sociocultural variables need to be included in any discussion of this phenomenon. Grief— whether it be antemortem or postmortem—is proportionate to the value the dying person enjoys within a family system. What the dying person knows and how he or she prepares for death with family members also affects grieving. Finally, the psychological and social supports a family has determines to a significant extent its ability to face death and dying in developmentally constructive ways.

To the extent that a society is thanatophobic—and American society is to a significant degree—it precludes the expression of many feelings related to death and dying and discourages efforts to psychologically prepare for loss. Opinions vary about the benefits of anticipatory grief. The majority opinion judges the conscious and unconscious efforts to be useful, not only to survivors but to the dying person as well. Some researchers have not been able to detect any significant differences in the reactions of individuals who did not do anticipatory grief work from those who displayed evidence of early grieving. Other differing perspectives on the assets and liabilities of anticipatory grief were discussed.

Adjustment to loss is a common goal shared by bereaved persons. This, likewise, is a concern of those who provide psychological, medical, and social support to widows and widowers. These professionals are interested in the physical and psychiatric morbidity of the bereaved. A number of important studies that researched this question were presented. These reports identify increases in medical and psychiatric consultations in the early months of bereavement. Conjugal loss appears to cause an increase in depressive symptoms as well as a wide array of psychophysiological complaints. Over time, the number and severity of these complaints abate. Psychiatric morbidity does not appear to intensify as a result of bereavement, though this does not be mean that widowed persons are not at risk for mental illness.

Suicide is one way in which some bereaved individuals act out their inability to cope with loss. For these widowed persons, suicide becomes an attractive solution to psychological despair. Age may be the most significant variable in assessing vulnerability to suicide. Older widows and especially widowers appear to exercise this option to take one's own life in the aftermath of a spouse's death.

Of interest are the mortality patterns among the bereaved. As stated above, widowers seem to be at a greater risk than widows, particularly during the first 6 months of bereavement. Although numerous investigators have reported increased mortality among the widowed, other researchers have challenged this position. Some explanations have been offered to reconcile these divergent opinions and to explain the basic pattern of increased mortality among the bereaved. Jacobs and Ostfeld (1977) have suggested that homogamy and environmental stress may be significant factors in explaining mortality statistics in this cohort. Other related factors have also been cited to explain the mortality data on widowed persons.

Since widowhood is not a disease and grief is not considered to be an abnormal response to loss, it is understandable that widowhood has not been identified as a medical-psychiatric priority. Yet, as underscored in this chapter, conjugal loss is an important issue of preventive psychiatry. The chapter concluded with a review of some of the specific issues involved in providing assistance to the bereaved. Age, stability of lifestyle, continuity of relationships, and religion were some of the variables considered. Competent care for and skillful intervention with bereaved spouses require comprehensive understanding of the multiple complex factors that underlie and diversify widowed persons' responses to conjugal loss.

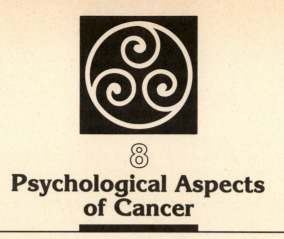

⑧ Psychological Aspects of Cancer

Brief Historical Overview and Introduction

Psychological Factors in Cancer Etiology

- Personality Traits
- Some Specific Psychosocial Predictors of Cancer
- Psychophysiological Mechanisms

Communication

- The Patient's Desire to Know and the Physician's Willingness to Tell
- Informed Consent and Communication Patterns
- Special Problems Encountered in Communicating with Cancer Patients

Iatrogenic Stresses

Defense Mechanisms and Coping Behavior

- The Crisis of Diagnosis
- The Crisis of Treatment
- Sexuality, Sexual Functioning and Self-esteem

Summary

Brief Historical Overview and Introduction

As early as the second century there is evidence of speculation that a close relationship exists between cancer and one's mental and emotional life. The Greek physician and medical scientist Galen (130–201 A.D.) noted that women with breast cancer seemed to have a melancholic disposition. Contrasting these women with those of a more sanguine, naturally cheerful, or even temperament, he concluded that physical pathology is somehow related to mental or emotional attitudes. This early hypothesis linking psychological factors to *carcinogenesis* remained virtually unaddressed for more than 15 centuries. The eighteenth and nineteenth centuries witnessed a renewed interest in the possible connection between psychological states and cancer. In a primitive form of retrospective analysis, or *psychological autopsy*, physicians began to observe a relationship between stressful life events and the diagnosis of terminal neoplasms.

Cancer research in the nineteenth century fell under the aegis of experimental pathology. Although research into the genesis of cancer principally involved study of cell physiology, the scientific community was nonetheless interested in what might trigger the particular tissue and cellular changes that are descriptive of cancer. While not actively engaged in exploring external conditions that might activate or precipitate these internal changes, scientists of the last century were at least attuned to possible psychophysiological causes. Medical and surgical textbooks and journal articles of that period reflect the growing awareness that certain personality factors may predispose to cancer. Environmental stresses were considered among the possible triggering mechanisms of cancer. Most of the conclusions current in late nineteenth-century medical sources were based on observational research, however. No matter how accurate these observations may have been, they do not in themselves constitute scientific proof.

Modern psychiatry emerged contemporaneously with these observational and experimental studies in pathology and oncology. Freud himself was trained in neurology in the 1870s and would have been interested in the hypotheses linking cancer to certain psychophysiological interactions. At the base of psychoanalytic theory is the principle that unconscious and unresolved conflicts are responsible for psychopathology. The unfolding of psychoanalysis during the early part of the twentieth century paralleled developing research in clinical medicine, but these fields did not collaborate effectively in searching the possible causal relations between psychological states and physical pathology.

A distinct cleavage between mental and emotional processes and somatic disease characterized traditional medical thinking in the early part of this century. Modern psychiatry has been viewed with suspicion by some and as an adversary by others. The medical community ignored the psychosomatic hypotheses of carcinogenesis proposed by such eminent nineteenth-century physicians as James Paget (1870) and Herbert Snow (1893). Greer (1979) has reasoned that the early attempts by Freud and his psychoanalytic contemporaries to bridge this gap in psychophysiological research contained a "mythology based on unfathomable, irrefutable insights" that did not attract or appeal to other scientists.

The major research studying the psychological aspects of cancer postdates the Second World War. Lickiss (1980) has suggested that studies of psychological factors in neoplastic development can be classified in 6 categories: (1) animal studies; (2) descriptive human studies; (3) human studies involving a control group; (4) studies concerning possible mechanisms; (5) studies concerning further neoplastic progression (including metastases); (6) studies concerning patient response to diagnosis and treatment. It is well beyond the scope of this chapter to summarize each of these major efforts.

This chapter will focus on the psychological mechanisms that are most frequently cited in contemporary research of cancer. In addition, psychosocial issues of relevance to cancer etiology will be discussed. Communication involving cancer patient, family, and the primary care physician will be examined, as will be the related issue of iatrogenic stresses, which are frequently noted in both the medical and psychological literature.

Diagnosis and treatment of cancer is judged to be crucial to controlling the progression of the disease; attention will be given to the psychological issues involved in cancer-related surgery, radiotherapy, chemotherapy, and immunotherapy. Because psychological defense mechanisms play such an important role in how a person copes with the crisis of cancer, these defenses will be reviewed. Suicidal ideation is not uncommon among cancer patients, although the rate of suicides is proportionately quite low among this group. It is important for those who work with cancer patients to have an understanding of how these people come to terms with the life crisis that cancer represents and what place time, belief systems, sexuality, and human relationships occupy in a cancer patient's hierarchy of values.

Psychological Factors in Cancer Etiology

Opinion sharply divides on the role mental processes play in the development of cancer. Some scientists dismiss entirely the participation of psychological processes, viewing cancer as an exclusive and autonomous biological mutation. For example, Burnet (1957, 1971) defends a theoretical position of cell transformation. He defines cancer as the product of randomly determined changes in a somatic cell that result in malignancy in that cell and in its mitotic descendants. Burnet reasons that cancer results from the body's inability to manage and control the virulent proliferation of these malignant cells.

No serious attempt has been made to put forward a theory of cancer that posits exclusively psychological processes as causes of the disease. However, renewed interest in holistic medicine, coupled with more effective collaboration in psychobiological research, has bolstered hypotheses that consider the role psychological processes may play in the development of cancer. If the random mutation model described above is plausible, then what specifically accounts for the body's inability to control the proliferation of the malignancy? Some scientists would look beyond mere biological functions for the answer and would widen the search to include things like emotional equilibrium, motivation and drive, volition and mental attitude. These psychological variables are considered by many to be *homeostatic regulators*; subtle shifts in these control variables not only affect mood, but also exercise influence over other bodily functions.

At one time it was thought that activities regulated by the autonomic nervous system were immune from external influence. Today, the scientific community is more receptive to the suggestion that the activities of organs like the heart and lungs can be influenced by psychological processes. *Biofeedback* is an outgrowth of this knowledge. By presenting an individual with visual or auditory information on physical functions like heart rate, respiration, blood pressure, or skin temperature, a person is able to marshal psychological resources to exercise some control over the physiologic variable being sampled.

It is reasonable to hypothesize that such control might be brought to bear in the effort to regulate the spread of a malignancy. While some practitioners of holistic medicine strenuously assert that people can thus cure themselves and describe cases in which self-cures have occurred, a shroud of skepticism surrounds this position within the wider medical community.

One difficulty in mediating the debate between the two distinct schools of thought is that there is scant research to support psychobiological theories of cancer etiology. Evidence of hormonal and immunological influences on the development of certain cancers is already advanced. Parallel research is simultaneously documenting the fact that endocrine and body immune functions are susceptible to psychological influence. The next logical step is to join these two lines of research in a collaborative effort. Greer (1979) notes that what has been postulated by certain researchers is not that psychological factors constitute a necessary or sufficient cause of cancer but that these factors can, by the way they exert their influence on homeostatic controls and on behavior, contribute to cancer susceptibility in some people.

Personality Traits

In his classic study, Gordon Allport (1937) suggested that *personality* is the "dynamic organization within the individual of those biosocial systems that determine his or her unique adjustment to the world." The biosocial systems to which he was referring are those personality traits, habits, motives, and values that are partially rooted in biological inheritance and partially related to social learning and human experience. The particular way in which these biological and social influences are organized and actively interact with the environment determines the way a person adapts to life.

If cancer is not an exclusively biological phenomenon but is related to psychological processes rooted in personality structure, it may be possible to identify those who are at greater risk. It was this hypothesis that inspired the 1946 longitudinal study of medical school students at Johns Hopkins Medical School. By administering psychological tests and yearly questionnaires about health and lifestyle, researchers hoped to identify certain traits that might be related to cancer. The study was not limited to studying the personality-cancer relationship but was likewise interested in other personality-related disorders, including coronary heart disease, mental illness, essential hypertension, and vulnerability to suicide.

Precancerous Personality

The profiles obtained from students in 17 successive classes at Johns Hopkins Medical School who later developed neoplasms revealed low mean scores for closeness to parents, whom the students described as remote and cold. The medical school graduates themselves tended to be emotionally unexpressive (Thomas & Greenstreet, 1973; Thomas & Duszynski, 1974). One problem associated with this type of research is that relationships are sought between specific personality structures defined in terms of particular traits and precise types of cancer, and studies are often conducted without the benefit of adequate control groups. Moreover, insufficient attention is paid to the ways in which a patient diagnosed with cancer responds to diagnosis and participates in treatment.

In a review article discussing psychosomatic aspects of cancer, Murray (1980) notes that the concept of *precancerous personality* has received little attention in recent literature. He is particularly interested in how significant losses contribute to the development of cancer. Though recognized as a legitimate field of inquiry, the potential linkage between personality and cancer has not been sufficiently investigated.

Greer (1979) studied women admitted for breast tumor biopsy. This study attempted to identify psychological factors associated with the development of breast cancer, and the interactive effects of psychological factors with hormonal and immunological variables. In following those patients admitted for biopsy ($N = 160$) who subsequently were found to have breast cancer ($N = 69$), the researchers were interested in identifying any psychological or biological factors that might be predictive of outcome.

The classic associative factors of denial, depression, or stressful losses appeared to be inconsequential in the Greer studies. The most significant main effect was related to the suppression of anger throughout the adult life; these women characteristically did not feel comfortable ventilating their anger but were more likely to conceal their hostile feelings.

Applying this variable in clinical situations, they were curious to discover whether pathological outcome might be predicted from evidence of suppression of affect. Surprisingly, diagnostic prediction made solely with the psychological variables proved to be 72 percent accurate. Routine clinical diagnosis of breast cancer is made by considering the size and outline of the tumor, nipple discharge, and inversion and palpability of ipsilateral lymph nodes. Results of this sort are certainly not conclusive, but they are impressive. This kind of research suggests that precancerous personality studies are not obsolete or useless.

Greer (1979) is cautious about the tendency to overgeneralize his research conclusions, no matter how impressive they may be. He is correct in exercising such caution. However, the implications for research in this direction are apparent. Since many developmental psychologists maintain that personality is relatively stable throughout the human life cycle, it may be possible to establish links between personality and certain cancer types and to identify persons at increased risk or susceptibility. This possibility provides an incentive for mounting carefully designed and controlled psychobiological studies.

Some Specific Psychosocial Predictors of Cancer

Psychophysiological research concerns itself not only with personality variables that may be preconditions of cancer but is also interested in identifying psychosocial conditions that may contribute to the outbreak of the disease. Foundational to this field of research is the hypothesis that specific psychosocial constellations may predispose to certain somatic diseases, including a wide variety of neoplasms.

Grossarth-Maticek (1980) reported on a 10-year follow-up study of 1,353 inhabitants of a Yugoslavian town. Employing a 109-item, interpretation-free survey instrument prospectively, the researcher sampled a variety of psychosocial variables, including psychosocial stress and the social expression of needs and feelings. The investigator was sensitive to "explosive behavior" that might be a reaction to such internal stressors as abuse of food, alcohol, tobacco, and medications. In addition, chronic depression and feelings of hopelessness were monitored as well as long-lasting hostile or angry feelings.

All of these data, once coded, were considered independent variables and not open to *ex post factum* interpretation in light of the dependent variables (i.e., the incidence or nonincidence of disease). Discriminant analyses yielded 93 percent correct predictions, suggesting that with early recognition as well as effective intervention, certain cancers may be preventable.

Schmale and Iker (1971) studied a number of patients with diagnoses of uterine cancer. Greene, Young, and Swisher (1956) studied a wide range of lymphomas and leukemias and reported their results over a number of years.

These and other similar studies have described certain psychosocial factors in cancer patients that suggest that those events (including experiences of loss and separation) which induce depression and feelings of helplessness and hopelessness may indeed be preconditions for the development of malignancies. In fact, the common denominator linking many of these independent research efforts is the conclusion that this constellation of psychological factors may be a key to carcinogenesis.

When the Schmale research was recently replicated by Spence (1979), not only were the results similar, but the conclusions were strengthened. Spence utilized an automated, computerized screening procedure that did a frequency count of the language used by a number of women presenting themselves for cervical cancer screening by *cone biopsy*. A cone biopsy excises an inverted cone of tissue from the uterine cervix for microscopic examination. By analyzing the conversations of these biopsy patients for "lexical leakage" he was able to identify positive diagnoses of uterine cancer at a level of significance less than .01. By lexical leakage, Spence meant the specific linguistic expressions used, including vocabulary and phrasing.

Bahnson and his colleagues have been studying the relationship of psychosocial variables to cancer for more than 20 years. In a 1980 report Bahnson notes that loss and separation are not sufficient preconditions for the development of cancer. He maintains from his clinical and experimental investigations that the loss must be accompanied by a history of childhood affective deprivation in order for the loss to be considered predictive of cancer. Bahnson thinks that the internalization of affect and the proclivity to loneliness, depression, and emotional rigidity may have their origin in isolation and inhibited affect during childhood.

Describing the psychodynamics of this process, Bahnson describes a centrifugal family of origin, wherein early individuation, mutual isolation, and distancing of members from one another become characteristic patterns of relationship. In this condition, a child is blocked in emotional expression and does not benefit from the sharing of feelings and experiences with parents and other family members. Defensive strategies that rely heavily upon denial and repression are commonly due to chronic inhibition of affect and the resulting frustration. Bahnson asserts a psychobiologic (narcissistic) regression in cancer; the psychosocial history of a cancer patient, he maintains, may often disclose evidence of loss and depression in early childhood.

Psychophysiological Mechanisms

Psychosomatic research attempts to identify those pathways by which neoplasms develop. Considerable attention has been given to the role that the *immune* and *endocrine systems* play in this pathogenesis. Are these systems influenced by psychological stimuli? Apart from the specific relationship of these systems to the development of cancer, empirical evidence has shown that changes in emotions are accompanied by changes in circulatory levels of *catecholamines* (e.g., dopamine, norepinephrine, and epineph-rine) and *corticosteroids*.

Since the mid-1960s, both clinical psychiatry and experimental biological psychiatry have suggested a strong link between affective disorders (depressions and elations) and changes in the central nervous system catecholamine metabolism. The *catecholamine hypothesis* proposes that some, if not all, depressions are associated with an absolute or relative decrease in catechol-amines, particularly norepinephrine. Elation, conversely, may be associated with an excess of such amines (Schildkraut, 1965).

The corticosteriods are any of the steroids (or synthetic equivalents) developed by the adrenal cortex in response to the adrenocorticotrophic hormone (ACTH) released by the pituitary gland. Their principal biological activities influence carbohydrate and fat metabolism, and regulate electrolyte and water balance. In clinical usage, the synthetic steroids are used in hormonal replacement therapies. They help to suppress ACTH secretion by the pituitary and are used as antineoplastic and antiinflammatory agents. They also suppress the immune response.

Endocrinological relationships to psychological changes are easily monitored and reported; endocrinological relationships with the body immune functions are not. *Immunopathogenesis*, a process in which the course of a disease is altered or affected by an immune response, is a new frontier in psychobiological research. Work with animal subjects points to the role of immune factors in the development of neoplasia.

Although research with humans is still immature, there is keen interest among scientists to identify a pathway to cancer originating in a psychological state and mediated via some immunological mechanism. It is known that certain psychological conditions can be immunosuppressive; whether this phenomenon is causally related to the incidence and development of cancer has yet to be established.

Greer (1979) has reviewed some of the more significant studies of the possible effects of psychological stimuli on endocrine and immune functions. Although none of these studies is conclusive, the emerging body of research suggests endocrine and immune system participation in cancer etiology.

Communication

Effective care of the cancer patient is not simply a matter of proper diagnosis and judicious surgical, chemotherapeutic, or radiotherapeutic decisions. Long-term survival may be as much conditioned by the psychological state of the patient and the psychosocial resources on which he or she may be able to draw. This section will discuss the specific role communication plays in the treatment of cancer, with particular focus on the participation of family and health care professionals.

As noted in the previous discussion of etiological factors in carcinogenesis, personality variables and coping strategies may predispose to neoplasm. Whether these hypotheses can be supported or not, there is sufficient evidence available to warrant continued study. Given the diagnosis of cancer, it is likewise important to pay attention to these same issues of personality and coping capacities when planning treatment protocols.

Allen (1981) emphasizes the importance of assessing psychological factors in the treatment of cancer. So often physicians and other health care professionals perceive their task in terms of controlling and eradicating a disease. While not consciously intending to exclude the patient's participation in this effort, their approaches can inadvertently ignore the importance of certain psychosocial variables. The exclusion of the patient from the critical communication process in planning for and implementing treatment can intensify the subjective feelings of helplessness in a patient and among family members and can negatively affect the outcome of therapeutic efforts.

The following retrospective case report documents the ways in which failures in communication, both between patient and physician and patient and family members, negatively affected the course of a terminal illness.

My mother died 5 years ago of brain cancer. She was hospitalized on the 26th of October and died the 17th of January: 10 weeks of illness. She was 68 years old.

It all began with what seemed to be a grippe, accompanied by overwhelming fatigue—around the beginning of October. Once, during the month of August, she had confessed to me: "I'm afraid to die."

Then one night, she was paralzyed on her left side and she lost her equilibrium when she attempted to walk. Our family doctor had her hospitalized immediately. . . . The transfer was done by ambulance since her condition was precarious. My father accompanied her and I went ahead to meet them at the hospital. It was there that I realized that she was going to die; I captured her sad expression, full of anxiety, a look of distress that I shall never forget. It was at that moment that I knew that I was going to lose her. . . .

Then the tests began and the x-rays. . . . There was no immediate diagnosis suggested, just the insecurity, the utter confusion. What did she really have?

She asked me: "Am I going to die?" I answered that she was in good hands and that they would do everything possible to help her recover from this illness.

The doctor told the family that it might be arteriosclerosis or a tumor—benign or malignant—that's the question!

Time passed; the visits, the members of the family and friends kept coming in a steady stream. It was like a reunion around her bed. One Sunday the whole family was gathered together, and she spoke and thanked us all for being there; she cried at the end saying that she would like very much to hear the *Ave Maria* of Schubert. Since she had always told me that that was the music she would like to hear on her death bed, we children were stunned and told her that it was not a question of dying, but of getting better! There was considerable discomfort among us. She was very lucid, content that her husband and her three children and their spouses were there along with her sister, brother-in-law, and other members of the extended family. It was a very solemn moment with all of us gathered around her bed. I felt that she had every reason to be thinking about her death, but none of us dared to say to her that we, too, were thinking that perhaps she was going to die. But we all thought it.

Our waiting was long and finally the diagnosis was communicated to us by an intern who met with us in a small room on the hospital floor. He told us that there was a tumor and that it was necessary to operate. My father, my husband and myself and one cousin were there together to hear the verdict. This young doctor was wonderful, very compassionate; he tried to respond to whatever questions we had and did not rush away.

He was silent and then he told us how much he admired how we handled the difficult news. . . . He said that the chief of surgery would speak with mother about the operation. We had never met this young doctor before, nor did we ever see him again.

When I went to see my mother the next day, I asked her if the doctor had spoken with her and told her that they wanted to operate. She didn't respond. I asked her again and told her that they wanted to operate; she finally answered: "All right! They're going to operate, that's that. . . . I did not know how to talk to her about it. There were so many heavy silences. Some days later I asked her. "You are not talking to me?" She replied: "What do you want me to say?" I answered: "Tell me how you are feeling? What's going on with you? You seem to be so far away!" Silence. Then I added: "Do you think that you are dying?" Complete silence. . . . I sensed that she was very depressed, in great pain. . . .

After the operation, I waited to see my mother. I tried to find out how everything had gone in the surgery. Yet I couldn't get any details from the staff and was unable to find a single doctor. . . . Someone gave me the telephone number of the surgeon. I called him around 8 P.M. that evening at his home. In a trenchant tone of voice, as if he were very annoyed that I would have called him, he told me: "The tumor was enormous and badly situated; we had no choice but to open and immediately close."

I excused myself for having disturbed him and I felt guilty that I was the daughter of a patient with such a villainous tumor. The "Good night, Madam" of the surgeon was rapid and striking: a 30-second message that basically said "your mother is lost." I would have liked to have known what to anticipate about the course of the illness, what attitude to take, what to say, what to do. I felt the doctor just did not want to be involved any further; this poor sick woman had been reduced to an object. The family was the one that was left to be involved with her. (Gazut, 1981, excerpted and translated from the French)

The Patient's Desire to Know and the Physician's Willingness to Tell

One issue that is keenly debated among health care professionals is how much should be communicated to a cancer patient and how and when information should be shared. Prior to the 1970s most surveys on the subject of communication with patients with life-threatening diseases indicated that the conspiracy of silence was unquestioningly upheld; that situation is no longer tolerated. Using the polling resources of the Gallup organization and supported by a training grant from the National Institutes of Mental Health, Blumenfield, Levy, and Kaufman (1978) surveyed the attitudes of normal adults in the United States.

They posed the question: "If you had a fatal illness would you want to be told about it, or not?" Nine out of 10 people personally interviewed ($N = 1,518$) indicated that they desired to be informed if they had a life-threatening disease. The polling strategy tried to develop a representative sampling of adult Americans, excluding those in prisons or hospitals. More than 300 sampling locations were identified in the study. It is interesting to note that 92 percent of the men and 87 percent of the women interviewed indicated a desire to know their diagnosis. This sex difference is statistically significant at the level of p less than .05. A smaller percentage of nonwhites (82 percent), those of lower educational background (85 percent), and those of lower socioeconomic levels (83 percent), indicated a desire to know. Taking into consideration these comparative differences, the overwhelming evidence points to the average person's preference to know the available information concerning diagnosis, prognosis, and treatment options.

In 1979, Novack and his associates at the University of Rochester Medical Center repeated a survey previously conducted by Oken in 1961 (Novack *et al.*, 1979). The original questionnaire completed by a sample of practicing physicians indicated that 90 percent of those participating in the survey did not favor telling a cancer patient of his or her diagnosis. Suspecting that attitudes have shifted, 699 university-hospital medical staff were asked the same questions; of the 264 respondants, 97 percent indicated a preference for telling the person the details of the diagnosis. What accounts for this change in attitudes?

Novack and his colleagues (1979) observe that of late the topic of communication with the cancer patient seems to be more regularly discussed in medical schools and in clinical training programs than in the past. Clinical experience also has a formative influence in shaping the health care professional's attitude toward communication with the cancer patient concerning diagnosis. It is very interesting that in both the 1961 and 1977 samples, both groups clearly cited personal and emotional factors as contributing to their own principles and policies about the communication of information to a cancer patient.

It seems that the medical profession is sensitized to the ethical right of a person to know. The values of honesty, sensitivity, and personal rights seem to be influential in shaping the attitudes of contemporary health care professionals toward communication with patients. Supporting these beliefs is the knowledge and experience that, in a considerable number of cases, cancer can be effectively treated and cured.

Love, Hayward, and Stone (1980) surveyed primary care resident physicians and medical school faculty members about their attitudes toward cancer medicine. In this study, faculty respondents in family-medicine reflected attitudes about cancer medicine significantly different from those of their peers in internal medicine and oncology. Family-medicine faculty placed considerable importance on the communication with patients concerning risk management, early detection and screening, and effective treatment. They placed a high premium on communication with the patient and the partnership forged in this effort. While internal medicine and oncology specialists may share these attitudes, the family practice approach appears to place greater emphasis on the intrinsic therapeutic value of patient-physician communication and is more optimistic about its benefits. However, the majority opinion in the health care professional community is that cancer patients should be informed of their condition.

Hardy and his associates (1980) reported on a survey of 185 practicing Tennessee physicians regarding their communication patterns with cancer patients. The results of this survey were similar to the patterns reported in the Novack study: 98 percent of the responding physicians indicated that they always or usually inform patients that they have cancer. From these attitudinal surveys, it is clear that a change has taken place in the ways in which the medical community perceives its responsibilities toward communication with patients.

Informed Consent and Communication Patterns

The concept of "informed consent" is inextricably linked to the discussion of patient-physician communication. According to this principle, the patient has the right to know his or her diagnosis and needs to be appropriately informed about options available for treatment. The government has established laws that attempt to ensure that the right of patients to know and to choose will be honored. Since many hospitals and research facilities depend heavily on federal support for primary medical research, these regulations affect policy. Individuals placed at risk by experimental medications and procedures must be effectively informed of the risk. To treat disease means that the patient must first know the scope and course of the disease.

Some physicians have resisted these controls, arguing that they interrupt patient care and mandate communication which may not always be in the patient's best interest. These same physicians maintain that some patients are not able to assimilate such information and do not wish to know all of the possible consequences of treatment protocols. They fear that the practice of medicine, much of which is experimental, is unnecessarily compromised by too many attempts at external regulation.

After testing a consent form with oncology patients in a Midwestern hospital, Kennedy and Lillehaugen (1979) made appropriate revisions and simplified the presentation. This form requested approval to use for teaching and research purposes the information gained from history, physical examination, and routine laboratory reports. The only permission involving an invasive procedure requested one test tube (10cc) of blood for research purposes. Fifty patients were given the consent form and 46 agreed to sign it; of this group, 34 signed it immediately without question—some not even reading it. When the researchers followed up one week later with these 46 persons who signed the consent form, 2 patients did not recall they had signed it. As suspected, the majority of patients had quite discrepant recollections about what was included in the form.

Kennedy and Lillehaugen concluded that the signed form needs to be recognized for what it is: evidence that consent has been obtained. It does not imply that the patient fully understands what is being permitted. That can only be assured through competent education of the patient so that he or she can make a free and informed decision. The open communication process this requires begins at diagnosis. Information is supplied and interpreted as it becomes available. Time must be taken to explain all procedures and answer all questions posed by a patient. The communicative environment is such that the patient senses a partnership has been set up between him or her and the physician and medical staff.

Negative information communicated at the time of diagnosis is emotionally upsetting to most patients. It is readily understandable why so few patients can recall the discussions they had with their physicians about proposed treatments; many do not recall giving their consent to these procedures. If such consent is judged to be the patient's right, then health care professionals should not view this consent as a duty to comply with certain regulations governing medical procedure but as a primary component of the communication that should exist between physician and patient. Although the process of providing honest, accurate, and complete information on the disease and proposed treatment is often difficult and time-consuming, it is essential if the patient's right to know is to be ensured.

Marianne Gazut concludes her narrative about her terminally ill mother:

I had many times asked to meet with the priest or chaplain who had seen my mother, but I never was successful in meeting him. The doctors were never available when I went to the hospital. . . . the nurses are changing shifts all the time and did not seem to be available to families. Maybe I am too demanding; they take care of the physical needs of the patient—they can't do more. How far does the role of the hospital extend?

My mother went into a coma and only slept. . . . I was in a pretty sorry state myself, my feelings were all mixed up. Had I done the right thing in letting them operate on her? Should I not have taken her home? But in this condition, that was out of the question. Was this a therapeutic choice to have made to ease her pain? Would hers be a humane death? Why did she have to be nourished artificially while she was dying? How conscious was she? The word "euthanasia" kept turning around in my head.

What was the use of my visits while she was in such a state of coma? The visits, after all, only made me ill. I asked them to let me know when she began to fail so that I could be at her bedside when she died. The hospital called me at 2 A.M. on the 17th of January to inform me that my mother had just died. . . .

In the first place I have written this story [of my mother's death] to "settle accounts" with the hospital, but in the second place because I appreciate the difficulties that medical personnel have in approaching a sick person and dealing with death.

My account of my mother's death is indicting; it is simply because of my need to be somehow in communication with doctors and nurses. It has become so clear to me now—something that wasn't so clear earlier on—that I would have liked a very different death for my mother. But I was afraid to confront the essential task— to tell her that she was going to die. (Gazut, 1981, excerpted and translated from the French)

Special Problems Encountered in Communicating with Cancer Patients

Telling a patient about a diagnosis and exploring options for elective treatment are not simple tasks of sharing information. The patient's emotional state and the physician's sensitivity and perception are crucial variables that affect the outcome of this attempt at communication. Communicating a diagnosis of cancer is often emotionally traumatic for the patient. Some experienced physicians find such communication difficult. Patients begin to ruminate about the physical aspects of the disease and are concerned about how disruptive they will be. They are disturbed by the thoughts of how cancer and its treatment will interrupt their familial, social, and professional life. A diagnosis of cancer excites concerns about the economic consequences of extensive surgical and medical treatments and the physical and psychological demands that will be placed on family and friends.

People have many misconceptions and misinformation about cancer. These can distort their perceptions and contribute to attitudes about their own diagnosis and treatment. They can become emotionally paralyzed by the fears frequently associated with the disease, including surgery, mutilation, invalidism, loss of function, and death (Allen, 1981).

Providing information to a patient with a life-threatening disease may communicate paradoxical messages. On the one hand, the patient receives verbal and nonverbal messages that convey the impression that although his or her condition is serious, there is hope of effective and often curative treatment. Simultaneously, the patient receives verbal and non-verbal messages that death may result. In their classic study of schizophrenia, Bateson, Haley, Jackson, and Weakland (1956) coined the term *double bind*. By definition, the double bind involves a communication between two or more individuals involved in a significant relationship. One of the individuals communicates a message that implies a threat to the other if a certain injunction is not carried out. At the same time, that injunction is negated by a secondary message. The recipient of these two conflicting messages is unable to step outside the context of the communication, and is not only confused and unable to resolve the conflict, but in some cases is paralyzed by the process.

Longhofer and Floersch (1980) applied this concept of the double bind to cancer patients. As applied anthropologists, they were interested in how persons are affected by this style of communication in medical practice. They hypothesized that some cancer patients are forced to perceive realities about their physical conditions, not as they might appear to them but as they are defined by those in their environment. They studied patients in a Boston research hospital who were to receive bone marrow transplants. By evaluating the various messages exchanged in the course of this experimental procedure, they noted evidence of the double-bind communication pattern. For example, a physician may assure a patient that a particular experimental procedure is safe and fairly routine. The patient observes that many of the staff preparing for the procedure seem anxious and unsure. When the patient asks questions about the procedure, those questions are unanswered and referred back to the physician. What was stated as safe and routine appears to be risky and experimental. Paradoxical communications of this sort can not only erode patient-physician trust, but can mobilize other forms of dysfunction, including anxiety and depression. A patient can grow distrustful of those charged with his or her care and can prematurely withdraw from treatment. What the Longhofer and Floersch research suggests is that health care professionals should work to develop patterns of communication free of destructive double messages.

Iatrogenic Stresses

In a sensitive article describing his personal experience with an embryonal carcinoma with pulmonary metastases, Neil Fiore (1979), a practicing psychologist, reviews the course of his diagnosis and treatment. He comments that fighting cancer involves more than surgery or chemotherapy; he maintains that both the patient and the medical professionals need to recognize that the patient's "mind and body are powerful factors in this fight." Unless these resources are identified and marshalled, the battle can be lost and the patient may not only resist necessary treatments but may become so depressed that his or her will to live diminishes.

While the patient is often willing and ready to assume responsibility for participation in this curative enterprise, that readiness may be compromised by certain stresses in the way medical care is provided. These stresses are termed *iatrogenic*, from the Greek root *iatros*, which means "medical treatment or one involved in providing healing." Iatrogenic stresses involve issues of powerlessness, impersonalism, blind faith, patient's suggestibility, and patient's lack of adequate knowledge about the disease, its predictable course, and its treatment.

As Dr. Fiore discovered, cancer patients are often willing to share their experiences with interested individuals. One woman commented on her experiences to a group of medical students (Trillin, 1981). She noted that we are raised in a cultural context where we believe in the "magic of doctors." By ascribing this magical power to a profession, we feel as though we have control over something we otherwise might fear. Trillin reflects a solid principle of clinical practice when she notes that the best physicians are the ones who find effective ways to share their power with their patients, providing them with the information they need to control their own treatment.

This ideal is not easily achieved in the practice of medicine, which has become so specialized and in some instances impersonal. Physicians are limited in the amount of individual support they can provide to any one patient and may tend to rely on other members of the health care team to make up this deficit. The routinization of treatment may block the effective delivery of necessary support, creating a condition of social isolation for the cancer patient faced with questions, doubts, and uncertainties about his or her disease. The use of technical explanations by physicians and other professionals may not be understood by the patient, who may be reluctant to seek further clarification from the doctor.

Patients are sensitively tuned to the attitudes of those who provide them with medical care. Because they recognize the vulnerable position in which they find themselves, they often try to please their doctors. Bean, Cooper, Alpert, and Kipnis (1980) report on 33 cancer patients receiving chemotherapy. Among the comments made by patients, one woman said: "If you're a nice person you get nice treatment." Another responded: "I have to be satisfied; my doctor put me here." It is evident from this limited survey that patients are concerned with the potential negative reactions of health care providers should any criticisms be voiced.

These feelings are linked with the sense of powerlessness patients have. For this reason, it is the physician who must invite questioning and explore ways in which to engage patient participation and patient involvement in strategizing treatment. The goals of medicine itself to control and cure disease are frustrated when patients' involvement in their treatment is diminished or precluded.

Although medicine has made significant progress in the diagnosis and treatment of cancer, the disease is still somewhat elusive and unpredictable— which can frustrate the physicians who are responsible for its treatment. The patient may somehow feel that he or she is causing the doctor additional trouble by not getting better. A doctor's anger or frustration, no matter how well masked, may be perceived by the patient and create unnecessary guilt. Unexpected side effects, setbacks, and relapses are all components of cancer treatment. Care must be taken to help the patient not to interpret a physician's disappointment with treatment in subjectively destructive ways.

Patients faced with the diagnosis of cancer and confronted with urgent choices concerning treatment options are highly suggestible. As was noted in the discussion of informed consent, some patients do not even read the description of those things to which they give their approval. Fiore (1979) has compared this state to that of a hypnotic trance. The patient is highly suggestible because he or she recognizes the danger represented by the disease and the need for help. A person in these circumstances sees the physician as the one who can respond most effectively to this need. For this reason, not only the manner but the words and gestures a physician uses can feed the patient's imagination with fantasies of a hopeful or a despairing outcome. Fiore remarks that the aware physician can use this suggestible state to therapeutic advantage both to calm the patient and to engage the patient in active participation in the treatment process.

Without intending negative effects, some physicians' descriptions of standard procedures and routine chemotherapies fail to underscore the positive aspects of these treatments. Fiore (1979) highlights this point in a single paragraph that merits reflection. He argues that the selection of language can not only foster patient understanding, but it can create positive or negative expectations and images in the cancer patient.

The positive statement uses the word *medication* instead of *drugs* to emphasize the helpful nature of chemotherapy, and uses *powerful* instead of *toxic* to emphasize the point that this is a strong ally to the body. The loss of hair and other side effects are presented as possible, and not certain, to avoid self-fulfilling prophecies. Most importantly, the statement allows patients to conceptualize the side effects as a sign that their powerful ally is working at killing rapidly producing cells. Without this kind of intervention, patients often conclude that the side effects are proof that they are dying—if not from cancer, from its treatment. (p. 287)

A patient's belief system about disease and health, which functions to gain control over the disease that may be threatening his or her life, is influenced by numerous factors. Of special importance is the information received through verbal and nonverbal cues from the primary care physician and other important care providers. Research is reinforcing the opinion already held by many people that one's belief system does influence the course of illness and health.

In 1959 in his presidential address to the American Cancer Society (cited in Sachtleben, 1978), Dr. Eugene P. Pendergrass concluded with a theme that emphasizes this important point. He said: "As we go forward . . . searching for new means for controlling growth both within the cell and through systemic influences, it is my sincere hope that we can widen the quest to include the distinct possibility that within one's mind is a power capable of exerting forces which can either enhance or inhibit the progress of this disease." Medicine must be careful not to neglect this important ally in its defensive armory. More importantly, it is incumbent upon physicians and others who assist in the care of a cancer patient not to allow their words and gestures to influence negatively the course of treatment.

Defense Mechanisms and Coping Behavior

The word *crisis* is frequently used to describe the events and circumstances surrounding the diagnosis of cancer. The healthy resolution of this crisis is contingent on a number of factors, including the interpersonal and intrapersonal resources a person can summon as supports as well as the environmental variables that come to bear on the situation. Concretely, these resources include family members, friends, and professionals. The ways in which a person perceives and understands the crisis, the ways in which such crises have been managed in the past, and the personal success one might have experienced in resolving these difficulties all influence the course of crisis resolution.

Because the diagnosis of cancer can involve a long process of treatment, it can be looked upon as an extended crisis. Ordinarily, crisis refers to a transitional, short-term event. Cancer patients frequently describe the course of the disease as a series of crises, each to be negotiated in a manner proper to the particular circumstances. Each of these crises requires different resources and coping strategies. We would like to consider some of these individual crises in the often prolonged course of cancer treatment.

The Crisis of Diagnosis

A life-threatening diagnosis severely constricts the boundaries of personal freedom and control. Some social psychologists (Brehm, 1966; Wicklund, 1974) have theorized that in such circumstances individuals become mobilized to restore control. This *reactance* behavior is predicated on the assumption that the stronger the threat or the more important the outcome, the greater the amount of emotional reactance. When this theoretical model is applied to a person's learning of a diagnosis of cancer, it is easy to understand and situate reactions of anger, hostility, and rage.

Some persons react to a positive diagnosis of cancer in a distinctly different way. They seem to lack motivation to engage in aggressive treatment and become passive. Seligman (1975) suggested that *learned helplessness* might explain this coping behavioral pattern. He and his associates found that exposure to aversive stimulation (e.g., information concerning diagnosis and prognosis) can interfere with the acquistion of subsequent adaptive learning (ways to treat and cure the disease). Reactive depression may be one specific clinical expression of this coping style.

Wortman and Brehm (1975) have attempted to describe a model that integrates both reactance and learned helplessness theories. They reasoned that a person's expectation of ability to control or influence a situation, whether the outcome is perceived as important, and how long they had failed to gain control all contribute to his or her reaction. Individuals who expect to control will react vigorously, strongly motivated to harness the crisis. If these efforts fail, then personal motivation may wane over time and these persons may conclude that control is impossible to achieve. This conclusion can lay the foundation for withdrawal, passivity, and depression.

For some time Fred had been fearful that his problem might be "cancer." He tried for a long time to ignore the symptoms. He was losing weight and periodically coughed blood. When his wife became aware of these symptoms, she insisted that he visit the family doctor. With great reluctance he agreed to the suggestion.

When the doctor began to explore the history of Fred's complaint, it became clear that a few months had passed since the first symptoms had appeared. Fred acknowledged that he had simply dismissed them as being of any consequence. But the symptoms were insistent and this gave Fred serious doubts about them, although he tried to hide his concerns from his wife. He told the physician: "I'm afraid it might be cancer, Doc."

After bronchoscopic examination and an exploratory thoracotomy, Fred's worst fears were confirmed. The doctor, aware of his apprehension, tried to present the information on the diagnosis and treatment program in the most direct terms. While Fred and his wife were very disturbed by the news, they were anxious about what could be done.

The diagnostic evaluation revealed an inoperable tumor within the lung. Radiation therapy (4500-6000 rads by continuous fractionation) was the treatment of choice. No adjuvant chemotherapy program was initiated since it was judged to be of little benefit in the definitive treatment of regional inoperable lung cancer. In the judgment of the thoracic team who evaluated Fred's case, the survival expectation was about 12 months with the radiation treatment protocol.

It was evident that Fred was experiencing deep anxiety; he confided to his wife that he thought that the doctors might be hiding something from him and that his condition was more serious than they were telling him. In fact his suspicions were well founded. Catherine had spoken with the thoracic surgeon and had pleaded that he not be told. She claimed: "He could not cope with the news."

Even though Fred was suspicious, he did agree to the radiotherapy treatments. He was very passive in his approach to treatment. He never asked the staff any questions about the radiation treatments or about his survival chances. It seemed that he did not want to know more about his condition. The radiologist offered to make available to him a videotaped program on lung cancer, but Fred declined to view the presentation. Whenever he did make reference to the disease, it seemed as if he conceived of the cancer as something extraneous to him.

Several months into the treatments, Fred did not sense much improvement and he felt that things were more serious. During one of his treatment sessions he asked the radiologist how he was progressing. The doctor tried to communicate gently that the program was useful, but that the most it could do was to buy him additional time. Fred nodded in a silent but knowing gesture of understanding. This was the first time anyone had directly acknowledged to him what he had long suspected. He was dying. The only other question he wanted to ask was how much pain he might expect; he did not ask how much longer he had to live.

Although the full truth of Fred's diagnosis was not communicated to him initially, he seemed to know the terminal nature of the findings. He submitted to the proposed program of radiation, but his behavioral response reflects a degree of regression, rejection of reality, and an isolation reaction. He only talked of the cancer as something apart from him. After 6 months of treatment, he came to the point where he could accept the inevitability of his diagnosis and that everything was being done; he was ready to invest his final energies in palliative efforts to manage any pain associated with the terminal stages of the illness.

Lewis, Gottesman, and Gutstein (1979) studied the course and duration of crisis in a group of patients undergoing surgery for cancer. They compared this experimental group ($N=35$) with a control group ($N=35$) of surgical patients with less serious illnesses. All of the people were tested for anxiety, self-esteem, depression, perceived locus of control, and general perception of crisis on 4 separate occasions: the night before surgery and postoperatively every 3 weeks. It is generally assumed in crisis theory that the healthy individual makes a reasonable adjustment within 6 to 8 weeks.

The experimental group was composed of individuals who were undergoing exploratory surgery to verify a suspected diagnosis of carcinoma. Those who had benign tumors ($N=6$) were dropped from the study as well as 6 others who elected not to continue. The final sample size of both groups was adjusted to 23 persons in each of the groups. Significant effects were noted on most variables considered. The cancer surgery patients either remained consistently high on most of the measures of pathological affect, or these traits gradually became more pronounced. The cancer patients initially displayed more anxiety and feelings of helplessness than did the controls. Postoperatively, when the diagnosis was confirmed, depression and lowered self-esteem were more characteristic. These reactions did not appear until several weeks after the crisis had been precipitated.

This research provides clinical experimental support to the theoretical positions of Wortman and Brehm (1975). The preliminary portrait of the cancer patient emerging from this study shows the person intially overwhelmed by feelings of anxiety and helplessness. A perceived inability to exercise effective control over the situation develops into a form of reactive depression and concomitant loss of confidence in self.

One of the most interesting findings reported in this study was the evidence that the anticipated adaptation to the crisis among the cancer patients was not achieved within the predicted 8-week period. This is not surprising, given what we noted earlier about the extended nature of the crisis of cancer. Adaptation was noted for some variables sooner than for others, even in the continued presence of the disease.

Garusi (1978) notes that the psychological problems confronting a cancer patient, more than with other diseases, makes it necessary for physician and patient to discuss the situation in a trusting environment. The patient needs time to adjust to the facts of the diagnosis, the suggested course of treatment, and the consequences that may result. In all of this, it is the health care professional who must be ready to adapt to the particular requirements of the cancer patient, providing simple and direct answers to multiple questions, avoiding complex answers and explanations that might only further confuse and intensify anxiety in the patient. Garusi speaks of the truth of diagnosis expressed with discretion and prudence, "graduated to his [the patient's] capacity of assimilation."

Robert O. Beatty (1978) was an executive with Boise Cascade when he was invited to assist the then Secretary of Health, Education and Welfare (currently the Department of Health and Human Services), Elliot Richardson. In 1971, at age 47, Beatty was diagnosed with incurable cancer of the prostate. The following describes some of his initial reactions to this diagnosis.

Derrick (Dr. Fletcher Derrick, head of the Department of Urology at George Washington University Hospital) is a refreshingly direct person. . . . "Bob, I don't like to tell you this, but you have cancer of the prostate, and it looks like Stage Four to me." Meaning what? I asked. "Meaning that it's probably spread to other places in your body, and I want to do some more tests". . . .

We meandered back to the room as Derrick explained and scratched out on paper for me the various stages of prostatic cancer. I didn't hear much of what he said because of all the other thoughts racing through my mind.

Predictably, my next question was, how long do I have to live? He answered, "In your case, I'd guess about three years. Generally it progresses faster in younger people, but some people make it for twenty years. There are lots of things we can try to slow it down, but for right now, I'd try nothing until you develop unpleasant symptoms."

I must say at this point that I was and am grateful for Dr. Derrick's candor. I think it's a terrible mistake for doctors not to be honest with their patients about this (or any other) disease, because sooner or later the patient will find out anyway—if he doesn't already sense it—and then all confidence between patient and doctor is destroyed. (Beatty, 1978, pp. 4–5)

The Crisis of Treatment

Surgery, radiation, chemotherapy, and immunotherapy are among the most common methods by which cancer patients are treated. The medical goal of these interventions is to arrest the growth of the malignancy. The psychiatric aspects of these treatments have received considerably less attention. Psychiatric sequelae of cancer treatment generally merit notice and discussion when neurologic disturbances are identified, or when central nervous system toxicity is at issue. In clinical practice, the most common psychiatric presentations involve organic mental disorders or affective disorders, not sequelae directly related to cancer treatment agents (Peterson & Popkin, 1980). In those specific instances where chemotherapy can be directly associated with psychiatric effects, these situations are usually reversible with a change in the medication protocol.

Depression

The clinician who attempts to assess the psychological status of an individual undergoing cancer treatment must make a careful differential diagnosis that considers the nature of the illness and the multiple factors involved in aggressive treatment protocols. One of the most common problems encountered in cancer treatment patients is depression.

Peteet (1979) suggests a framework in which to consider depression among cancer patients. He distinguishes three types of depression: (1) tran-

sient stress reactions, (2) major psychiatric disturbances that require immediate attention, and (3) other depressive reactions often mistaken for the
other two.

The first category is related to the crisis of diagnosis and the affective reactions that follow in its wake. These reactions were explored in the previous
section. An effective strategy for dealing with this type of depression is to present the diagnostic information in a way that provides some degree of hope
and comfort. The physician needs to show empathy for the difficulty the patient has in accepting the news and needs to be available for whatever support, help, and clarification is desired.

Finally I called the nurse for a pen. I wrote on the backs of some clinical charts,
the only paper available, my initial reactions to the knowledge that I had this dread
disease. Here they are, pretty much as I wrote them:

It couldn't happen to me, but it has. Dr. Derrick has informed me that I probably have three years to live. Of course, he could be wrong. Doctors, being human,
often are. And then again, he could be right. Doctors, being doctors, often are.

The kaleidoscope of thoughts that come crashing into one's head with a revelation such as this is astounding. I'm not afraid, particularly, but I have a sort of
eerie, chilly feeling, as though I were floating through some unreal world, not
really attached to anything.

The first thoughts are of what will happen to Louise, and how do I plan for that.
Others immediately follow. Since this is centered in the prostate, with perineal-
nerve invasion, I have some questions about my sex-life. That's kind of odd, I
guess, because all sex, beyond procreation, is a form of pleasurable communication
between man and woman.

I—we—are going to have to remake our lives and our life plan. There are so
many factors involved, I don't know where to start. Should I waste another year at
HEW? Whom should I tell, if anybody? What's the status of my company insurance? Would my company take me back if they knew I had cancer?. . .

I'm also thinking of all the things I would like to do with my life which had been
sort of vague because I always figured I'd have plenty of time to do them. How can
one change one's life plan with this kind of revelation, if true?. . .

Oh God, please help me not to become a person who consciously or unconsciously seeks sympathy because of this and tries to use it for selfish ends. Please
help this experience make me move more in service to Thee and to others in Thy
sight. Please watch over, guard and care for my beloved wife, children and grandchild, and please help me to make these last years the best of our lives. (Beatty,
1978, pp. 6–7)

Beatty's initial reactions were controlled and rational. He approached his
terminal diagnosis with a positive and hopeful attitude. In the course of his
final illness, he became invested in living, rather than narrowly focused on
dying. In his own words "the more I've learned about cancer, the more my
fears have subsided." Some individuals faced with a similar bleak diagnosis
may not respond as positively. They may exhibit more evident signs of depres-

sion. However, even these reactive symptoms are quite distinct from more serious behavioral dysfunctions, which include eating and sleeping disorders, serious affective disturbances, and other classic symptoms. In these instances, referral for more definitive psychological diagnosis and treatment is generally indicated.

The third category is the most relevant to the patient involved in cancer treatment. This type of depression is characteristic of the *extended crisis period* of prolonged treatment and is characterized by persisting anxious symptoms. The fact that these symptoms continue may indicate that adjustment is not occurring. Peteet (1979) advises some ways of responding to a person who displays these symptoms. An empathic interview might disclose important characterological issues or lifestyle concerns. Exploring some of these issues and concerns may begin to address the source of the depressed affect and afford some relief to the patient. In the course of discussion the patient may also see some effective ways to regain control and mastery over his or her problems. The success in this type of intervention establishes a good foundation for assisting the patient in working with other family members or in other adjustments as the treatment of potentially fatal disease progresses.

Martha Fay (1983) has written a most illuminative book on 8 patients treated for various cancers at Memorial Sloan-Kettering Cancer Center in New York City. Her stories of cancer diagnosis, treatment, recovery, and dying highlight many important dynamic issues concerning both the patient and the family. These comprehensive chronicles of the course of cancer treatment help one to understand some of the inner psychological experiences of individuals being treated for cancer and of their families as well.

Suicidal Ideation

The literature on the topic of suicide continues to grow. Despite this fact, there is little that specifically focuses on the relationship between cancer and suicide. Maxwell (1980) has commented on this empirical lacuna in the scientific literature. She has speculated that in a culture that has come to understand cancer and the burdens of treatment often associated with it, the thought that such a person might take his or her life is less disturbing. If cancer is perceived as synonymous with terminal illness and death, then, for some persons, suicide represents little more than an acceleration of this inevitable outcome.

Cancer can seriously disrupt a person's life, interrupting important marital, familial, and other interpersonal relationships. The attempts to conquer the disease may involve aggressive drug therapies and painful surgical procedures. These not only physically alter important aspects of bodily image and functioning but can psychologically erode self-esteem. When all aspects of the disease are considered, one might suspect that the statistics of suicide would be high for cancer patients. The fact is that the number of suicides among cancer patients is surprisingly low.

Forman (1979) acknowledges that cancer is counted among other taboo subjects like suicide and death. Although some important research is being done on cancer and suicide, society is reluctant to delve too deeply into this area and researchers perceive a subtle professional stigmatization. Admittedly, as in the general research on suicide, the methodologic problems are extremely complex; data are not easily accessed nor can the reliability of available data be assured.

Although the original studies are dated, the work of Farberow, Shneidman, and Leonard (1963) continues to be clinically relevant and helpful in identifying the cancer patient with an elevated risk of suicide. The composite portrait of the person with the greatest vulnerability for suicide was derived from a comparative study of the records of 32 cancer patients who suicided and a comparison group of 32 nonsuicidal cancer controls. The picture that emerged from this analysis is the following.

The mental life of the suicide group disclosed anxiety, mood swings, and depression. These affective disorders reflect significant emotional disruption and agitation. These patients required and demanded much from the hospital staff; they constantly sought attention and reassurance and often complained bitterly. Although they demanded much from staff, they were often uncooperative in the treatment programs, refusing medications or other therapies.

As a group their threshold for pain was low; they did not tolerate the discomforts that accompany some cancers and treatments. Not only were they stressed by the disease and its treatment, but there was also evidence that they felt other pressures not specifically related to their diagnosis and treatment. These included marital difficulties, financial concerns, and problems with children at home. Their emotional resources were insufficient to handle the combined psychological and physical stresses associated with their diseases. Finally, these individuals had previously entertained suicidal thoughts, and some verbalized threats and made actual attempts on their lives.

Susan was 36 years old when she was diagnosed with malignant hepatocellular tumors. She had been taking oral contraceptive steroids for the past 12 years. She had presented with severe abdominal pain. There was hemorrhage into the tumor, but without rupture of the liver. Ligation of the hepatic artery was accomplished and a partial lobectomy was performed.

Although Susan survived the emergency procedures and her prognosis was judged favorable, a psychological consultation was requested because she spoke of suicide. In speaking with her it was clear that her thoughts about suicide were more general than specific. In fact, she confessed that she had not seriously thought about this prior to her hospitalization for the pain in her stomach. The thought of "cancer" had frightened her.

Susan was unmarried, though she had been involved in two long-term relationships that terminated prior to a marital commitment. The experience of a cancer diagnosis had triggered fears in her not only about her future but about her attractiveness to men as a possible mate. She was distrustful of the guarded optimism of the oncologists and surgeons. She had little confidence that she would get well. She was afraid that the cancer would spread and that she would be in terrible pain that would require more surgery, more hospitalizations, more restrictions, and ultimately death.

These thoughts were preoccupying her and she saw suicide as a peaceful way to resolve the problems. When the consultant expressed an understanding of the ways in which she felt, she became even more responsive. She seemed relieved to think that someone appreciated her reasoning. The consultant gently reinforced the conservative prognosis earlier offered to her by the house staff physicians. She listened more intently. Each of her concerns were explored, and she became actively engaged in the discussion. Her depression began to lift as the conversation progressed.

She thought that some opportunity for counseling after her discharge might be beneficial, and she expressed gratitude to the consultant for helping her to get a hold on her life. Her preoccupation with thoughts of suicide quickly subsided, although she still had fears about the cancer and more pain.

Clinicians working directly with oncology patients seem to agree that suicidal ideation does not correlate significantly with high lethality (Forman, 1979; Maxwell, 1980). Suicidal ideation, threats, and attempts can be efforts to cope with the stresses associated with the disease. Reich and Kelly (1976) report on two terminal cancer patients who attempted suicide at Boston's Peter Bent Brigham Hospital. Both of these cases were women who acted impulsively in response to information that the curative attempts to treat the cancers were proving unsuccessful. This information about the failure of the treatment program crushed their remaining defenses of denial; suicide was but an effort to cope.

If suicidal ideation and attempts are signals of the inadequacy of personal coping resources, professional intervention may be necessary and beneficial, as evident in the case of Susan noted above. Suicidal responses in cancer patients frequently have their genesis in the perception that they are being rejected by health care professionals and family members. In the cases cited above in the Reich and Kelly (1976) study, both women attempted suicide when they perceived that the doctors had tried everything possible and that they could do nothing more. Among the danger signals that professionals need to recognize in a cancer patient who may be highly vulnerable to suicide is the perception that he or she has no one to turn to. The lack of social supports—real or imagined—can be a decisive factor in a person's choice to end his or her own life. In Susan's case, she felt some genuine relationship with the consultant who listened and accepted her feelings. By demonstrating a willingness to discuss the issues that were triggering her suicidal thoughts, she was able to unburden herself and consider options other than self-destruction.

The issue of helplessness has surfaced in various contexts throughout this discussion of psychological aspects of cancer. It has its particular relevance to the topic of suicide. Helplessness, as we have seen, is tied to the issue of control. Too frequently, a patient who gives evidence of feeling helpless is treated with antidepressants. While this strategy might suppress affect, it does not deal at all with the psychological issue that the patient feels alone and helpless; pharmacologic treatment has the ironic effect of reinforcing this sense of being alone and misunderstood. Forman (1979) remarks that this type of intervention can possibly increase suicidal thoughts and further suicidal risk in the cancer patient.

In addition to careful efforts to reinforce and keep intact the psychological defensive mechanisms of the cancer patient, a supportive and collaborative team approach to care is the best insurance against the patient's attempting suicide. The team approach benefits from the comprehensive information that various individuals can provide about a patient. With knowledge about the specific physical, social, psychological, and spiritual needs of the individual, more effective ways to support the individual can be planned. In sum, this may be the best way to assist a cancer patient who may be at risk for choosing and attempting suicide.

Sexuality, Sexual Functioning, and Self-esteem

Cancer, its diagnosis and treatment, can be a mortal foe to the self-esteem of its victim. Perhaps this is no more apparent than in the way it can affect a person's sexuality. Human sexuality is not a simple variable. It describes not only physiological needs and drives but is a mirror of how a person feels about himself or herself. Sexuality is an important conduit for social expression and an important vehicle for significant human communication. Sexuality serves an important integrating function in ongoing personality development; somatic, emotional, intellectual, and social aspects of the self find an appropriate medium of expression through an individual's sexuality.

In the case cited earlier, Robert Beatty (1978) alluded to sexual issues in his initial reactions to his diagnosis of Stage Four prostatic cancer.

I had already told Louise, on the way home from the hospital. I don't think she said over a hundred words in response, but I do remember that when we returned to our apartment we spontaneously and tenderly made love, perhaps to prove to ourselves that there was still a lot of living for us, and that this wasn't the end of everything as we had known it. . . .

But I needed answers to a lot of things . . . Would there be any new treatments available soon? (None except experimental drugs.) Would I lose my potency? (In all likelihood.) What were my differing life expectancies if I followed different treatments, from doing nothing to immediate surgery, radiation, or chemotherapy? (All about the same.)

Scant attention has been paid to the effect that the presence and treatment of cancer may have on a person's sexual behavior. The resistance to talk about cancer is already very strong; to add another topic that traditionally has also been repressed in public discourse compounds resistivity. Whatever explains the reluctance to explore the impact of cancer on sexuality does not justify ignoring the issue, however. Human sexuality is too crucial a dimension of the human personality to be ignored or dismissed from discussion.

Lamb and Woods (1981) have broken the silence in an excellent treatment of sexuality and the cancer patient. They suggest that sexuality may have a particular meaning to a cancer patient. If sexuality and sexual expression convey being human and being alive, then interruptions or cessation of this mode of expression may communicate messages of dying and death to the individual. Older persons will not uncommonly supply such interpretations to the cessation of sexual interest and sexual expression. In a jocular communication an aging person might comment: "When I'm no longer interested in sex then you will know that I'm dead!" Somehow, sexuality symbolizes basic vitality, even though the particular meanings associated with it vary with each individual. Many of the jokes about losing one's sexual interests or ceasing one's sexual activities are attempts to reconcile the conflicts associated with death.

Sexuality as Support and Validation

If sexuality involves communication, then it requires receptivity and response. Cancer patients frequently speak about the withdrawal they sense from others. This involves not only those directly responsible for their care, but it can often include friends and family members. This withdrawal has many faces. On the most basic level, it may be avoidance or the unwillingness to be involved in more personal discussion and sharing. Open and free communication is a facet of sexual validation. With spouses, physical intimacy is a more profound expression of this personal validation. A gradual or sudden withdrawal of these sources of validation can intensify the personal pain and doubts of the cancer patient.

Sexuality, understood in this way, has either positive or negative potential. The negative outcome is evident; a person who perceives a withdrawal of support from significant others is vulnerable to depression and hopelessness that can thwart other therapeutic efforts. But human sexuality can be a powerful ally to both curative and palliative efforts. Not only does human responsiveness communicate acceptance and support, but it can sound a strong, humanizing chord in the otherwise cacophonous symphony of disease and its treatment. Persons with cancer may be seeking these forms of validation and support in the testing and demands that they frequently make of their doctors and nurses.

Because the diagnosis and treatment of the disease or a questionable prognosis may be eroding self-esteem, a cancer patient's demands for validation may be overstated and may be perceived by others to be unreasonable and alienating. It is precisely this issue of vulnerability of self-esteem that is the fundamental issue. Demanding behavior on the part of a cancer patient requires attention, interpretation, understanding, and response. Too frequently, the behavior is too quickly assessed and a strategy of behavioral modification through avoidance is adopted. While the behavioral objective might be secured, the patient might read the staff response as rejection and interpret this to mean, "No use being involved with me anymore; they've given up on me because I'm a goner." A cancer patient shared this interpretation with a consultant who was asked to speak with her because of her perceived emotional withdrawal and noncooperation with treatment. This may be a common perception among patients who appear depressed and withdrawn.

Sexuality and Self-esteem

When psychologists speak about *self-esteem*, they intend to describe the totality of the ways in which an individual thinks and feels about himself or herself. As such, it is a dynamic, comprehensive concept embracing facets of the self. These include a person's thoughts and feelings about his or her body and the ways in which it functions and how those features are perceived and judged by others. Self-esteem involves the ways individuals perceive themselves in relationships with other persons. These relationships include the most intimate and personal affiliations as well as relations with family, friends, professional, and business associates. Appreciation of self is measured in terms of what one does, by successes and failures. All of one's ethical principles, religious or spiritual values, and moral choices form a backdrop against which self-esteem is assessed.

Appreciation for the individual quality and comprehensive nature of self-esteem is important in assessing the ways in which the diagnosis and treatment of cancer can challenge it. This is of special importance in considering sexuality, since in many ways a person's sexuality is an important vehicle of self-esteem. It is important to note that the totality that is termed "self-esteem" is greater than any one of its component parts. In addressing this issue, Schain (1980) compared the psychological self-esteem system to a commercial banking system. She suggests that an individual is capable of establishing assets, recording debits, and rearranging his or her psychological currency to ensure operating at a profit.

There are infinite arrangements and permutations in which an individual can put in (deposit) and take out (withdraw) from his/her self-esteem bank account. Sometimes, however, the individual (patient in this case) seems fixated: restricted to an equilibrium (self-esteem balance) which works only fairly well and which may be subject to an impending major withdrawal as a result of radical cancer surgery. Such a crisis as this might require a sudden traumatic realignment of emotional currency due to changes in actual functioning. In addition, the patient may experience a depreciation or dimuntion of feelings of value and competence and should be encouraged to draw upon other resources to regain emotional equilibrium . . . (Schain, 1980, p. 17)

Cancer diagnosis and treatment and the life-death threats it presents to a person are often experienced as major drains on personal and familial psychological reserves. This extended crisis can quickly deplete resources and negatively affect self-esteem. Any efforts to assist a cancer patient need to be focused on realigning "emotional currency" and helping the person regain emotional control of remaining resources.

Cantor (1980) views cancer as a potentially devastating blow to a person's self-esteem, the proverbial "straw that breaks the camel's back." He correctly observes that cancer and the ordinary protocols used to treat it assault the private self-image that anchors self-esteem. Not only are these consequences seen in the fears of abandonment and withdrawal discussed earlier but they are also manifest in sexual dysfunction.

Cancer and Sexual Functioning

Despite the greater knowledge people have about cancer, some individuals may avoid intimate contact with their spouses for fear that they might also contract the disease. Women with cervical, endometrial, ovarian, or vulval cancer report that their husbands may be reluctant to be engaged in intercourse because they are afraid either of being infected by the cancer or of being harmed by the potential effects of the irradiation that is being utilized in its treatment. If the cancer requires a surgical intervention that creates a significant change in body appearance, as in the case of a radical vulvectomy, mastectomy, colostomy, or cystectomy, the person may sense some resistance in the sexual partner.

When diagnosis is terminal and aggressive treatment is not begun or suspended, people tend to assume that the dying person has no interest in or desire for sexual intimacy. While great variation will mark the patient's feelings about sexual relations during the terminal days and weeks of life and some of these feelings will be directly related to the site of the cancer and the extent of physical pain and discomfort, people should not necessarily conclude that the dying person has no need or desire for sexual expression.

The *well* spouse is understandably hesitant to be the initiator of sexual involvement with the *dying* partner. In some situations, the physician or the nurse who is caring for the dying person may discreetly explore this issue with the patient and provide counsel and encouragement to the patient. The patient may have to become the *initiator*, inviting the spouse to become sexually involved and providing information, understanding, and support for whatever fears and apprehensions might be blocking response. Occasionally, some of these issues can be anticipated in couples' groups that are routinely part of many inpatient education programs in hospitals and clinics. Lamb and Woods (1981) appropriately observe that for people who are dying, sexuality can be a "part of being alive, a means of enriching a cherished relationship" (p. 140).

Assisting cancer patients and terminally ill individuals with sexual needs and concerns is not something that many nurses or doctors are comfortable in doing. Some would question the prudence and appropriateness of such interventions. Stereotypes about human sexuality and personal biases may effectively block interventions. Obviously, therapeutic discussions of this issue with a cancer patient and/or his or her spouse require their trust and respect and much discretion on the part of the one providing the counsel.

Hospitals are not normal environments; a patient's privacy is frequently invaded and routine delivery of care interrupts a family's attempt to restore a degree of normalcy to relationships with the ill or dying person. To encourage sexual expression in this milieu requires significant effort on the part of the hospital or nursing home staff. In addition to providing the basic requirements of privacy and time, health care professionals must help couples to explore alternate ways of expressing physical affection that take into consideration the physical limitations of the sick or dying person. Lamb and Woods (1981) have presented some reasonable and useful guidelines for nurses involved in cancer patient care; their work could be of service to anyone similarly involved. To benefit from these practical suggestions, the nurse or physician must first assess their appropriateness and determine the place that sexuality and sexual expression have in the psychological life of a cancer patient. In any effort of this sort by a health care professional, the needs and desires of the patient in relation to his or her spouse are of paramount importance. The most important service the caregiver can provide is to seek the most appropriate ways in which the needs and desires of the cancer patient can be fulfilled.

Summary

The history of medicine documents an abiding interest in the relationship between physical pathology and psychological functioning. In modern and contemporary medicine, this relationship continues to invite speculation and research. As the exploration goes forward to determine the origin of cancer, the psychophysiological hypothesis provides a rich avenue for research.

Opinion varies concerning the role that mental processes play in the etiology of cancer. Some scientists deny any role at all to psychological factors, claiming that cancer exclusively and autonomously involves cellular transformation. Others entertain the hypothesis that psychological processes may function as homeostatic regulators, exercising influence not only over mood and affect, but over other somatic functions as well. Research using biofeedback methods lends some support to this line of reasoning. However, little controlled psychobiological research data exist to support a psychophysiological hypothesis of carcinogenesis.

One of the theoretical approaches to the study of the relationship between psychological variables and cancer is grounded in the study of personality. Allport (1937) defined personality as "a dynamic organization within the individual of those biosocial systems that determine his or her unique adjustment to the world." Adaptation—physical and psychological—depends to a great extent on the ways in which biological and social influences are organized and interact with the environment. Personality may be a key to understanding why some people may be more susceptible than others to cancer.

The concept of a *precancerous personality* inspired the longitudinal studies in the 1940s of students at Johns Hopkins Medical School. The data from these studies continue to be analyzed retrospectively in the hope of identifying certain traits that might be linked to the development of particular forms of cancer. While this type of research is intriguing, it has failed to maintain active support from many scientists. Although the few studies that continue to be published strongly suggest a relationship between personality and cancer, it would be imprudent to overgeneralize their findings (Greer, 1979).

Other researchers have systematically attempted to isolate certain psychosocial predictors of cancer. Issues of stress, expression of needs and feelings, experiences of loss and separation have been studied in relationship to cancer. Although the various studies discussed in this chapter are inconclusive, they do underscore the potential importance that psychosocial factors may play in the development of cancer. None is judged to be a sufficient precondition for the development of cancer.

Psychosomatic research continues to consider the role that psychological stimuli may play in altering the activities of the body's immune and endocrine systems, as illustrated by the *catecholamine hypothesis*. There is evidence that a link exists between changes in CNS catecholamine metabolism and affective disorders. Study of the biological activities of the catecholamines and corticosteroids leads one to consider the role such psychologically induced physical changes might play in the development of cancer. Immunopathogenesis is a new frontier in psychobiological reseach.

Not only are psychological issues important in the genesis of cancer, psychological factors play an important role in the control and management of the disease. The chapter reviewed a number of important topics related to the care and treatment of the cancer patient.

Communication is both a science and an art. It is a science inasmuch as it involves a body of information that is shared and received. It is an art because it relies upon interpersonal abilities, nuance and sensitivity, timing and method. Many health care professionals find it extremely difficult reconciling the scientific and artistic aspects of communication with a victim of cancer. Numerous specific questions challenge the success of this important communication.

The issue of what, when, and how much to tell the cancer patient has been regularly debated among physicians. Traditionally, physicians have been reluctant to share much information with a patient. Recent surveys indicate that physicians are more inclined to be open with a cancer patient; whether they are more communicative in clinical practice is difficult to assess. Adults express a strong preference to know the available information concerning diagnosis, prognosis, and available options for therapeutic or palliative care.

The issue of *informed consent* continues to attract much attention in medico-ethical discussion. According to this ethical principle, a patient has a right to know his or her diagnosis and must be appropriately informed concerning treatment strategies. Informed consent implies effective and successful communication, not simply the presentation of information to a patient. Studies have demonstrated that the emotional disequilibrium experienced by a patient confronted with a serious medical diagnosis may effectively block communication efforts. Professionals need to take these psychological reactions into consideration as they attempt to ensure that a patient is completely and appropriately informed and freely consents to proposed treatment plans.

Communication about cancer can be obstructed by the misinformation and misconception already surrounding the disease. These distortions in knowledge and experience can color a person's perceptions and responses. A patient may likewise fall prey to the ambivalent, mixed messages coming from physicians and nurses, from family members and friends.

Other environmental stresses complicate the world of a cancer patient. Some of these are directly associated with the practice of medicine and are generally described as *iatrogenic*. Medicine commands a significant power and physicians are perceived agents of this power. For a patient with cancer the patient-physician power equation can be imbalanced to such a degree that he or she feels powerless. This situation can become the catalyst for still further negative reactions, including withdrawal, doubts, resistance, and compliance.

Medicine, as currently practiced in its many specializations, can be quite impersonal. This context of clinical practice may prevent patients from properly understanding various aspects of their treatment and contribute to their feelings of isolation. In an effort to cooperate with and please a physician, a patient may become increasingly passive and dependent. Each of these stresses can mentally cripple a person, thus weakening the important psychological component of healing.

Psychological defenses serve an important function in helping an individual to cope with a critical situation. The specific repertory of coping strategies used by a person is unique to that person. However, a person's style of coping will be influenced by the experience the person has gained in previous efforts to manage crises. This chapter considered some of the ways in which people manage cancer in its various stages: the period of initial diagnosis and the often extended period of treatment.

Two important sociopsychological theories were reviewed with respect to the crisis of diagnosis: *reactance theory* and *learned helplessness*. Each of these theoretical constructs can help to explain what contributes to a particular behavioral response to a perceived threat. If a person feels in control, he or she may respond positively to the threat. If, conversely, the person feels out of control, then withdrawal, passivity, and depression may be the behavioral consequence. The reactive depressions frequently observed among cancer patients may be partially explained by reactance theory.

The psychological aspects of cancer treatment have received far less study than the medical factors. When certain therapies produce pronounced neurological side effects with behavioral disturbance, psychiatric consultations are often requested. Two of the more common disturbances are depressions and suicidal ideation. The chapter explored both of these topics as they touch on the diagnosis and staging of treatments for cancer. Both of these psychiatric problems can be attempts by the cancer patient to cope with the stresses associated with the disease; they must be understood in this important context. They can either be efforts to cope or signals of the inadequacy of personal coping resources. It is vital to ascertain the meaning of the behaviors before embarking on a therapeutic program.

A final issue explored in this chapter is sexuality. Sexuality is an important conduit for social expression, for human communication. Somatic, emotional, intellectual, and social aspects of the self seek expression through one's sexuality. Our discussion has explored some aspects of the impact of cancer and its treatment on sexuality, sexual functioning, and self-esteem. We have considered the important ways in which sexuality can help to support and validate a cancer patient. The link between sexuality and self-esteem is important, since self-esteem is tied to the ways a person thinks and feels about himself or herself. Since cancer puts significant stress on a person's self-esteem (both physically and psychologically), it is important to assess how sexuality may serve to maintain self-esteem during this extended crisis.

In surveying the psychological factors that have some bearing on the etiology and treatment of cancer, this chapter has highlighted issues that are currently the object of research and related some of these issues to problems encountered in clinical practice with cancer patients and their families. From these various analyses, it is evident that the individual psychology of the patient must be given appropriate consideration in the whole process of providing care. An individual's psychological organization may have contributed not only to the development of the disease but may be likewise crucial to the success or failure of efforts to treat it.

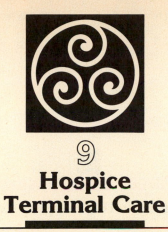

⑨
Hospice
Terminal Care

Introduction: The Hospice Concept

The Management of Terminal Disease

- Palliative Versus Curative Care

- The Polypharmacology of Hospice Care

- Related Physical, Psychological, and Spiritual Concerns of the Terminally Ill

Flexible Approaches to the Care of the Terminally Ill

- Psychosocial Needs of the Dying Person

- Family Members: Primary Hospice Workers in a Home Care Setting

- Continuity of Care: the Inpatient Hospice

Hospice Bereavement Services

- Initial Viewing of the Body after Death

- Funeral Rites

- Contacts with Surviving Family Members

Closure to Hospice Care

Summary

Introduction: The Hospice Concept

In 1947 an English medical social worker encountered a 40-year-old man with inoperable cancer. He was in considerable physical pain, and depressed by the realization of what he judged to be an unfulfilled life. In the course of their relationship during the final weeks of his life, David Tasma and Cicely Saunders shared many dreams. They spoke of the kind of a place and the quality of care that would best respond to his needs. From these conversations and shared experiences, Saint Christopher's Hospice was born, founded on a philosophy for the care of the terminally ill that has since taken root in many other countries.

David Tasma bequeathed 500 pounds sterling to Cicely Saunders to be a "window in your home." In 1967 that home opened its doors to the public and since that time more than eight thousand terminally ill patients and their families have gazed through its windows and have benefitted from the care of Dr. Saunders and her dedicated staff. Reflecting on the original inspiration she received from her relationship with David Tasma, Dr. Saunders wrote these verses in the Hospice poetry workshop:

STARTING POINT—FOR DAVID TASMA

Only forty years old—
No one to leave,
Nothing done for good or ill
For the world to remember.
A leaf floats down the river
And is lost forever,
No trace left behind.

Someone comes to listen,
I find I have something to say.
I remember—a child in Warsaw—
The Rabbi, my grandfather,
Calls me down from bed,
Makes me talk far into the night
Search out the ways of God.

Somehow,
In the years between
I lost all thoughts of God—
And I never found myself.

In the busy ward
I come to the end of life
I find a friend
Who offers mind and heart.
A window opens
And, gently, the God of my fathers
Calls me home.
Now only—I begin.

So I will leave a window.
Who will look through it
And find there
His own starting point?

Although modern comprehensive care of the terminally ill has its roots in the concepts and procedures developed at Saint Christopher's, this is not the first organization to arise from a humanistic concern for the dying. Stoddard (1978) provides a careful survey of the many precursors of the modern hospice movement and documents the numerous efforts by religious groups in the United States during the early part of this century to provide care for the terminally ill.

This chapter will discuss the principal components of the hospice philosophy of comprehensive care for terminally ill persons, not only as it relates to their physical needs but also as it relates to their emotional, psychosocial, and spiritual needs and those of their families. Since pain control is of paramount importance, considerable attention will be devoted to this topic. Home care is an important dimension of a hospice program. This will be discussed with particular emphasis on the practical issues involved in making it possible for a person to live the final days of his or her life at home. Finally, the bereavement follow-up program with families of hospice patients will be examined and evaluated.

The contemporary hospice movement has been viewed with caution by the medical community in the United States. It is fair to observe that medical education has not only neglected the topic of death and dying in its curriculum, but it has resisted a serious engagement with the principles of palliative care explicit in the hospice philosophy. The trend in contemporary American medicine toward holistic care may narrow the gap that exists between traditional approaches to terminal care and those represented by the hospice principles. It is the purpose of this chapter to attempt to bridge that chasm, providing health care professionals with an opportunity to consider terminal care from an enlarged perspective.

The Management of Terminal Disease

Palliative Versus Curative Care

One of the most difficult realities that physicians must confront is that, despite their best efforts and the most sophisticated procedures and technologies, nothing more can be done to cure the disease processes threatening a patient's life. Some physicians resist this conclusion and will not accept the fact that their science is finite. Determined to keep the patient's hopes alive, they may elect a course of treatment that is often experimental, painful, costly, and of dubious potential benefit. Contrasted with this approach is *palliative care*, which attempts to marshall the best medical wisdom to alleviate symptomatic pain associated with certain terminal diseases (Buckingham, 1983; Butterfield-Picard & Magno, 1982; Cohen, 1979; Garner, 1976; Gotay, 1983; Koff, 1980).

Doris Morrison is a 52-year-old married woman with breast cancer with metastases to the lungs and bones. A radical mastectomy was performed, followed by an adrenalectomy [removal of the adrenal glands] and oophorectomy [removal of the ovaries]. She received radiotherapy to the bony metastases as well as chemotherapy.

Upon consultation with her physicians and spouse, she has elected to discontinue aggressive treatment. She desires to be at home, and has requested the services of a hospice home care team. Her physical complaints principally involve great difficulties in breathing, and relatively constant pain in her chest area. She is very aware of the nature of her illness and is open in discussing it with her doctors and husband, but she is reluctant to deal with her diagnosis with her children. She reasons that until her condition deteriorates further there is no need to burden them with the fact that she is going to die.

The hospice team made a careful assessment of her condition and, in consultation with her doctors, discontinued the prescription of codeine and Demerol that she had been taking for pain management. In its place they began a program of morphine (5 mg) and prochlorperazine [Stemetil] (5 mg), 4 times a day. In addition, they provided a portable oxygen set to assist her breathing.

The hospice philosophy, which emphasizes the importance of the quality of life for the dying person and his or her family, recognizes that certain diseases are resistant to curative efforts and as such require different care and management. It is important to note that even when curative efforts fail, appropriate treatment is still required.

Too often physicians feel a certain degree of personal failure when their curative efforts do not succeed; effective palliative care continues to challenge their skills and abilities as long as the patient continues to live. The termination of curative efforts should not be seen as the *surrender* of the physician. That decision simply refocuses the goals and objectives of care from cure to assisting the person to live whatever time remains in the most comfortable and supportive way possible.

Perhaps the hospice concept has been misunderstood as an adversary of the traditional goals of curative treatment efforts. Decisions governing treatment of life-threatening diseases are the privileged domain of *both* patient and physician. In arriving at determinations concerning treatment, they must balance the potential of success against the risks, pain, side effects, and economic and emotional costs. It is only when reasonable curative efforts have been attempted and exhausted or when the patient and physician mutually agree to discontinue treatment that hospice care is undertaken. Humanistic terminal care champions the patient's right to be informed concerning the strategies of curative treatment and his or her ultimate and decisive prerogative to accept, discontinue, or refuse such treatment. Patient advocacy of this sort may be the point of conflict dividing traditional curative medicine and hospice methods of care.

Palliative care is dedicated to the goal of ensuring that dying persons maintain whatever control is possible during their final days of life (Garner, 1976). To this end, every effort is made to alleviate the physical pain that frequently accompanies the terminal phases of certain diseases. Experience with many terminally ill persons has confirmed the fact that the greatest fear of dying persons is not death, but the pain that accompanies dying (Glassman & Popkin, 1980). Saunders and Baines (1983) contend that terminal pain is often treated ineptly and that the fears of terminally ill individuals are not illusions but have grounding in fact.

When a person is diagnosed with a life-threatening disease, acute care strategies for treatment are frequently administered. The patient, feeling powerless, surrenders control and accepts invasive and often painful treatments. These are understood to be the short-term costs for the long-term benefit of cure. The calculus is quite different in palliative care. Care is no longer focused on the disease itself but rather on the ways in which the progress of that disease is affecting the dying person and his or her family. The emphasis in palliative care is not on the treatment of the disease but on continual efforts to treat the symptoms and effects of an incurable disease. By attending to the nature of the patient's pain, the specific sites where it is felt, and the possible causes for it, health care professionals can plan effective ways to manage and alleviate such affliction (Ryndes & Brown, 1981, 1982). Twycross (1981) and others believe that lack of training and experience may explain some physicians' inadequacies in responding to terminally ill patients. These same physicians may be unaware of the state of the art in pain control (Baines, 1984; Barber & Gitelson, 1980; Bonica & Ventafridda, 1979; Doyle, 1982; Lipman, 1979; Mount, Melzack, & MacKinnon, 1978; Noyes, 1981; Saunders & Baines, 1983; Twycross, 1980a,b).

The Polypharmacology of Hospice Care

Neoplastic disease may not be initially painful, but as it progresses in its terminal course, the level of both physiological and psychological pain tends to increase (Noyes, 1981; Twycross, 1978a,c). There are many reasons why the physical pain of terminally ill persons goes untreated. When aggressive curative treatment is aborted, some afflicted individuals may believe that everything possible has already been done, including the management of their pain. They may engage in efforts to mask the extent of their physical suffering in order to protect their families from additional upset (Bass, 1983; Krant & Johnston, 1977).

On the other hand, a physician may neither perceive the extent of the individual's pain nor be aware of effective ways to manage it (Baines, 1984). Some may too quickly resort to some standard drugs prescribed on a *pro re nata* (p.r.n.) basis, that is, as circumstances require. Instructions for use and determinations of standard doses of drugs that are derived from clinical studies may be judged effective in ordinary medical practice, but they may not be generally efficacious in the management of terminal cancer pain.

Analgesics

The initial goal of pain management is to *titrate* the analgesic with relation to the dying person's pain, modulating the dose until the person is pain-free. Specifically, **titration** means finding out how much of a certain substance is contained in a solution by measuring how much of another substance it is necessary to add to the solution in order to produce a given reaction. In the context of titrating a drug to relieve pain, the given reaction is a pain-free state in the suffering patient. Concomitant objectives are that the person be alert and that the effect of the drug endure as long as possible. To achieve the end result may require several days of trial adjustments, but never at the cost of the principal goal of pain control. The timing of drug administrations is crucial; regular medications in anticipation of need replace orders "as required" or "on demand." In this way, the patient is never faced with the situation wherein medication has worn off and pain returns (Saunders, 1963).

Shortly after Doris began the new medication protocol she acknowledged that she had pain and discomfort. She was still anxious about shortness of breath, particularly when she exerted herself in the slightest way. She also noted that she was experiencing some problems with bowel movements. A stimulating agent [bisacodyl] was prescribed, since bulk-producing cathartics were not effective for her.

Her chest X-ray revealed new destructive lesions on her ribs and a small pleural effusion. Further irradiation was not indicated since this area had already received maximum dose.

Within a week, the pain was returning within 3 hours of the ingestion of the medication. The morphine mixture was titrated to 10 mg. q4h.

The preferred route of medication is by mouth rather than by injection. Apart from the obvious differences in these two approaches, the oral medication has distinct advantages. As mentioned earlier, it is important to safeguard whatever control the dying person can maintain. Injections foster dependence and are often experienced as invasive, emergency responses to critical situations. They provide immediate response to the re-emergence of pain. The oral preparation, taken in anticipation of a "crisis of reemergence," puts pain control and management into the hands of the terminally ill person and his or her primary caregivers and avoids medication becoming psychologically associated with crisis.

Some physicians are reluctant to become involved in the prescription of *analgesics*, especially the more potent of this group. In classic usage, analgesics, or *pain killers*, have been grouped under three categories, graded according to their efficacy: nonnarcotic, weak narcotic, and strong narcotic. Aspirin or an alternative nonsteroid antiinflammatory drug (for example, flurbiprofen) may be useful in treating a mild terminal pain throughout the course of an illness. Dextropropoxyphene with paracetamol (Darvon) continues to be used for this purpose. Just as aspirin has been successfully used in the treatment of pain related to osteoarthritis and rheumatoid arthritis, it is likewise helpful in managing some bone and joint pain in terminal disease.

Because aspirin is such a common drug in the experience of many people, there may be some doubt in their minds about its potential to manage pain. Gentle encouragement to use aspirin, along with careful attention to any gastric upset that a regular regimen of aspirin ingestion may cause, not only can adequately manage the pain but may also respond to deeper psychological needs for assurance and care.

The weak narcotic group of drugs is useful in controlling moderate pain. A wide variety of effective, approximately equianalgesic preparations are available, often combined with codeine (for example, dihydrocodeine). One frequent side effect of these combined drugs is constipation. Darvon is less constipating than dihydrocodeine. Experience at Saint Christopher's and other hospices has been that the use of pentazocine (Talwin), an agonist-antagonist, has little usefulness in terminal pain management. Not only is the drug relatively short acting, but too many patients experience psychotomimetic effects, including hallucinations, distortions of perception, and schizophrenic-type behaviors.

Some physicians are reluctant to utilize strong narcotic drugs (diamorphine, levorphanol, methadone, morphine) in the treatment of terminally ill persons. These doctors may harbor fears that the patient will become physiologically addicted if such potent narcotic analgesics are prescribed. Terminally ill persons in chronic pain have different physiological and pharmacological responses to drugs; moreover, the fear of addiction is considered by many professionals to be a moot point in the discussion of the pain control of terminally ill persons. Twycross (1974) reported that when narcotics are administered on a regular schedule, there is no psychological dependence. This same conclusion has been reported by others (Saunders, 1963). Controlling pain pharmacologically, even with potent narcotic analgesics, does not appear to trigger drug-seeking behavior commonly observed in non–terminally ill drug-addicted persons. Even when abrupt withdrawal occurs, withdrawal symptoms are mild and do not mimic those noted in drug addicts (Walsh & Cheater, 1983).

Cautious physicians may choose a less potent drug that may prove to be too weak to alleviate the pain adequately. However, oral morphine and dia-morphine (5–10 mg oral morphine) may prove to be the most valuable cur-rent drugs used to control pain (Saunders & Baines, 1983). Twycross (1981) considers morphine sulphate in solution as the most versatile drug; when in-jections are necessary, diamorphine or another opiate of high solubility is often the drug of choice. Sustained-release morphine sulphate has been dem-onstrated to remain effective for 12 hours without accumulation during contin-ued therapy.

Morphine (2.5–180 mg every 4 hours) is absorbed well when taken orally and reaches a peak blood level between 90 and 120 minutes after ingestion (Walsh & Cheater, 1983). Morphine sulphate and morphine hydrochloride are both available and Baines (1983) reports them as interchangeable. One ob-vious benefit is that the drug can be easily increased to respond to the pa-tient's needs without significantly increasing either the volume of intake (usu-ally about 10 ml) or the medication schedule (every 4 hours). Morphine is often begun when mild, nonnarcotic or weak narcotic preparations are judged to be inadequate to control pain.

Walsh and Cheater (1983) note that between 85 and 90 percent of patients with pain from advanced cancer can effectively be helped with an oral admin-istration of morphine. An initial dose of 5 mg of morphine in a 10 ml aqueous solution may be satisfactory. For some this may be a suboptimal dose, but it can be adjusted to need while providing an improvement in pain manage-ment. Drowsiness may accompany the shift to stronger narcotics, but within a short period of time the person will adjust to the drug. Adjuvants of the phenothiazine family (chlorpromazine [Thorazine], prochlorperazine [Com-pazine]) are useful in counteracting the side effects of chemically induced nausea and vomiting, which frequently accompany morphine usage. Twy-cross (1981) often uses haloperidol (Haldol) because it is nonsedative and does not cause the mouth dryness associated with other similar drugs. An-other side effect of morphine, already noted, is constipation. Twycross (1981), in discussing the use of laxatives and bowel softeners (for example, Dorbane), observes that unless carefully monitored, constipation may be more difficult to control than pain.

Arthur Lipman, an American clinical pharmacist, was an early associate of Dr. Saunders and Dr. Twycross at Saint Christopher's and has become an expert in pain management of terminally ill persons. He maintains that phar-macology has traditionally taught that oral morphine sulphate is poorly ab-sorbed; while this may be correct, it is important to note that morphine sul-phate is consistently absorbed (Lipman, 1979). The more recent findings of Walsh and Cheater (1983) claim that, used correctly, oral morphine is a reliable, safe, and effective analgesic in patients with advanced malignant disease.

Lipman expresses a preference for methadone (Dolophine) for hospice pa-tients, especially because of its long-acting nature, even though certain phar-macokinetic research does not seem to support his own accumulated clinical experience in 15 years of association with a number of hospice programs. The doses titrated for certain patients' needs may seem to be high, but megadoses are common. Terminally ill individuals in chronic pain seem to have more demanding biochemical needs that require such considerable doses. One concern is that methadone accumulates and is not as easily excreted as are morphine and diamorphine.

The course of a particular disease process may prevent a patient from taking oral medication. As noted before, injections are avoided whenever possible. Certain effective analgesics are available in rectal suppositories; these are particularly beneficial to those who are caring for the terminally ill person at home. Oxymorphone hydrochloride (Numorphan), hydromorphone hydrochloride (Dilaudid), and oxyocodone pectinate (Percodan, Tylox) have been reported to be effective.

Twycross (1981) notes that with cancer, one is confronted with a *progressive* pathological process. As such, one must be vigilant for the emergence of new pains or the reemergence of ones previously controlled. The pharmacology of cancer does not simply mean increasing a once effective analgesic. Hospice care demands constant reassessment and evaluation done in close consultation with the patient before new pain control protocols are mounted. Any change in medication can effect a change in lifestyle. These changes are not undertaken without careful consideration of all of the implications of such a program. The patient's well-being and comfort always remain the paramount concern of care.

Mrs. Morrison's disease was progressing rapidly. Although the increase in the morphine mixture seemed to contain the pain, she did complain of difficulties sleeping during the night hours. To address this problem, the morphine was increased to 15 mg at 11 P.M. and the other 3 daily administrations were left at 10 mg. This seemed to help her sleep better and she often did not awake in the morning with any pain.

The symptoms of shortness of breath continued and she relied frequently on the oxygen.

It is not velleity of hospice medical personnel that decides that pain be controlled. The goal of a pain-free state is achievable in more than 85 percent of the patients treated (Twycross, 1979).Dr. Balfour Mount and his colleagues at the Royal Victoria Hospital Palliative Care Unit in Montreal judge their success rate in pain management to be similar to that of Twycross but report that within their inpatient service their success rate may rise to 90 percent (Mount, Melzack, & McKinnon, 1978). With demonstrated success of this sort, patients can and must be told that to a significant degree their pain will be effectively managed. Although the pain control process may take some time, most patients will feel some alleviation within the first 24–48 hours after treatment has begun.

Nerve Blocks

In some situations, for example in nerve compression pain, the patient's suffering is best addressed by performing a **nerve block**. Not only does such a procedure frequently lessen the need for high doses of narcotics, but such a procedure may facilitate the return of some degree of normal functioning. The nerve block can produce dramatic relief from pain without significant side effects (Doyle, 1982a, b). These blocks tend to interrupt the nerve pathways that mediate pain. Because the peripheral nerves in most regions of the body can be blocked, this procedure is useful in treating specific areas of pain that may not be responsive to certain forms of drug treatment.

Palliative Irradiation

Saunders and Baines (1983) comment that palliative irradiation may be beneficial. Unlike aggressive curative radiotherapeutic treatments, the goals of **palliative irradiation** are quite different. The sole purpose of these interventions is the relief of pain, for example in certain metastases of the bone or in tumor reduction. One of the most attractive aspects of this modality of treatment is its noninvasive quality. However, the anticipated effect of such a procedure must be balanced against the cost to the patient in terms of time and side effects.

If the intended results can be accomplished with relatively few treatments, then radiotherapy may be a most helpful resource in pain management. Irradiation can also retard the growth of tumors. Saunders and Baines (1983) utilize irradiation to relieve **hemoptysis** (expectoration of blood) and **hematuria** (blood in the urine), which can be distressing not only to the patient but to family members who are unaccustomed to blood discharge. Finally, x-rays may effectively treat fungation and vaginal discharge. Because of its potential benefits, irradiation may be a very useful procedure for terminally ill persons.

Related Physical, Psychological, and Spiritual Concerns of the Terminally Ill

Pain is a comprehensive term describing many aspects of the terminal disease process. Hospice care concerns itself with all of the interrelated sources of pain, which may be specifically related to the physical dimensions of the course of disease or linked to psychosocial or spiritual problems. Physical discomfort is more readily identified and effectively remedied than psychosocial or spiritual stresses, which may be difficult to recognize and address. Some pain may be psychophysiological. Since hospice care is committed to total response to the various needs of terminally ill persons, it attends to all of the varied sources of pain.

Breathing Difficulties

An individual may suffer from difficulties related to breathing. As in ordinary medical practice, care must be taken to isolate the cause of the **dyspnea** (for example, difficult or painful breathing) and to undertake appropriate treatment. The causes of breathing difficulties may be cardiac, exertional, expiratory or inspiratory, or renal, to name a few. Saunders and Baines (1983) have identified a number of drugs that they have found useful in treating breathing difficulties in numerous terminal patients. Included in this list are glucocorticosteroids, antibiotics, opiates, and hyoscine. In addition, the phenothiazine and benzodiazepine tranquillizers can be useful in calming the person who is anxious because of problems encountered in breathing.

Complications that affect normal breathing patterns can symbolically represent for the patient the closeness of death and thereby entail much emotional energy. While the specific group of drugs mentioned above may adequately ease or relieve a specific breathing difficulty, the patient may require additional support to process what the experience means.

As the weeks passed Mrs. Morrison developed bronchospasms. She told the hospice nurse that these bronchial contractions really frightened her; she often wondered if she would be able to catch her breath or whether this would be the way she would die. She admitted that these episodes concerned her greatly. Ventolin inhalations seem to address this problem and appear to considerably relieve the anxiety associated with these attacks.

Breathing, for many persons, is the primary evidence of life. Having difficulty with breathing may be doubly painful; not only does it cause physical stress, but the psychological pain may be even more stressful. It is not sufficient, as hospice practice has verified, simply to address the physical source of distress: it is equally important to provide some specific support to the person who may be troubled by the psychological meanings linked to the physical pain.

Insomnia

An oft-repeated wish expressed by many people is that they die peacefully in their sleep. In fact, sleep is a poignant paradigm for death—the poets have often referred to the "sleep of death." A terminally ill person, even one who has accepted diagnosis and prognosis, may harbor some residual fears about sleeping and never awakening. The wish to die peacefully in one's sleep addresses a preference to be free of pain and free of consciousness. However, for a person who *knows* that death is imminent, the act of falling asleep can be fraught with anxiety. While resisting sleep, dying persons may become anxious about not being able to sleep. Desire and fear pull equally in their trying to fall asleep or remain awake. One way in which some patients resolve this conflict is by taking many short naps.

Constant pain may also deprive a person of an integral night's sleep and may make him or her despair of ever being able to find refuge in sleep. Since pain is not only physical but also psychological, the quiet of night and the diminished involvement of others in providing care and support may intensify the suffering of the terminally ill person and prevent sleep.

It would be a facile solution to seek immediate resolution of the problem of sleep disruption in the prescription of **hypnotics**. Direct pain relief is the first-order priority; unless a patient specifically requests one of the long-acting benzodiazepines (for example, Valium), these should be avoided. The goal of pain management, as has been mentioned before, is to minimize the degree of sedation while alleviating the pain. If the physical source of the painful symptoms has been successfully managed, the patient may simply require a bit of personal reassurance and encouragement. A short-acting benzodiazepine may be helpful owing to its anxiolytic action, but interpersonal contact may more effectively diffuse the anxiety that is disrupting the patient's sleep.

Anorexia

A lack or loss of appetite for food may be a problem for some terminally ill persons. This can be explained by a variety of reasons. Choosing not to eat may be a sign that an individual has given up a desire to continue living or may be a side effect of medication. Since the hospice, in principle, sees little place in its philosophy of care for nasogastric tube feeding or intravenous fluid treatments, the problems associated with eating are of particular interest and concern to hospice programs.

Certain drug protocols can cause nausea and induce vomiting. For this reason, great care is taken to include antiemetics in treatment programs. Thorazine and Compazine are often quite effective if the vomiting is related to biochemical alterations. Occasionally, a person has difficulty in gastric emptying; metoclopramide (Reglan), taken before meal time, can effectively respond to this problem. If the vomiting is more difficult to manage, the use of an antihistimine such as cyclizine (Marezine) may be effective. Regardless of other reasons for lack of appetite, a person is unlikely to be receptive to meals and eating unless nausea and vomiting are under control.

During the early weeks of her home care program, Mrs. Morrison retained her appetite. Her children assumed responsibility for preparing her meals and the family often enjoyed informal eating together in her bedroom. As the disease progressed, she ate less and preferred to eat a softer diet.

Fortunately, throughout the entire course of her terminal period, she was not troubled with either nausea or vomiting.

Another common side effect of certain medication protocols and certain disease processes is a dry or sore mouth. Oral hygiene is a primary concern of hospice nursing. A foul-tasting mouth does not make eating a pleasurable experience. Mouthwashes can be used effectively to prepare an individual before mealtimes.

Hospice dieticians are acutely sensitive to the problems of their patients and are creative about enhancing the eating experience. At Hospice, Inc., in Branford, Connecticut, the culinary department is headed by a chef who has distinguished herself for artistic achievements in her profession. She has brought her skills to bear on the specific problems encountered by her patients and has devised numerous ways to respond to the specific eating problems of terminally ill persons. All of the meals served to patients are attractively presented, incorporating different textures, colors, and garnishes. The goal of the dietary department is to make mealtime as pleasant an experience for the patient as is possible.

Body Image and Self-esteem

The way a person looks can subjectively affect the way he or she feels. These feelings, in turn, can affect experiences and behavior. Neoplastic disease, in its terminal phases, can significantly alter body image. Such alteration is an added source of stress to the dying person. Not only does this include major changes in the body resulting from cancer and its treatment but superficial changes that can be very noticeable.

Excessive sweating and discharging wounds or sores can create unpleasant odors that are not only offensive to the afflicted person but may make it difficult for family and caregivers to relate to him or her. Aggressively treating sources of odor can do much to boost the person's morale. Besides presenting specific problems in effective nursing care, a fungating lesion, vaginal or rectal discharge, poor bladder control due to weakening muscle control, and diarrhea or more chronic incontinence can have a demoralizing impact on the terminally ill patient.

Shaving, grooming, and the application of cosmetics and perfumes can provide a tremendous boost to a person who is terminally ill. Not only does the attention and care make the individual feel better, but the effect of the care may elicit positive and favorable reactions from other family and other staff. It is important to maximize the potential of the terminally ill person; whatever can be done to keep the body image intact should be attempted. As long as a person is able to perform cosmetic functions independently, he or she should be encouraged and assisted to do so. Otherwise others should continue to address them. Since personality tends to be stable throughout life, even to death, it is imperative to assess how important certain aspects of body image are to a given individual. What may be unimportant to one person may be vitally important to another. To the degree that these aspects of self can be maintained, a person will feel better about himself or herself and be more satisfied with life.

When the hospice volunteers arrived Mrs. Morrison was very depressed. She had lost considerable weight and her complexion was quite sallow. As a result of the earlier chemotherapy program she had lost her hair and the new growth was slow and spotty. Although she had a wig, she was not wearing it.

After the volunteers had assisted her to bathe, they suggested that they might help her to apply some cosmetics. Although she resisted the suggestion at first, she agreed. They combed and arranged her wig, gave her a facial, applied makeup, and gave her a manicure and pedicure.

When her daughters arrived later they each commented on how much better their mother seemed to them and how much improved her spirits were. She joked with them that she was "Queen for the day."

Spiritual Pain

A discussion of the pain associated with terminal illness might not ordinarily include the topic of religion and spirituality. However, when pain is considered comprehensively, not only are physical and psychological dimensions germane to the dialogue, but religious components also require attention and response (Gibbs & Achterberg, 1978).

Spiritual suffering of some terminally ill persons cannot be managed in the same way as biochemical and biophysical processes that cause pain. Analgesics and nerve blocks will not be effective in managing this kind of pain. In fact, the way in which this form of suffering is relieved is by appropriate, sensitive, and effective interpersonal intervention. Twycross (1980a, b) maintains that the control of chronic pain has as much to do with the spiritual and psychological concerns of the dying person as it has to do with what drugs are administered.

Although many individuals can be helpful relieving spiritual pain, a hospital chaplain, rabbi, minister, deacon, or priest may be the most appropriate one to make this effort. In some cases, the expressed need may be minimal, if dying is situated in the context of a life of active religious faith and practice, for dying has its legitimate place in the continuity of personal religious experience and belief. In other cases, the dying person may not have been significantly involved with organized religion for many years. Proximity to death and the comprehensive life review it often evokes sometimes reawakens religious feeling.

Terminal illness, as a crisis, may set in motion a coping style that is regressive. This is particularly important in trying to understand the spiritual suffering of some dying persons. Individuals may have been alienated from the practice of religion at some earlier moment of their lives, an event that may be connected with some unfinished work. Regression may cause the dying person to relive this unresolved religious conflict, which is at the heart of his or her spiritual pain.

Regression can also be identified in a dying person's retreat into the safety and security of rites and rituals that may not have had any significant place in the person's adult life. In the face of death, the dying person may seek some consolation in the assurance these religious practices seem to provide.

Too frequently, ministerial interventions with dying persons are restricted to the recitation of precribed formulae and the performance of appropriate rituals. In some instances, even this kind of religious response can be comforting. However, this hardly represents the ideal of pastoral care of the dying. Dying persons may vacillate between hope and despair, faith and doubt, consolation and desolation. They may seek spiritual support or reject it. The expressed religious need may mask other important human and spiritual conflicts that are pressing for resolution. The chaplain who engages in providing spiritual support to the dying person must be prepared to be involved at many levels of diverse needs, grouped under the common umbrella of spiritual pain (Corr & Corr, 1983).

It is to this quality of pastoral care that the hospice aspires. While preserving a respect for the individual's personal religious faith and practice, hospice workers are cognizant that many people, both those with formal religious affiliation and those without, experience some degree of spiritual pain in their final days of life. Hospice care attempts to create an environment that is responsive to this source of suffering. Just as it is so careful to identify and treat the sources of physical pain, hospice care likewise accounts for the way in which spiritual and religious issues can be burdensome to the dying person. As part of the hospice's multidisciplinary team approach, the religious professional has an important role to play in either providing direct service to the dying person or in facilitating contact with those who might best respond to the spiritual needs of the terminally ill individual.

Flexible Approaches to the Care of the Terminally Ill

Whenever possible, the hospice encourages home care of a terminally ill person (Brann, 1983; Creek, 1982; Lamerton, 1979; Koff, 1980; Rossman, 1977). The concept of home care was first introduced at Saint Christopher's in 1969. In order to make this ideal a possibility, carefully coordinated support services must be made available to the primary caregiver and the family of the terminally ill person. This section will discuss the components of the care program that permits families to care for their dying relatives in the home until such care is no longer appropriate or feasible.

The Psychosocial Needs of the Dying Person

When professionals engage in discussion about the psychosocial needs of dying persons, loneliness, isolation, and abandonment are frequently cited as the major concerns. This supports Freud's assertion that the fear of death actually represents the unconscious fears of helplessness, physical injury, and total abandonment. Whether one subscribes to this assertion or not, it is reasonable to assume that dying in the familiar context of one's home, with the support and assistance of family and friends, is preferable to dying in an unfamiliar, institutional setting. Dying is a developmental crisis; it makes specific demands on the individual and involves specific tasks. The "work" of dying is greatly facilitated if the environment is held constant.

The home, even with its limited care facilities, provides the least disruptive environment for the dying person. Dr. Saunders maintains that in her experience, a patient's bed is the most secure environment for a terminally ill individual (personal communication, November, 1983). Inpatient hospice staff are acutely aware of the added burden that the transition from home to institutional care can present to the dying person. When such a transfer of care is required, every effort is made to minimize the negative effects of this move. Such sensitivity may not always characterize the care provided to the terminally ill in a general hospital setting.

Considerable attention has been focused on the maintenance of the dying person's dignity. Independence is a key component of the preservation of personal dignity. The environment of the home makes it possible for the dying person to remain involved in family concerns and activities. While involvement may be reduced because of the progressive course of the disease or side effects of pain control medications, participation in family life is never entirely eliminated.

Home care provides quality time for dying persons and members of their family. The privacy of the home is better suited to the kinds of conversations and terminal preparations that are frequently on the agenda of dying persons. Because family members are often the ones who provide primary care, these interactions provide opportunities for interpersonal sharing that are not only beneficial to the dying person but are of incalculable value to the surviving family members. Sometimes the family needs the assistance of hospice staff members to facilitate this important sharing.

From the beginning of her illness, Doris and Bill Morrison maintained an open communication. Bill was by nature an introverted personality; Doris was the stronger personality in the marriage. It was evident that Bill had great difficulty expressing his feelings about her prognosis. He respected her wish not to share the full details of her diagnosis with their three children.

The children all sensed the seriousness of their mother's illness. From the time of her initial mastectomy through the year of follow-up therapies, they were quietly apprehensive.

The presence of the hospice team helped them enormously. On different occasions each of the children, singly or together, spoke with the team members about their mother's condition. When one of her daughters asked the direct question, "How much longer does my mother have to live?" the hospice nurse was able to say that it was probably weeks rather than months. The daughter seemed relieved to have this confirmation of her own estimate.

As her condition worsened, Mrs. Morrison asked the hospice nurse how she might talk to her children. The nurse suggested that both she and her husband should talk to the family together. They rehearsed what they wished to communicate and they were able to talk about the facts of her condition openly.

Separately each of the children confessed how relieved they were that their parents could share this information with them and how much easier it made talking with both their mother and father. Now they felt freer, as if a big burden had been lifted from their shoulders.

This was one of the observations made by Kassakian, Bailey, Rinker, Stewart, and Yates (1979) who compared the benefits of home and hospital care of the terminally ill. They reported that terminal patients who received home nursing care during the final months and weeks of their terminal illnesses maintained greater involvement in social activities and were more involved in satsifying hobbies and crafts. They were more mobile and were able to retain independence in bathroom activities significantly longer than their hospitalized counterparts. They reported significantly less pain than those who were cared for in hospital settings. The researchers concluded that the real advantage of home care is not simply economic, but psychological.

Family Members: Primary Hospice Workers in a Home Care Setting

The literature on hospices frequently begins by describing their historical ancestry in medieval Europe. A hospice was a house or shelter for strangers, soldiers, and pilgrims who were engaged in a variety of journeys. Often these refuges, which provided a place for rest and nourishment, were administered by religious orders who saw them as a concrete expression of fraternal charity. While the contemporary concept of the hospice has preserved some of the characteristics of the medieval shelter for wayfarers, there are some notable differences in both definition and purpose (Aiken & Marx, 1982; Bayer *et al.*, 1983; Buckingham, 1983; Butterfield-Picard & Magno, 1982; Corr & Corr, 1983; Gotay, 1983; MacElveen-Hoehn & McIntosh, 1981; Rizzo, 1978; Stoddard, 1978; Twycross, 1980).

Although some people do seek out the inpatient services of the residential hospice—whether it be in a separate facility or one incorporated into a community hospital—the majority of patients receive primary care in their own homes (Creek, 1982; McPhee, Arcand & MacDonald, 1979; Ward, 1978). The hospice team goes out to them rather than vice versa. The journey of dying often concludes in the patient's own home or in the home of the primary care provider, assisted by the interdisciplinary services of the hospice team (Ward, 1978).

Peter Mudd (1982), who formerly directed the Home Hospice Program in Evanston, Illinois, has reflected on the problems encountered in facilitating a home care program for the terminally ill. He notes that much of the literature that discusses hospice home care tends to gloss over the doubts, conflicts, and stress that are a normal and anticipated part of providing home care for the terminally ill. The success of any home care effort depends on the degree of mutual respect and trust that is fostered between the family and those professionals and volunteers who make up the hospice team. In Mudd's experience, this relationship is rarely ideal.

Mudd believes that hospice home care works best when the family and the hospice team members confront the frightening reality of death together. Family members need to clarify their role in this process gradually, and hospice team members must assist in this role clarification. The family members are the ones who primarily provide care; in this task, they are supported and assisted by physicians, nurses, physical therapists, clergy, and a whole cadre of other volunteer assistants. This role of primary care provider must not be usurped or undermined by the hospice home care team.

It is important that hospice team members do not disturb the dynamics that provide a certain degree of cohesiveness to the family structure. Professional and other supportive services to families who have elected to care for a dying relative at home must be harmonized with established familial routines and customs. Some families are openly affectionate and intimate; others may be characteristically private and undemonstrative. Some family systems include extended relations with numerous other relatives while other families tend to limit themselves to the nuclear unit. Home care may be more easily realized in certain families and fewer outside resources may be required. Some families, given the physical and emotional health of the primary care provider, may need more frequent and more extensive assistance than others. All of these factors need to be delicately assessed and balanced if effective service is to be provided to the family caring for a terminally ill relative.

There is a danger for professionals and volunteers to attempt to do too much for a family and not exercise sufficient restraint. It is a different modality of care to see one's professional role in terms of doing something *with* another rather than *for* another. Mudd (1982) noted that well-intentioned hospice professionals and volunteers can unintentionally cripple a family in its efforts to care for its dying member.

Mr. Morrison arrived home one day while the hospice nurse was providing routine skin care to his wife. The nurse pointed out to him the reddened areas on her back and buttocks and described what could be done to alleviate these problems. He readily accepted her invitation to continue the skin care treatment and Mrs. Morrison seemed pleased that he was so quick to respond.

Home care is predicated on maintaining *normality* to whatever degree possible. If too many well-intentioned services are precipitously provided they may not only exacerbate the crisis experience of a family, but they may inadvertently give the family the message that they are not capable of caring for the dying member. External professional assistance that can be interpreted in this way may not only foster a sense of helplessness within the family but may also jeopardize the potential of a family to carry out its primary care functions.

The services of a hospice must be tailored to the specific needs of a given family. Furthermore, they must be carefully assessed not only in terms of actual need, but also in terms of whether they are furthering or detracting from the objectives of the family.

Since families are often reluctant to refuse assistance offered, team members must be vigilant in monitoring the psychological impact that services have on the dying person and his or her family. The best service a hospice team can provide a family is the encouragement that the family itself has the resources to provide the best care for its dying member. To the extent that these family resources require auxiliary assistance and specific support, hospice services can effectively supplement the family's primary efforts (Cohen & Wellisch, 1978).

Continuity of Care: the Inpatient Hospice

Saunders (1978a) remarked that although home care is a preferable environment for many dying persons, it must always be considered as one option among others. Some families are not prepared to provide the kinds of services mandated by a decision for home care. Certain terminally ill individuals may prefer to be cared for within an inpatient facility. They may not want to subject their families to the degenerative aspects of a terminal disease, or they may judge that home care would be too physically and psychologically draining on the limited emotional resources of their families. In some situations, a dying person may have no family to provide home care.

It is important not to place so much emphasis on home care that families feel guilty because they do not elect to provide this kind of care for their dying member. Dr. Saunders notes that not every terminally ill person has a family and not all families can support this kind of care. If a family has attempted to care for its dying member at home and concludes that it is not able to continue this care, assistance must be provided in preparing for the transition to an inpatient service. While many of the services formerly provided by the family may be taken over by professionals, the family needs to be encouraged to remain actively engaged in the delivery of care to the extent that this is possible.

The Morrisons continued to care for their dying mother at home. Her condition progressively worsened. Although they were all committed to keeping her at home until her death, the number of consultation calls to the hospice team increased. Her medication protocol was increased to 15 mg of the morphine mixture to address the increasing chest pain. It became increasingly difficult for her to eat solids; her diet was almost exclusively liquid.

Her coughing and breathing problems intensified, and it became clear that the family was greatly disturbed by these episodes. They openly questioned, as Doris herself had often asked, would she choke to death? For the first time Mr. Morrison told one of the hospice volunteers that he was not sure how much longer he could cope with the pressures of his care. He had a hard time verbalizing these feelings, but he seemed relieved to have expressed them. He also said that the children were finding the daily responsibilities to be very difficult.

After extensive consultation within the home care team and with the family, it was decided that Doris should be moved to the inpatient hospice.

When a family decides on inpatient service in a hospice, the same principles that governed home care must be maintained. It is important that the family remain in control. Residential hospices try to create an environment that is noninstitutional. Because sophisticated medical monitoring and life support equipment is not necessary to palliative care, the association with the hospital milieu can be avoided to some extent. Family members are welcome on a 24-hour basis. Small family living rooms provide comfortable places to relax when individuals wish some distance from the patient's bedside. Kitchen facilities encourage family members to continue to prepare meals or snacks for the dying patient. If spouses wish to share intimacy, residential hospices try to respond to this desire by providing private rooms for a couple.

All of these details underscore the primary care function of the dying person's family. When family are not available or unable to provide caring services to the dying person, the hospice volunteers and professional staff assume many of them, always respecting the wishes of the patient and the boundaries he or she might establish. In a real sense, the inpatient hospice team becomes a "family" to the dying patient. The success of these interactions depends to a large extent on how effectively the team members become a community, united by a common purpose and a shared commitment. Just as natural family members share the responsibility for care, relieving each other when stresses become overwhelming, so too the hospice team members exercise this responsibility in the same way.

Mrs. Morrison seemed content to be in the hospice. The family was visibly relieved to know that their mother was receiving the best attention possible, even though they had done an excellent job caring for her at home. With the assistance of the hospice staff, each of the children was able to spend some private time speaking with their mother. She told one of the nurses: "I know the end is near now, but I feel content that the family is OK."

Two days after her admission to the inpatient hospice, Mrs. Morrison's respiration became more labored. In the presence of her husband and children she died peacefully.

Hospice Bereavement Services

The hospice attempts to provide care for the family of the deceased. It does not see its work concluded with the death of an individual patient. Provision of comprehensive bereavement services may be the most difficult organizational problem faced by many hospices. Often these services have no external sources of support; they are not reimbursable through any third-party repayment structure. Even though they are judged to be important to the comprehensive program of hospice care, they often are relegated to a lower priority in the actual organizational hierarchy of needs and services. Despite fiscal and managerial problems, bereavement services continue to be included in the delivery of services. The next section will review briefly some of the principal components of a hospice bereavement program and explore the potential benefit of such interventions to the post-mortem adjustment of the surviving members of bereaved families.

Initial Viewing of the Body after Death

The first visit by family members to view the body of the deceased is of great importance. Whether a person dies at home or in a residential hospice, it is advisable that the family be provided with the opportunity to spend some time with the body of the deceased before arrangements are concluded for transfer to a mortuary. In residential hospices, viewing rooms are available. This space is designed to resemble a bedroom. The body of the deceased is washed, groomed, and clothed in clean garments and placed in an ordinary bed. Family members are invited to spend whatever period of time they wish in the presence of the body of their deceased relative.

The work of bereavement may have begun during the final days and weeks of terminal care; whether or not this is the case, the death of the person becomes an important index event in the bereavement process. For some families this first encounter with the body of the deceased may be the catalyst for the necessary processes of grief, bereavement, and disengagement. Because death is contextualized by culture and rituals, families are often swept up in the dynamic of transition rites. The quiet opportunity to say good-by provided in the early moments after the loved one's death may be the most significant time for individual family members. This time is free from the demands and expectations of others and may contribute significantly to the way in which the death is remembered and integrated. In no way should families be distracted during these private moments; they have important bereavement work to do and require time and privacy to conclude it.

Depending on their religious beliefs, the family may welcome the presence of a chaplain or member of the clergy during the final moments of the initial viewing period. Although some formal religious services may later be planned as part of the funeral arrangements, what is celebrated in the private and intimate family moments may be of greater significance to the family.

Clergy who are privileged to participate in these moments need to recognize the importance not only of their liturgical and sacramental function but also the potential their ministry has to assist bereavement and adjustment. Their intervention should be sensitive, responsive, and personal. Their very presence is supportive and reassuring. Admitted to these most intimate moments in a family's life, they need to respect the family's feelings and be careful not to transgress any boundaries the family may have established. Clergy are dedicated to a role of service; nowhere is this more important than in ministering to the needs of a bereaved family.

Funeral Rites

The presence of a member of the hospice care team or bereavement team at the funeral of the deceased patient is of symbolic importance to the bereaved family because of the relationship of trust that was developed and nourished during the terminal phase of the deceased individual's life. At this critical point of transition, the continuity of both care and trust is made manifest by the presence of the hospice community at the funeral rites. Not only do members of the hospice team want to participate in this way, but their presence and support is desirable and beneficial.

While extended family and friends provide a certain quality of support, it is important to underline the distinctive role of the bereavement team. Sharing in the important passage ritual the funeral represents enables the team member to continue the relationship that has been fostered throughout the terminal care period. The focus of care naturally shifts from concern for the dying person to the support and care of the bereaved family. Most families are receptive and responsive to this kind of follow-up care.

Contacts with Surviving Family Members

Home visits and telephone contacts were an ordinary part of home care during the terminal phase of the patient's life. The family is accustomed to this approach. Therefore, these methods of follow-up present little difficulty to most families and provide opportunities for reflection, ventilation, and exploration. For the trained bereavement counselor, contacts and discussions provide important data for assessment of bereavement reactions and coping abilities. Home visits where direct observation of family dynamics are possible may uncover certain problems among some members that might require more specialized professional asssistance. Appropriate referrals can be suggested.

Some of these potential difficulties may have been identified and begun to be addressed during the final phase of the terminal illness. However, emotional involvement with the dying family member may have precluded effective treatment of these issues. Postponement of appropriate treatment may seriously impact the course of bereavement. Included in the problems a family may have to face are the incomplete resolution of prior losses, dysfunctional relationships within the family system, ineffective psychological defenses, inadequate personal coping styles, and insufficient sources of interpersonal support and poor communication within the family. A keen hospice team may recognize these potentially troublesome problems and be in a position to assist the family in finding effective ways to address them.

Although potential adjustment difficulties may be identified and hospice bereavement team members are ready to respond to needy family members, intervention efforts may not be successful. Studying this problem, Parkes (1979) noted that in high-risk families with some of the problems noted above, the interventions of a hospice bereavement team does not significantly lower the incidence of morbidity and mortality.

For example, an elderly woman who may have depended almost exclusively on her husband for planning and decision making may be virtually unable to make the adjustment to independent living. Even with encouragement and assistance, she may not be successful in assuming the various roles formerly performed by her spouse. As a result, she may add nutritional and health deficits to the ordinary psychological losses associated with bereavement. Even a bereavement team may not be successful in altering the negative direction of this process.

Some families are able to utilize the supports available to them. Other families, who may have accepted help during the terminal illness, may not be as receptive to the offers of assistance made by the bereavement team.While a family may not desire to have visits from hospice workers, however, they may be receptive to occasional telephone conversations. Some families may themselves initiate telephone contact during the bereavement process. It is important to stress that individual persons and individual families vary in the kinds of external assistance they require and permit. A hospice bereavement program must be flexible in offering and providing services suited to this diversity of need.

Closure to Hospice Care

Involvement with a terminally ill person and his or her family depends, as we have seen, on establishing effective communication. To the degree that hospice workers succeed in this goal, the family is assisted in the bereavement work of the final days spent with a dying or deceased member. Everything continues to be done to manage the physical, psychological, and spiritual pain that may be associated with terminal disease and dying. These efforts to assist are never at the expense of taking control away from the dying patient and the family. Responsibility for pain control and decision making is a collaborative enterprise, and the patient's and family's role in these endeavors are of paramount importance.

While a program with such clearly articulated humanistic objectives as those of a hospice may be of great benefit to the palliative care of a terminally ill person and his or her family, this quality care is not without its costs to both caregivers and familial survivors. Lattanzi (1982) remarks that work with terminally ill persons and their families forces caregivers to face the inevitability of losing, through death, all the individuals to whom energy and effort is directed.

One of the mutual benefits of post-mortem associations that can exist between hospice team members who provided care, the bereavement team members who follow up, and the surviving family members is the opportunity to benefit from reflections about the meaning and value of their investment in terminal care. To achieve closure it is important to be able to see that what one invested in terms of time, energy, emotion, and care was all that one could have done. It is consoling to recognize that what was attempted proved to be helpful.

Families need opportunities to acknowledge this judgment; they need to hear others reinforce it. Likewise, professionals and volunteers who invest their skills and energies in hospice care thrive on the gratitude and appreciation that families so often desire to communicate to them. Bereavement followup provides family members and hospice workers the opportunity for this important closure activity. It is an added source of comfort to know that the choices made and followed through on added to the dignity and peaceful death of the terminally ill family member. Significant relationships are built and deepened between hospice workers and families through the common commitment to care. The final act of sharing that closure represents confirms surviving family members and hospice caregivers in their strength and unity.

Summary

The contemporary hospice movement, begun in Great Britain in the mid-1960s, has undergone remarkable growth and has attracted widespread interest and support in the United States during the past decade. In significant measure, the success of this concept of care for terminally ill persons and their families is responding to a social trend to allow dying to be a more humane experience. Hospices are likewise filling a void that has existed for some time in medical care for the terminally ill.

Criticisms of established medical practice with the terminally ill come not only from within the health professions themselves, but also from ethicians. Bayer and his associates (1983) raise the question whether current expenditures on dying patients are disproportionate, unreasonable, and unjust. Extended hospitalizations and the sophisticated technologies required to care for the terminally ill are costly. Contemporary ethical discussion does not assume that such costs are necessarily a misuse of society's resources, but it does demand closer study of cost/benefit analyses. Among their recommendations, Bayer and his colleagues at the Hastings Center suggest that a patient and his or her family have greater autonomy with regard to decisions to begin or discontinue certain kinds of treatment. They favor alternatives to institutional care such as hospice care.

A major resistance to the hospice concept among some physicians has been focused on the issue of palliative versus curative care. Hospice is dedicated to the support and care of the terminally ill. By definition, terminal illness implies that competent medical diagnosis has determined that a disease has progressed to such a degree that death will result. Some physicians refuse to suspend curative efforts until a patient has died. These physicians believe they have a responsibility to preserve life at any cost, including the use of new experimental drugs and procedures. Others believe that quality of life is the most important variable in planning interventions in the terminal phase of an illness.

Palliative care uses medical science to manage the often painful symptoms of terminal illness. It sets as its primary objective to assist the dying person to remain pain-free and alert. Palliative care is attuned to the holistic concerns of the dying person and uses a variety of resources to respond to his or her needs. It focuses on the quality of the life remaining to the dying individual.

Comprehensive hospice care requires the effective collaboration of a patient's physician as the goals shift from curative treatment to palliative care. Medical and nursing education—both at the medical or nursing school level and in continuing education programs—needs to provide improved professional training in the care of the dying. Hospices provide unique opportunities for physicians to confront the role conflicts and ethical issues related to terminal care while learning new skills in the use of drugs to manage intractable pain. The hospice can assist the physician in forging an effective partnership with a dying patient and his or her family. It can help the physician to relinquish certain controls to the patient and family members who assist in providing care.

One consistent criticism of hospice programs is their preoccupation with pharmacology and other technical details. This is a legitimate criticism, since so much of the mission of hospice intervention depends upon the use of drugs to manage pain. Because most of the patients who are supported through hospice programs are dying of neoplastic diseases, physical pain is an important issue. This chapter reviewed some of the major ways in which analgesics, nerve blocks, and x-rays have been utilized in the management of pain associated with terminal illness.

In the use of analgesics, emphasis is placed on putting control into the hands of the patient and those assisting in his or her care. A broad spectrum of analgesics—from nonnarcotic to strong narcotic preparations—is currently used in hospice care, raising important issues of drug titration, addiction, psychological dependence, and effective antidotes to drug-related side effects. In dealing with these issues, hospice care demands continual reassessment and evaluation, in conjunction with the physician, health care team, family, and patient. The patient's well-being and comfort are always the primary objectives of care.

Nerve blocks are useful in alleviating regional pain and providing a patient relief from high doses of narcotics and their negative side effects. The relieving of pain by a nerve block is secured by making extraneural or paraneural injections of anesthetic drugs in close proximity to the nerve whose conductivity is to be cut off. In patients for whom more conventional analgesic treatments are not successful in managing pain, nerve blocks may be useful. Likewise, x-rays also can be beneficial in managing pain associated with certain tumors and metastases, as well as in certain other distressing symptomatic conditions associated with various cancers.

Considerable emphasis has been placed on the concept of *pain*. This term not only describes physical discomfort but includes the psychosocial and spiritual stresses some terminally ill persons experience. The chapter described some of the physical, psychological, and spiritual concerns of dying persons and showed how they are interrelated. Difficulties in breathing and sleeping are not only physical issues, but psychologically these are intimately connected to the issues of death and dying. Some aspects of effective pastoral care of the terminally ill were also reviewed. Twycross (1980) is correct in his observation that the control of chronic pain has as much to do with spiritual and psychological concerns of the dying person as it has to do with what palliative drugs or procedures are utilized.

As a philosophy of care, hospice embraces many different programmatic applications. Each of these models shares the same goal of providing the most humane care possible to the terminally ill. Some of these different models include free-standing in-patient facilities (such as St. Christopher's in London and Hospice, Inc., in Branford, Connecticut), hospital-based programs, day-care programs, and home care services. The most common application is the home care model. Each of these various models is effective in providing comprehensive quality care to dying persons.

The home care program, as it is discussed in this chapter, has special advantages. Within the familiar environment of one's own home, the patient and family are assisted in their task of preparing for death. Professionals and lay volunteers assist the family in meeting all of the dying person's needs. The home environment insures maintenance of the patient's autonomy. The community ideology of the hospice is well-implemented in a home care program through applications of effective team work. The home care program maintains proper focus on patient and family as the primary unit of care; there is an appropriate blurring of roles among the professionals and volunteers from the wider community who assist the patients and families in their tasks.

Hospice care, as it has been demonstrated in this chapter, is above all comprehensive care. Not only are medical issues of concern, but psychological and spiritual issues command equal attention in the provision of care. Further, the responsibilities of hospice care do not terminate immediately upon the death of a patient. Recognizing the important partnership that has been forged between hospice staff members and a patient's family, hospice assumes some responsibility in assisting the family in the important work of bereavement.

While initial assessment of the impact of hospice care on the bereavement of surviving family members is encouraging (Cameron & Parkes, 1983), a conclusive assessment is difficult. Some reports note fewer psychological symptoms and shorter duration of grief and anger among the relatives of hospice patients than among those who participated in conventional hospital-based treatment programs. Reasons which support these trends in adjustment include the following: patients died virtually pain-free; there was an open and free discussion of death within hospice families; families were given support after the patient's death by hospice bereavement teams. The chapter concluded with a brief discussion of the ongoing relationship of hospice programs with the families of persons who were assisted in dying by hospice personnel.

Hospice care has provided a new challenge to the humanisitic practice of medicine. Its success suggests that dying is most easily managed within the dying person's community, and that the best care is family-centered. Hospices have helped to resituate death and dying in their proper interpersonal and intrafamilial contexts. It is encouraging to see that the windows Cicely Saunders helped to open for terminally ill persons and their families have attracted the support of medical, governmental, and educational institutions that, collectively, are so instrumental in determining the quality of care for dying persons.

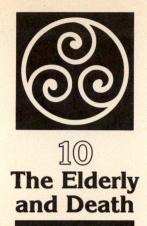

10

The Elderly
and Death

Introduction

Some Dimensions of Death in the Later Years

- The Context of the Dying Process
  - Expectation of Death
- Environmental Events Predicting Death

Terminal Drop Theory

- Cross-sectional Analysis of Longitudinal Data
- Longitudinal Analysis of Longitudinal Data
- Terminal Drop Versus Terminal Decline

Disengagement Theory

Psychology of the Dying Older Person

- Preoccupation with Death
- Role of Regression in the Dying Process
- Life Review as Developmental Process
- Physical Illness, Depression, and Death
  - Care of the Dying Older Person

The Process of Dying and Ethical Considerations

- The "Right-to-die" Question
- Voluntary and Involuntary Euthanasia
  - Active and Passive Euthanasia
  - Direct and Indirect Euthanasia
- The American Medical Association's Policy on Euthanasia
  - The Elderly and Euthanasia

Summary

Introduction

People commonly associate *old* with *death*. There is an understandable and reasonable connection between these two concepts in popular thinking. As an individual ages, he or she becomes more vulnerable to disease and to other processes that seem to foreshadow death. However, aging and dying are not synonymous. As an individual ages the approach of personal death may become a conscious concern and may influence certain other developmental processes. This still does not mean that it is natural or expected that people will die simply because they are old.

Awareness on the part of older persons of the approach of death may stimulate some discussion of this fact by the elderly. Such conversation and related behaviors does not necessarily mean that older people are fearful of impending death. It is more likely that older people are merely preparing for this final, human developmental event. However, this can excite death fears and anxieties in some younger persons with whom the elderly may communicate their thoughts and feelings.

This chapter will explore some of the issues related to dying in the final stage of the human life cycle, such as the notion of the **dying trajectory** introduced by Glaser and Strauss (1965), who attempted to describe a terminally ill person's awareness of impending death. Their classifications of awareness are useful in describing older persons as they approach their own deaths. The chapter will also examine the ways in which an older person predicts his or her own death. Environmental events that may precipitate death will also be considered, including death of a significant other, relocation, and retirement.

In the 1960s terminal drop theory was introduced. It suggested that dying precipitates a decline in intellectual functioning. The chapter will look at some methodological problems encountered in testing the assumptions of terminal drop theory and the implications of these assumptions. The distinction between **terminal drop** and **terminal decline** will be noted. Another popular aging theory of the same decade is **disengagement theory**. Its application to an older person's approach to death will be discussed.

Is there a particular "psychology" of the dying older person? Discussion will focus on certain issues that may help to elucidate this psychology, including the older person's preoccupation with death and the role of regression in the dying process. Familiarity with some of the ways in which an older person faces death may aid in providing care for the dying elder.

The chapter will conclude with an exploration of the "right-to-die" question. Of particular interest in this discussion are the attitudes of older persons toward the controversial medico-ethical-legal issue of euthanasia.

Some Dimensions of Death in the Later Years

The Context of the Dying Process

In their celebrated study of the awareness of terminally ill persons, Glaser and Strauss (1965) spoke of the "dying trajectory." Operationally defined, this *trajectory* refers not to the actual course of a person's dying, but rather to the socially perceived course of that process. While this research specifically addressed the issues that surround dying in hospital settings and was not limited to the population of older persons, the principal insights of the study have relevance to those who die from what might be simply called "old age."

The Glaser and Strauss report identifies four types of awareness contexts: *closed awareness*, *suspected awareness*, *mutual pretense awareness*, and *open awareness*. Each of these distinct postures toward communication with the older person can influence the way in which the normal tasks of dying will be negotiated.

The *closed awareness context* describes a situation in which a dying person is unaware of impending death. In an effort to spare an older person the pain of facing this reality, important factual information may be withheld. This assumes that the older person does not desire to know the facts and is fearful of death. On the contrary, an older person is generally aware of the possibility of death because of advanced age; this may become a more focused awareness because of a particular disease process. The older person with normal cognitive functioning is able to understand detailed medical data. Death is a natural process and many older people are in fact prepared to face it (Marshall, 1975).

Frequently older persons pick up on the behavioral cues that attend efforts to withhold important information from them. The *suspicion awareness context* describes a situation in which an older person intuits that he or she is dying and searches for verification of this suspicion. This can be a very frustrating project since it frequently runs counter to simultaneous efforts to mask the evidence that would confirm the suspicion.

The charade of denying the fact of death, which unfortunately isolates a dying person from important information and contact with significant others, is termed *mutual pretense*. It is understandable that some older persons reason that their death is too difficult for others to face, so they at least tacitly consent to participate in the game of mutual pretense. The dying person and those who surround him or her behave as if death were not imminent and avoid any conversation that might disturb the mutually guarded secret.

My poor son and daughter-in-law! They think that I don't know that I am dying. After living a full life these past 82 years I think I've learned something. This body of mine and I have become good friends over the years and I know what's going on; it's tired and it is wearing out.

I know my son finds it hard to think about my death. He seems so sad each time he comes here. To listen to his conversation you would think that I had another 20 good years ahead of me. That isn't so! I'm dying and I am quite content with my life. I let Richard and Catherine tell me their encouraging stories through their glassy eyes. I simply nod agreement to spare them the pain of having to admit that their old mother is on her last legs. . . . .

Finally, **open awareness** may be considered to be the most natural, the most beneficial, and the most desirable context in which many older persons would elect to face death. It creates an environment in which death is accepted as a natural conclusion to a human life. Emotionally healthy older persons generally view death in this way. In the case noted above, there is clear evidence that the 82-year-old woman was comfortable with the knowledge of her impending death. Her preference would have been to share this openly with her family. Her accurate perception of their discomfort with the facts of her dying forced her into a posture of protective silence.

The one expressed fear of some older persons is the fear of dying alone (Butler & Lewis, 1973). An open, comfortable communication with an aging person about his or her death represents the best and most supportive environment in which the process of dying can take place. In the case cited above, the older woman shared this information with one of the nursing home staff members in an informal chat. It was noted that the woman was comfortable and free in talking about the irony of her position. She was humorous in describing what poor actors her children were. It was likewise clear that their discomfort put certain burdens on her to maintain the "secret." She seemed content at least to let someone know that she was aware of what was happening and that death presented no great fear to her.

Expectation of Death

Although death is a normal and natural expectation during the **senium**, or advanced old age, mental health professionals have observed a phenomenon whereby persons who were not emotionally disturbed predicted their own death. Weisman and Hackett (1961) referred to this as **predilection to death**. While this phenomenon is not exclusively linked to the situation of the elderly, it may be more common among this cohort than is reported.

Jensen (1980) reports what happened to a 91-year-old great-grandmother who lived in a comfortable retirement home in a large metropolitan urban center and was both alert and physically well.

Her grandson, a successful professional, visited her daily. For a number of months before her death, he spent up to an hour a day visiting with her, making her feel needed, touching her and giving her hugs. He explained, after her death, that he felt she would have died months earlier if he had not made her feel needed by him. About 2 months prior to death, she learned that her daughter had cancer of the breast and this deeply concerned her. She talked for the first time and from then on, about "putting her things in order" and designated her possessions to be inherited by various family members. One morning she could not walk due to an unexplained paralysis of both lower extremities. Her mind was clear and she seemed concerned but resigned. She was admitted to a general hospital for a diagnostic evaluation. Three days later she stopped eating and acted increasingly withdrawn. Two days later she died quietly at 7:00 A.M. There was no positive diagnosis of disease, nor an obvious cause of death. (pp. 199–200)

In discussing this case, Jensen comments that the most probable explanation for this woman's conscious or unconscious choice to die at that precise point in her life was her daughter's malignancy. She simply did not wish to risk the possibility that her daughter might predecease her. Another explanation may be the older woman's perception that she was impeding the development of her grandson by the emotional burdens her care was placing on him. Death may have been viewed as a loving way to release him to pursue other important personal goals.

Whatever the psychodynamic explanation that best explains the fact of her death, it is evident that there was some self-determination involved in the process. Jensen concludes that death expectation may play a more significant role in the deaths of older persons who otherwise might be thought to die simply of old age.

Reynolds and Nelson (1981) have come to similar conclusions. In a study of the attitudes and behaviors of institutionalized chronically ill elderly patients, they explored the likelihood that certain attitudes about living and dying may be associated with behaviors that hasten death in an indirect, but regular, way. These instrumental behaviors, which might accelerate the natural process of dying, were termed by the investigators as *indirect self-destructive behavior* (ISDB). Included in the description of such behaviors are self-injurious eating and drinking, abuse of medication protocols, or noncompliance with treatment programs.

A number of interesting personality and life situation variables were found to be significant in the Reynolds and Nelson study. One finding of their research is of special interest to the present discussion. The nonsurviving group in the study was observed to have engaged in 50 percent more indirect self-destructive behavior than the other similarly aged persons who outlived them.

If this observation reflects the influence of conscious and unconscious choices, it is evident that an older person's will to live or die can determine survival or death.

This conclusion raises an interesting issue in the provision of health care for an older person who seems unwilling to continue living. Storlie (1980) reports on the case of a 66-year-old obese white woman who was admitted to a general hospital emergency room after a motor vehicle accident. As her acute medical problems were being addressed, she developed cardiopulmonary complications and other difficulties that extended her hospitalization to 72 days. She seemed to develop a new problem every time an old one was managed. In the assessment of one nurse, "she seemed to be getting better *by systems* but not getting well as a person." The patient was depressed and uncooperative in her treatment. She refused to eat or to cough. She did everything in her power to prevent the staff from caring for her.

The staff determined to change her attitude and adopted an assertive program of care. Although they encountered much resistance, their intervention strategy worked and she did recover. The point of the case underlies the fact that people can hasten their death by certain attitudes and behaviors. Had the staff not intervened, this patient would have certainly died.

Environmental Events Predicting Death

Practitioners in the field of psychosomatic medicine have long maintained that certain stresses in a person's life can be responsible for precipitating the death of the individual. They have assumed that these sources of stress are so intense that they effectively command the person's attention and cannot be ignored. An individual's response to these stressors may be in one of two extreme directions: hyperexcitation or complete surrender. Both of these responses can set in motion the mechanisms that precipitate death. These environmental events therefore have a special interest to those who work with older persons who may be subjected to these stresses. The principal research in this area (Engel, 1971; Weisman, 1972; Seligman, 1975) expresses consensus on the point that certain environmental events bear upon the health and possibility of death of a stressed individual. When attention is focused on the aged as a group, the potential number and frequency of stresses may increase at a moment in the life course when the reservoirs of physical and psychological resources may be ebbing.

Rowland (1977) has carefully reviewed the studies of three events that frequently have been cited as major threats to the lives of older persons and that continue to command attention in gerontology: death of a significant other, relocation, and retirement. She narrowed her investigation and focused only on those studies in which death was the criterion variable; she investigated only natural deaths and not those that were accidental, homicidal, or suicidal. As might be expected, studies that met the established criteria were generally naturalistic in design. Subjects were those older persons who had experienced one of the three main stresses; they formed the experimental group. Others who had not experienced them formed the control group. This naturalistic design sacrifices many of the controls necessary for rigorous scientific research, which seeks to establish causal relationship between variables.

Additionally, Rowland noted that much of this type of research is mounted after considerable time has elapsed since the stressful experience. She correctly concluded that when persons are not interviewed and observed immediately after the event, it is possible that those who might be most vulnerable to the effects of the stress may actually die. Those who do survive and adjust become subjects of the studies and so may be contributing little to the understanding of how death can be predicted from environmental events. For a thorough discussion of these issues, a careful reading of Rowland's report is suggested.

Death of a Significant Other

It terms of dynamics, the loss of a close lifelong friend can be compared to that of a spouse. To examine the impact of the death of a significant other—close friend or spouse—on older persons, as noted above, the only data available can be found in prospective studies that compare the mortality rates of recently bereaved persons to those of controls with intact marriages. It is interesting to note that this method of study frequently defines the deceased spouse as a significant other, ignoring the role that the death of other persons (for example, a child or grandchild, sibling, lifelong friend) may play in precipitating death in the aged survivor (Steuer et al., 1981).

While certain trends in demographic data indicate a particular vulnerability during the first year of bereavement for some persons, it is not possible to conclude what role the death of a significant other plays in the complex interactive psychophysiological processes that may end in the death of the surviving older person. The major longitudinal studies currently under way offer the greatest promise for illuminating the role that this environmental event plays in accelerating the death of the surviving individual.

Relocation

It is not an uncommon event that an older person may either choose to or be required to change residence. Housing plays a vital role in the emotional well-being and adjustment process among the aged. From an economic perspective, housing responsibilities and costs place considerable burdens on the elderly. Approximately half of those over age 65 own or have equity in their place of residence. As the principal asset of many older persons, it can be the source of the principal drain on current income or other assets through taxes, repairs, and operating expenses. For many older persons, particularly those living alone, their own homes become economic liabilities. Sale of a home can provide money for living expenses, but it also requires significant changes in lifestyle (Deak & Smith, 1979).

Those who seem most vulnerable to the economic and psychological pressures of relocating are older persons in poor physical or mental health. If lifestyle changes are precipitated by the death of a spouse or live-in companion and are coupled with economic demands, the transitional pressures are compounded. It is not easy to determine whether older persons are at risk because of the more obvious economic hardships to which they are exposed or because of the emotional consequences of the disruptions due to forced or elective relocation. The following excerpt of an interview with a widowed, 83-year-old woman underlines how disruptive relocation can be.

After my husband died (8 months earlier) my children and my grandchildren were all worried about me. They did not want me to stay alone in my own home. In many ways their arguments were right, but I did not want to leave my home; I certainly did not want to move in with any of my children, even though they all extended me invitations. I did not want to disrupt their families and their lives.

Finally I gave in to their pressures and accepted to come to this "senior citizen" apartment. I had to break up my large house and get rid of many of my lifelong possessions. Now my life is contained in these two and a half rooms. I'm very secure here and my family is very content. However, I must confess to you that I am not adjusting to this place very well.

There were so many important memories attached to my old home. While this apartment is very nice and everyone here is lovely, it is not home. I miss my old neighbors very much. I used to be able to walk to the store. Now I have to wait until one of my children comes to take me out. I've lost most of my independence, if you know what I mean.

I'm starting to feel like a real "old lady." That might seem a bit funny to you, since I'm well beyond 80 years old, but I never used to feel old. After Ed's death the children became concerned that I couldn't manage on my own. Although I realize their concerns were well-intentioned, I regret that I gave in to their pressures and sold my house.

My son-in-law is an investment banker, and he persuaded me that this was the only sensible financial decision at this stage of my life. He's probably right, but I am embarrassed to tell him that all the money in the world is not worth the loneliness and isolation I am feeling now.

Maybe in time I'll adjust to this place. However, right now, I regret that I moved out of my home. It's too late in my life to begin making friends again in a new community. I feel like an exile in a foreign land. These two rooms, nice as they are, at times feel like a prison. You should never force an old person to make a decision like this.

Relocation can be for many people a traumatic event, symbolizing the termination of important associations and relationships with individuals and an environment that may have been quite supportive. In addition to the surrender of certain interpersonal ties with friends and neighbors, the older person is frequently required to dispose of many possessions as he or she prepares to move into often smaller living quarters. Adaptation involves adjustment to many new stimuli and, in some cases, to considerably less independence and restrictions in functioning.

Much research on the effects of relocation notes physiological changes that accompany relocation. That older people display physical reactions indicates that the event is experienced as inherently stressful. Although mortality rates for older persons have been seen to increase after they relocate, it is not possible to conclude that relocation in itself is responsible for the subsequent death. It may be that relocation is a marker event that brings together a number of related factors that, taken together, account for the older person's death.

Retirement

Fewer empirical data exist on the issue of retirement than on any of the three environmental events selected here for comment and discussion. Studies of the effects of retirement on mortality do not permit any important conclusions to be made. The variables of health status and employment status have frequently been confused in studies of this sort, making it virtually impossible to tell which are more important in precipitating death. In fact, the decision to withdraw from work may be made as a result of major change in health status (Champlin, 1983; Strahan, 1980).

What is least known about the impact of environmental events on the mortality of the elderly is the interactive process between these events and physiological response. Engel (1971) has suggested that stresses such as those in question here may so arouse certain sympathetic and parasympathetic functions that the rapid shifting between them may precipitate death. Whether this in fact is the case, it is a reasonable hypothesis.

Terminal Drop Theory

In 1962, Kleemeier introduced a theory into the field of gerontologic psychology that proposed that factors related to the death of a person also cause a decline in intellectual functioning. He assumed that it would be possible to document the course of this decline, in some instances several years before the actual demise of the individual. Basic to Kleemeier's hypothesis is the assertion that a variety of human functions are not specifically linked to chronological age but rather show a demonstrable decline in the days, weeks, and years prior to death. For most physical and psychological functions, a certain balance is maintained throughout the human life cycle. This balance is thought to be disturbed by whatever combination of genetic, environmental, and psychophysiological factors precipitate death in a person. The shift in this balance is thought to trigger a marked decline in functioning, particularly intellectual functioning. Rather than being an age-related change, this shift is considered to be linked with the presence of the *death factor* (Kleemeier, 1962).

Riegel and Riegel (1972) further explored Kleemeier's hypothesis that decline in intellectual performance is related to the death process. It would seem axiomatic that survival should depend on the maintenance of intellectual functioning, but this is hard to prove. The Riegels noted the difficulties in effectively mounting research that could test Kleemeier's broad assumptions about dying and decreased intellectual functioning in the aged. Despite the inherent difficulties in studying this question, terminal drop theory has attracted considerable attention in academic circles.

Palmore and Cleveland (1976) explain why the theory has been so seductive. They note that it describes quite well the actual patterns of some older people who succeed in maintaining most of their functions until shortly before their death. Observation of these individuals supports this theory. Palmore and Cleveland further comment that the theory helps to explain the discrepancies reported in cross-sectional and longitudinal studies. Often cross-sectional research notes progressive decrease in functioning with age while the longitudinal studies seem to contradict that pattern and report stability of function in the oldest cohort who survive into the later years. Finally, Palmore and Cleveland suggest that the theory paints a portrait of aging and dying that mirrors the ideal of many people who prefer to think of their later years as a relatively stable period of life, with decline evident just prior to death. This is far more attractive than a picture of aging that is dominated by a progressive erosion of physical and mental functioning, terminating in death. For this compelling psychological reason, the theory has immense popularity, despite its methodological problems or the weak evidence to support it.

Siegler (1975) has done an impressive job in reviewing the findings from several major studies that test the terminal drop hypothesis. Her report merits further consideration since it carefully analyzes the data of these studies, the statistical techniques utilized, and in numerous cases, the gigantic inferential leaps from data to conclusions. Two principal observations should be noted.

Cross-sectional Analysis of Longitudinal Data

The majority of the terminal drop literature is based on data from longitudinal research that does not, of its nature, ensure the integrity of strategies seeking to evaluate change over time. Siegler (1975) has described the utilization of these data sets by some researchers as a "cross-sectional analysis of longitudinal data." In analyzing the data, information from one period in time is grouped according to two variables: distance from actual death and survivor/nonsurvivor status. Mean differences form the basis of comparison and evaluation. Obviously, such an approach reflects little about changes over time, although some researchers would like to disagree.

Longitudinal Analysis of Longitudinal Data

Longitudinal analyses of longitudinal data are the only true test of the terminal drop hypothesis since changes in performance over an interval of time as related to the length of survival or distance from death become the focus of investigation. This method depends on the number of measurements taken and careful analysis of the resultant curves. Comparisons between and among groups may illuminate individual differences and lend further intelligibility to the terminal drop hypothesis. While this approach itself is not without its own particular problems and flaws, it represents the best strategy for documenting the existence of a terminal drop among older persons prior to death.

Terminal Drop Versus Terminal Decline

Palmore and Cleveland (1976) suggest that the inconclusiveness about terminal drop derives not only from the sources alluded to above in Siegler's observations, but even more fundamentally from a conceptual confusion in the use of the terms "terminal decline" and "terminal drop." They suggest that the steady linear decline prior to death be labeled *terminal decline* and the curvilinear or accelerating drop before death *terminal drop*. Utilizing this precise distinction between terminal decline and terminal drop and taking into consideration different aging effects, they report on an analysis of the subjects of the first Duke longitudinal study of aging.

The results of this study could document no substantial terminal drop effects, although intelligence did show a statistically significant terminal drop. The researchers note that this represents only 2 percent of the variance and therefore can hardly be considered a substantial effect. The variance in the other measures of function is explained by aging or linear declines before death.

Palmore and Cleveland's study notes a slow but progressive physical deterioration as a function of age. They did not find that the approach of death accelerates this deterioration. Not finding evidence in support of the terminal drop hypothesis, Palmore and Cleveland suggest in distinct opposition to it, that the changes noted, rather than being related to the imminent approach of biological death, are age-related phenomena.

Although the terminal drop theory has merit and appeal, it is as yet doubtful whether it accurately describes the complex psychophysiological processes that attend the natural death of an older person. As more sophisticated analyses of longitudinal data are reported, the terminal drop hypothesis may gain greater clarity and support as an explanation for non-age-related changes in function.

Disengagement Theory

One of the earliest theories of aging to attract wide attention in the field of social gerontology was disengagement theory (Cumming & Henry, 1961). Foundational to the theory is the assumption that the later years represent a distinct phase of the life course with specific developmental goals. It suggested that adulthood was too generic a concept to describe adequately the specific tasks and maturational goals of older persons.

Cumming and Henry (1961) viewed aging as an "inevitable mutual withdrawal or disengagement, resulting in decreased interaction between aging persons and others in the social system they belong to." This perspective on aging has generated considerable debate among gerontologists. Many of these researchers (Palmore, 1968, 1975; Shanas *et al.*, 1968; Neugarten & Havighurst, 1969; Kalish, 1972; McMordie, 1981) have challenged the inevitable decline and withdrawal it suggests. All of the studies that object to the conceptual premises of disengagement theory focus on the comparison between activity and withdrawal from activity, between social participation and nonparticipation.

After almost two decades of lively challenge of disengagement theory, Sill (1980) reconsidered the usefulness of this theory in trying to explain an older person's awareness of finitude. He recalls that central to Cumming and Henry's original thesis of disengagement is the awareness of impending death, a fact which has attracted little attention among the critics of the theory. In his own reconsideration of disengagement, he attempted to evaluate the function of this awareness of dying. Sill assumed that this awareness would provide a better index of disengagement than simply a person's chronological age. Marshall (1975) argued this same point. He presented data to demonstrate the weaknesses inherent in any effort to substitute age as a measure of awareness of finitude.

Awareness of finitude is defined to be the amount of time the aging person believes he or she has left before death. Working with a sample of 120 institutionalized elderly persons, Sill theorized that among this group, awareness of finitude would be a significant intervening variable between age and activity level. He reasoned that those who believe they have less time to live would be more likely to refuse participation in activities than those who judge they have more time ahead of them.

This study noted a significant relationship between awareness of finitude and activity count; those high in awareness of the imminence of their deaths were 3 times below the median in activity count. The relationship was constant and similar within subsamples dichotomized by age and by perceived health. Although Cumming and Henry (1961) did state that the older person's awareness of closeness to death and declining physical energy were of paramount importance in determining disengagement, they did not pursue these factors. In the case cited earlier of the woman persuaded by her adult children to sell her home and move into elderly housing, some of these characteristics can be noted.

Up until my husband's death I used to be a fairly active person. I kept my driver's license until I was 80 years old. Even though I didn't do much driving, it was a sign to me that I was free. Now I rely on others to take me everywhere.

There are many days when I wonder how much longer I have before I join Ed in heaven. To be perfectly honest, I hope that it isn't too long. For my age I'm in pretty good health, but there is not much more to live for. Occasionally I say things like this and my children become very upset with me. They say: "Mother, you've got the world to live for." I have become more careful not to talk about this in front of them, but I do think about this many times and I am ready to die.

I've noticed that I've lost a lot of my pep and energy. I have little interest in many things. I told you that I miss my old neighbors and friends, but I have no great desire to go back to the old neighborhood even though they have invited me many times. I seem to be brooding away here. My granddaughter said I'm becoming a recluse. She is right in many ways. Sometimes I think when I wake up early in the morning, "Well, maybe today will be my last day." One of these days, I'll be right.

Sill (1980) has recognized that chronological age has been correlated with awareness of finitude and poorer health in much of the earlier research. He has attempted to consider these two factors as discrete and not necessarily related to age. The results of his study suggest that a person's awareness of dying may set in motion a genuine process of disengagement, which may in fact be developmentally significant. Of course, if this is true, a mistaken conclusion about closeness to death may set in motion this disengagement process and may result in premature death. Should this disengagement factor prove to be linked with awareness of finitude, it may assist intervention with those who may have a distorted awareness of their closeness to death and who may be prematurely preparing for death.

Sill's research supports an earlier study reported by Chappell (1975). In her review of the literature on disengagement theory, Sill noted that most developmental gerontologists agree that the factor that appears to trigger the disengagement process is awareness of death. This awareness involves not only the knowledge of the closeness of death but also the meaning that this knowledge has for the person's future. She studied 40 hospitalized older persons. Evidence of knowledge of death and expressions of readiness to die were identified in these subjects. The author noted that almost half of these people saw themselves as having a future whose simple goal was to wait for death. These were observed to be socially withdrawn. The other half of the sample defined the future as a time for continued living. These remained active and socially invested. The factors that seem to account for these two different approaches to the future were the degree of specific involvement in social activities, versus social disengagement. While awareness of death may trigger disengagement to some degree, the ways in which a person conceptualizes future time may contribute more to social withdrawal than the fact that he or she is approaching death (Woods & Witte, 1981).

Psychology of the Dying Older Person

If death is a natural conclusion to the human life course, then certain normal psychological processes might be expected to be manifest in the dying person. Kubler-Ross (1969) has suggested a number of stages through which a dying person may progress. She proposes that *denial*, *anger*, *bargaining*, *preparatory depression*, and *acceptance* are five psychological stages in the process of dying and that everyone encounters them although not everyone experiences each of them in a predictable temporal or chronological sequence. What these stages describe are the psychological processes that assist a person in coping with the developmental task of dying. Like other tasks a person must negotiate in life, success or failure in dying is frequently linked to the adequacy and function of a person's psychosocial resources.

These psychological coping strategies can be described as *defense mechanisms*. The principal function of defenses is to assist a person in meeting the challenges represented by a particular crisis situation. During a person's lifetime, the particular constellation of these defenses is defined and strengthened. As a person ages and prepares for death, it is reasonable to expect that these same unconscious mechanisms will be called upon to assist in this last task in the human life cycle. Among the specific issues concerning an older person facing death, of particular interest are the ways in which lifelong patterns of coping either assist or inhibit effective management of this final task.

Preoccupation with Death

Unlike younger persons, the elderly have had considerable life experience with death. These experiences have included the deaths of their own parents and siblings, perhaps the death of a child or spouse, and the deaths of many lifelong friends and associates. In advanced old age, they are at least temporally closer to their own death. It is reasonable to expect that many older persons think about death and may express some fears about it (Roth, 1978; Sanders, Poole, & Rivero, 1980). Some people might consider an older person's preoccupation with death to be pathological. However, dying is a normal developmental task. In late life, it becomes a significant conscious issue requiring time, emotional processing, and preparation, just as any other developmental issue earlier in life.

In a continuation of the interview with the 82-year-old widow, this natural preoccupation with death becomes apparent. She describes some of the ways in which her thinking on death is maturing.

Since Ed has died I have found myself thinking about death much more. There was a time in my life when I must confess the thoughts of death troubled me. I was a person who was afraid to fly in an airplane for fear the plane would crash and I'd be killed. My late husband used to get upset with me; he reminded me that you could be killed just as easily crossing the street.

As I'm older now and alone, I think more frequently about death and I'm surprised myself how peaceful those thoughts are. It is as natural as being born, but somehow people seem to think being born is more natural. I think a lot about how it will feel to die; I hope I'm spared the pain that some people have to endure. My husband was blessed; he went to bed as he normally did and died peacefully in his sleep. That's the way I'd like to go.

I have a lot of pictures in my mind of what it's like to die and go to heaven. I like to think that I'll be reunited with my husband and my mother and father and all our other relatives and friends. It's sort of like a homecoming. This will seem a bit strange to you, but I sort of look forward to dying. Maybe that's why I find myself thinking about it more often now and praying that the Good Lord will take me soon.

It appears that this woman spends a considerable amount of time thinking about death and fantasizing about afterlife experiences. It is also clear that she enjoys a considerable degree of life satisfaction. Woods and Witte (1981) studied Erikson's final stage of ego integrity versus despair. They sampled 71 women and 29 men (aged 61–89 years) using measures of life satisfaction (ego integrity) and death anxiety (despair). They found an anticipated positive relationship to exist between life satisfaction and the way in which a person looks at death. Rather than being an index of despair, an older person's preoccupation with death may be one way in which many earlier developmental events are integrated. This issue will be discussed again when the developmental importance of the *life review* is examined.

Role of Regression in the Dying Process

Weisman (1972) has suggested that regression may be the most common defense of the dying person. While the term **regression** frequently refers to a turning back of the libido to an early fixation at infantile levels because of an inability to cope with reality, this is not the sense in which Weisman uses the concept. Rather, he views regression in the older person as a complex of behaviors, not just a psychological reversion or atavism. This normal adaptive process may be misunderstood and misdiagnosed by those who deal with the elderly. The grouping together of these behaviors may be thought to be either manifestations of dementia, the secondary effects of medication, or the attendant features of illness.

To aid in understanding the normal functioning of regression in the terminal older person, Weisman has described the complex of regressive behaviors. Characteristically, the older person may display disordered communications, including confusion or misuse of words, fragmented utterances, and misinterpretation of what is said to them. It may appear that their minds are not tracking what is said and that they are only partially attentive to what is being said to them. Thinking may appear to be faulty, even with the processing of what would otherwise be judged to be simple functions. To these disturbed communication processes may be added significant denial, projection, and externalization.

I have many times caught myself drifting off into these thoughts while other people are talking to me. I hope I have not appeared this way to you. I suspect that I have not since we have been talking about these precise things. I hope I am not boring you with these ramblings. . . .

I find that I get distracted by my random thoughts very often. My children frequently say: "Mother, are you all right?" I smile and say: "I'm fine." They probably think I'm a bit senile, because I drift out of their conversations and into my own private world of thinking. I frankly have very little interest in many of the things they are discussing. I even find this true when I watch television. If you asked me what was important in the news I often could not tell you, even though I was just watching Dan Rather on CBS. . . .

It is easy to understand why many observers might conclude that such behavioral manifestations could be related to senile psychosis or to the side effects of medication. Because these may be normal coping strategies, it is important that careful differentiation be made of these behavioral cues in terminally ill adults. Tatro and Marshall (1982) have addressed the importance of this question of differential diagnosis in providing care for the dying older person. They focus on three basic issues in making such an assessment: general information, history of the illness, and normal coping patterns.

General information about the person, including everything that routinely would be included in a comprehensive history, enables the assessor to make some determination as to whether the older person's reasoning processes are normal and typical or clearly abnormal and atypical. If they are judged to be the latter, then there may be reason to suspect they may be related to regression as discussed above.

The history of the course of a person's illness not only considers the particular pathology but also considers how the disease process is known to affect higher mental functioning as well as physical functioning. By reviewing the treatment protocol, including medications, it may be possible to compare normative reactions to the specific behavioral responses of the individual. It may happen that no apparent physiological cause for the behavioral shifts can be found to explain the change in the person's mental functioning.

Finally, assuming relative continuity of functioning throughout the life course, it is important to try to determine what constitutes a particular individual's normal coping pattern. This investigation should include an attempt to understand the person's general self-image. Family, friends, and coworkers are invaluable resources in piecing together this picture. Since death represents the final in a series of losses throughout life, this ultimate loss may be negotiated in ways similar to the strategies used in facing other losses. Therefore, it is also useful to understand how the person dealt with previous losses. The more enriched the data base is, the more possible it is to compare the current crisis with the ways in which previous developmental crises were managed.

When we started this interview I told you that I didn't think I had much to tell you, but I have been surely talking to you for quite a long time. Your tape must be running out. It has been helpful to me to say all the things I have, even if they don't all make much sense. . . . My children are very good to me—don't get me wrong—and I appreciate everything they do for me. However, they don't realize that there is little meaning left for me in life and I am ready to die. They are having a hard time recognizing that I'm preparing myself for this end which I feel is very near. I think you do understand what I am saying. . . . It's not a fearful thing to die.

Tatro and Marshall (1982) suggest that understanding the role of regression in the overall dying process will help the caregiver and family member to provide more realistic and supportive assistance to the older person. They underline the importance of patient listening and physical touch in encounters with the regressed older person who may be preparing for death. Additionally, they note the importance of preserving whatever controls a person can exercise in simple decision making. Finally, the safeguarding of a person's human dignity in the face of what may be perceived as cognitive and perceptual disorganization is of paramount importance. This may require helping those who may be prone to misread these signs to realize that what is observed is not bizarre psychopathology but rather normal adjustment to dying. If the ultimate developmental purpose of such behavior is keyed to the maintenance of self in the face of imminent death, then those who attend the elderly dying person need to be aware of this objective and respectful of the function such behavior has in the adjustment strategies of the dying person.

Life Review as Developmental Process

Some people have come to understand an older person's retreat into reminiscence and past memories to be another aspect of regression. Yet, Robert Butler, a psychiatrist and former director of the National Institute on Aging, suggested that this behavior might have a positive developmental purpose. Butler (1974) described this behavior as *life review*. He suggested that the life review is characterized by "a progressive return to consciousness of past experience, in particular the resurgence of unresolved conflicts which can now be surveyed and integrated." As in the dynamics of disengagement, Butler believes that the life review is mobilized by the older person's awareness of approaching death. The life review is the "unfinished business" to which Kubler-Ross frequently alludes.

Sullivan (1982) has studied the literature on the life review and notes a growing awareness among those who work with the aged of the positive function this kind of reminiscing serves in older persons. Rather than seeing these activities as psychologically dysfunctional, many clinicians are coming to appreciate the life review as an adaptive strategy of the elderly. The life review provides an important vehicle for resolving, reorganizing, and reintegrating the conflicts of later life.

The product of an older person's reminiscences presents a challenge to the clinician attempting to interpret the developmental significance of this material. Greene (1982) claims that the data of the life review can be used in creating a therapeutic milieu in which an older person can be helped to work through some of the important themes uncovered in this retrospective activity. Interpretation can help the older person gain clarity and deeper understanding of important topics, such as the dynamics that governed his or her family's functioning over the life course. This knowledge not only helps the older person to reconcile earlier life experiences, but it may assist the older person in facing the present dynamics within a family with greater understanding.

Romaniuk and Romaniuk (1981) conducted a study on reminiscence functions and triggers in a sample of 91 older persons (aged 58–98 years old).

Utilizing the Reminiscence Uses Scale (RUS) and the Reminiscence Triggers Scale (RTS), they attempted to determine whether functions can be predicted from triggers. Using multiple regression factor analysis, the researchers found empirical evidence to support earlier theoretical views on reminiscence and aging.

The Romaniuks found that the realization that principal goals of one's life were accomplished was a predictor of a positive image of self. Also, death awareness and resignation triggered problem-solving functions: old people seemingly appeared to set to the practical tasks of getting things in order (wills, personal belongings, funeral arrangements, relationships, and so on). Changes in body and threats to bodily integrity triggered functional self-understanding. Noting past and present differences in the way one's body functions helps a person be more accepting of inevitable physical changes. The Romaniuks also assessed the relationship between the triggers of reminiscence and functional behaviors in later life. Their findings suggest a relationship between contemporaneous experience and memories and provide empirical evidence to bolster the validity of the life review construct.

The life review has great potential for use in work with older persons. Westcott (1983) describes how this natural developmental process, which may be related to preparation for death, can be used in counseling older persons about interpersonal and intrapersonal conflicts. Some of the specific problem areas she mentions are: low self-esteem, intergenerational difficulties, preparations for continued living, and preparation for dying.

Physical Illness, Depression, and Death

Some geriatricians suspect that certain systemic diseases, particularly cancers and endocrine disorders, may be related to depression in older persons (Ouslander, 1982). In exploring this proposition, Ouslander reasons that depression may result from an older person's being in chronic pain having lost certain functions. Both of these factors can contribute to a weakening of self-esteem and may necessitate the older person's becoming dependent on others for care and support.

Depression may also be related to personality variables (Bromberg & Cassel, 1983). Some people cope well with illness and treatment; others seem to have less effective resources. The premorbid personality is an important key in predicting what effect a particular illness might have on an individual. Older persons who are subject to more illnesses and longer periods of hospitalization and treatment may be more prone to become depressed by the extent of their illnesses and the course of their recovery.

Many of the drugs used in the treatment of the diseases common to older persons have unpleasant side effects that affect psychological as well as physical functioning. Some of these effects mask as depression. It is crucial to diagnosis to determine whether depressive symptoms are psychogenic or stem from the illness itself or some pharmacologic agent.

Depression, whether psychological or physiological, can create a particular problem for the older adult. It can contribute to a loss of a will to continue living (Maizler, Solomon, & Almquist, 1983). Such a situation presents special challenges to those who provide care for older persons. Some ethical implications of this issue of the "will to live—the wish to die" will be reviewed in the concluding section of this chapter.

Care of the Dying Older Person

Americans tend to favor segregating the dying from the rest of society, preferring to shield themselves from any encounter with the symbols or the reality of death. If this accurately describes the posture of many Americans toward death, it is undeniably true of their unconscious attitudes toward older persons, whose very age symbolizes death.

For an older person, the process of dying can be a prolonged experience. Dying is not simply an event, it is a process involving complex physical and psychological components. While death is ultimately a solitary act, the preparatory process is both intrapersonal and interpersonal. The more isolated an older person is in the final stages of this process, the more difficult dying can become (Krant, Doster, & Ploof, 1980).

Health care providers are directing considerable attention to these issues and their implications. The hospital or nursing home frequently is the place where the elder retires in order to die. In this particular setting, the context and quality of physical care assume special meaning. McMahon and Miller (1980) emphasize the importance of the way in which physical care is provided to the older person who is dying. Routine positioning and skin care, attention to the older person's diet and medication needs, and regular monitoring all communicate to the dying person that he or she is important and is not alone. These normal health care services promote active verbal involvement with the person. Such personal engagement, which is possible to the extent that the patient is comfortable with the prospect of death, requires sensitivity and respect for the realistic boundaries the older dying person may establish in communicating about death.

McMahon and Miller (1980) discuss two responses that can characterize either professional staff or family reactions to the dying older person. At one pole is the underreaction, which either avoids the dying person or maintains a safe physical and psychological distance. This avoidance has its basis in feelings of fear and powerlessness. Few family members have had any experience with the dying and do not know how to interact with someone facing death. Conversation can tend to be banal or inappropriate and may ultimately yield to silence and withdrawal. Similar problems can exist among physicians and nurses who may have more experience in the presence of dying persons. It is easy to retreat behind medical jargon and patronizing assurances; it is far more difficult to respond in appropriate affective ways. An attitude of underreaction tends to reinforce the lack of importance a dying person may feel. The dying carefully attend to the whole repertory of verbal and nonverbal messages they receive from family and health care providers and are prone to interpret underreaction or inattentive behavior to be signs of their minimal worth.

At the other end of the spectrum is the tendency to overreaction. The genesis of this behavior can be similarly grounded in fear. A way of compensating for fear is to mount a frontal attack, which tends to dismiss the seriousness of the dying person's condition and treats things with casualness and humor. This kind of behavior may be intended to cheer up and to distract the older person, but it can have the opposite effect. The older person may conclude that he or she is not valued and his or her death is of little importance to those who share in its preparation.

The Process of Dying and Ethical Considerations

The "Right-to-die" Question

The previous discussion highlights the issue of death with dignity. Although the issue is certainly not restricted to death in the later years, older persons may be more vulnerable to attitudes and behaviors that tend to devalue the meaning of their deaths. Improvements in health care, nutrition, and other environmental supports have continued to extend longevity in Western societies. However, added years do not guarantee quality of life for older people. On the contrary, a greater number of older persons look forward to an extended period of *living death*, characterized by increasing dependence upon others for ordinary maintenance. The requirements of care sap the physical and psychological resources of other family members and quickly deplete economic reserves.

It is important to note that an older person is often a less powerful member of the social order. He or she may be relegated to a passive role in decisions that affect his or her life and death. This reality has contributed to an increasing interest in the issues that affect a person's right to control his or her state of dying as much as he or she controlled the course of living. Although contemporary medical science supports a philosophy of human life that emphasizes the care of the whole person, in practice this integrative understanding is frequently ignored in favor of the concern for treatment of biological processes and specific organ systems.

The majority of persons involved in the medical and allied health professions are women and men of sensitivity, compassion, and good judgment. Some of these, nonetheless, perhaps due to unconscious fears of death, may seek merely to maintain the biologic existence of several organs or the overall organism in itself. In the process of preserving life, they can lose sight of the person being treated and fail to develop a comprehensive understanding of the patient. Some doctors never seem to grasp how a patient may think about his or her life.

The issues of preserving maximum integrative function at a rational human level and defending a person's right to die with dignity are important ethical concerns (GAP Report, 1973). The controversy surrounding these issues in medico-ethical, philosophical, and theological debate centers on how the objectives they outline are pursued. The arguments are framed in a variety of ways. In many discussions, "death with dignity" is synonymous with indirect or passive euthanasia, although the term *euthanasia* is frequently avoided.

Euthanasia is defined in a number of ways in contemporary usage. Its basic meaning describes a quiet and painless death. Other definitions focus on the means for ensuring or procuring a peaceful death. Yet another definition stresses the action of inducing a painless death; a synonym in this sense would be "mercy killing." In general, euthanasia can be understood to emphasize the *manner of dying* or those *actions* (or failures to act) that facilitate a person's death.

Voluntary and Involuntary Euthanasia

A primary distinction in the definition of euthanasia involves an individual's free choice in bringing about his or her own death. Euthanasia is *voluntary* if the person himself or herself requests it. Today many individuals are verbalizing this preference in a *living will*. This document asserts a desire to live a full life, but not at any cost. It specifies that in the event that death is near and cannot be avoided (for example, in the case where a person has lost the ability to interrelate with others and where there is no reasonable chance of regaining this ability, or where suffering is intense and irreversible), the person does not wish his or her life to be prolonged. In many instances, this document specifies that mechanical life support efforts should not be undertaken, nor should other life-prolonging medical procedures be employed, including the administration of transfusions and medications. Only procedures that can provide comfort and support in the normal process of dying are authorized.

This expression of the wish to die is legally recognized in a number of jurisdictions in the United States. The law shields the health care professionals as well as the health facility from liability in responding to an individual's directives. Clear expressions of an individual's carefully considered intent, Living Wills are ordinarily executed at a time when the issues surrounding this intent can be rationally assessed. Because people do change their minds, some states require that these documents be routinely updated. What these Living Wills provide is documentation of a person's long-term desire that he or she be permitted to die without life-supporting interventions.

Occasionally, such a statement of intention is signed in extreme circumstances. Under these conditions, it is advisable that a proper attestation as to the individual's competence be provided to assure the validity of the document. The validity of this statement of volition resides in consciousness and mental competence.

Often the question of *involuntary euthanasia* arises when a person is comatose or judged to be too mentally incompetent to advise medical personnel about desires for care. More precisely, the term should be *nonvoluntary euthanasia*. *Involuntary* ordinarily means "against a person's will or without a person's permission." Strictly speaking, *involuntary* describes an act against a person's will, whereas *nonvoluntary* implies an act carried out without explicit permission. In any event, consciousness and competency are the *sine qua non* variables distinguishing voluntary and involuntary actions (Lauter & Meyer, 1982).

In practice, involuntary euthanasia becomes an issue when a person has not left any explicit directives to guide medical interventions after he or she has lost consciousness. Since the patient cannot exercise judgment in an unconscious state, the family and physicians act as they assume the patient would have desired. They act without the subject's permission, but presumably not against his or her will.

Active and Passive Euthanasia

The most controversial aspects of the euthanasia debate center on the distinction between active and passive euthanasia (Rachels, 1975). *Active euthanasia* involves a conscious and positive action to cause death. In common parlance, this active intervention is frequently termed **mercy killing**. *Passive euthanasia*, as the term suggests, means refraining from doing anything to sustain life; ordinarily, it is defined as "letting a person die" or "letting nature take its course."

Although the classifications are clear in the contrasts they serve to establish in terms of action and nonaction, some ethicians do not consider the distinction between active and passive euthanasia to be decisive. Being *passive* involves being *active* in a certain way, that is, in refraining from beginning or in discontinuing some life-sustaining procedure. Other ethicians consider the distinction between *killing* and *allowing to die* as morally significant.

Direct and Indirect Euthanasia

A third tier of distinctions in the definition of euthanasia involves direct and indirect action. *Direct euthanasia* implies the deliberate use of some specific means intended to cause a person's death. This might involve the lethal administration of some drug, the infliction of a mortal wound with a firearm, or some similar violent intervention. *Indirect euthanasia* involves providing treatment intended for a specified therapeutic or palliative purpose, the side effect of which may contribute to the individual's death. An example of this indirect euthanasia might be the administration of morphine to manage excruciating pain caused by cancer; the requisite dose to alleviate the pain may be toxic and may in fact accelerate the patient's death.

The American Medical Association's Policy on Euthanasia

More than a decade ago, the American Medical Association (AMA) issued an official policy statement on the topic of euthanasia. The purpose of this statement was to provide some guidelines for physicians who found themselves tangled in the language, distinctions, and presuppositions of the euthanasia debate, and to the assertive positions being taken by many of their patients and their families on this issue. On December 4, 1973, the House of Delegates of the AMA issued the following statement.

> The intentional termination of the life of one human being by another—mercy killing—is contrary to that for which the medical profession stands and is contrary to the policy of the American Medical Association.
>
> The cessation of the employment of extraordinary means to prolong the life of the body when there is irrefutable evidence that biological death is imminent is the decision of the patient and/or his immediate family. The advice and judgment of the physician should be freely available to the patient and/or his immediate family.

Active and direct euthanasia—doing something specifically designed to terminate a person's life—is absolutely excluded in the AMA's policy statement. In fact, whenever euthanasia is introduced into medical debate, it is to this specific sense of the term that reference is made. For many physicians, euthanasia is synonymous with the popular notion of "mercy killing." For these same physicians, the issue of euthanasia is not a debate over distinctions but over what actions are professionally (and legally) acceptable under the AMA guidelines.

A more acceptable classification for voluntary, passive, and indirect euthanasia would be "death with dignity," mentioned earlier. This concept aims to educate people about death, to help people to become comfortable with dying persons, and to assist persons to die in a humane way. This does not mean that the debate about euthanasia is nothing more than a question of semantics or terminology. The debate hinges on fundamental moral differences that are not simply matters of emotion but are rooted in philosophical and theological traditions that are part of the bedrock of Western civilization.

Complicating the issue is the fact that medical knowledge and technology have developed at such a pace and to such a level of sophistication that it is possible to prolong human life despite the presence of serious illness and an unfavorable prognosis for recovery. In the case of some elderly and terminally ill persons, physicians may not always consider whether the benefits of such prolonging life outweigh its liabilities in terms of cost, inconvenience, and inability to return the patient to normal health and functioning. Convinced that life must be preserved in all cases and at all costs, some physicians minimize the importance of these considerations and consider the ethical debates to be irrelevant to their task. Others, however, maintain strongly that discussion of the "quality of human life" is indispensable to appropriate terminal care.

The Elderly and Euthanasia

Ward (1980) analyzed the 1977 data from the annual General Social Surveys conducted by the National Opinion Research Center (NORC). These surveys sample representative cohorts of Americans aged 18 years and older living in noninstitutional settings. In the year selected for analysis, two questions were included about the issue of euthanasia. In analyzing responses to these two questions, Ward attempted to assess variations in acceptance of euthanasia across major demographic groupings—age, sex, and race. He was interested in whether age is a discrete variable influencing attitudes toward euthanasia. To accomplish this he constructed separate path models for two age subsamples: 18–59 ($N = 1193$), and 60 and older ($N = 330$).

It appears from this analysis and other evidence that public acceptance of euthanasia, at least passive euthanasia, has continued to grow over the past 30 years. The Ward report indicates that this acceptance appears to vary across the major demographic groupings in society. Women seem to be less accepting of euthanasia; in part, this trend is attributable to educational and religious differences. A significant racial difference was also noted; nonwhites were less favorable to euthanasia than their white counterparts. Ward suggests that this trend may be explained by the weakened institutional power exercised by nonwhites in society and the fear that they might not be able to control the way in which life-death decisions would be made in their regard.

Perhaps because of lower education and increased religiosity, the aged were less accepting of euthanasia than were the younger persons surveyed. Ward concluded that religious practice may play the strongest and most direct role in forming older persons' attitudes toward euthanasia. It is important to note, however, that the question raised in the survey suggests *active* and *direct* intervention ("end the patient's life by some painless means"), a position that most Judeo-Christian religious traditions have never supported.

Ward suggests that some older persons may be less accepting of active euthanasia because of their particular position in the human life course. For these elders, euthanasia might be psychologically linked with a concern about gerontocide. However, in the sample analyzed from the NORC survey, the older persons who were most accepting of euthanasia were those who were the least satisfied with their current lives (deteriorating health, shrinking income, and so on). Ward concluded that when one's death is set against that of many older people, the acceptability of choosing or hastening that death seems to be contingent upon the quality of the alternative, that is, continued life.

In conclusion, the findings appear to corroborate evidence that among older cohorts declining fear of death is attributable to aging effects, while rejection of euthanasia is related to education and religious factors. Death and euthanasia seem to be distinctly different issues, at least in the way that many older people relate to them (Devins, 1979; 1981). In the Ward analyses (1980), this distinction was evident since the patterns of predictors were quite different.

There are numerous interesting discussions of the topic of the elderly and their attitudes toward euthanasia. One insightful case report of a group of older people discussing the topic of euthanasia is found in Saul and Saul (1977). Another useful analysis of ethical issues related to euthanasia and older persons is found in Meier and Cassel (1983). Although the literature on the ethics of euthanasia is vast and varied, two useful sources are Ladd (1979) and Ramsey (1978).

Summary

The most frequent association people make with the word *death* is *old*. The life-cycle orientation of this book has attempted to correct a skewed perception that death is the unique concern of the elderly. However, death is a reality for older persons and dying is a developmental task of the last phase of the human life course. This chapter has explored some topics that relate to the task of dying in the senium.

The scheme Glaser and Strauss (1965) developed to describe awareness contexts of terminally ill persons was applied to the discussion of older persons' awareness of death. The closed awareness context addresses the issue of paternalism, of protecting the older person from important factual information about health. Older people often intuit that information is being withheld: this describes the suspicion awareness context. Or medical personnel, families, and the older person can engage in a game of mutual pretense whose objective is "to keep the others from knowing what I know." Finally, the most constructive approach to death and dying is the open awareness context, whereby death is acknowledged and accepted as a natural conclusion to life. Many older people acknowledge that their most strong death-associated fear is that they will die alone. The open awareness context helps to assure an older person of presence and support throughout the final stage of dying.

Death is a familiar topic to older persons. Some seem to have an ability to predict their own demise. This has given rise to the hypothesis that older persons exercise some self-determination in the process of dying. Mental health practitioners are interested in what variables may contribute to an older person's wish to die.

A number of environmental variables can precipitate death in an older person. Three of these contextual variables were reviewed: death of a significant other, relocation, and retirement. While the various studies that report on these variables have established their importance in relation to the physical and psychological well-being of the elderly, the most significant data is yet to come from longitudinal aging research.

Terminal drop theory hypothesizes that factors related to the death of a person can cause a decline in intellectual functioning. A drop in IQ (intelligence quotient) is thought to be an early warning sign of approaching death. Although this theory has attracted much interest, research has failed to demonstrate that terminal drop exists. The existence of this phenomenon is questionable.

The fact that an older person is aware of death and is psychologically preparing for it may catalyze the *disengagement* process (Cumming & Henry, 1961). The merits of this theory have been actively debated for more than 20 years as applications of disengagement theory have been made to gerontological practice. Current research places far more emphasis on the temporal proximity of the older person to death than did the original proponents of disengagement theory. Awareness of dying may set into motion certain disengagement processes that are developmentally significant. Traditionally, disengagement has been conceptualized as a social process. Some contemporary research views it from a psychodynamic perspective.

Specific psychodynamics of the dying process in the later years were reviewed. It is important to understand the psychological defensive organization of the older person since personality normally remains consistent into late life. The time that some older persons devote to thinking and speaking about death provides evidence that preparation for dying is under way. Since this preparation is an integral developmental task in later life, older persons must be helped to complete this work.

The term *regression* has been used to describe an adaptive process of older persons facing death. While some manifestations of regression may appear on superficial observation to be pathological, a more careful differential diagnosis of these symptoms may help to establish the beneficial aspects of regressive behaviors for the older person. The importance of differential diagnosis (general information, history of illness, and normal coping styles) must be stressed.

One of the most useful conceptual tools for working with older persons is what Butler (1974) termed the *life review*. The life review is a "progressive return to consciousness of past experience, in particular the resurgence of unresolved conflicts which can now [in old age, and prior to death] be surveyed and integrated." This process has a positive functional value to older persons, and may be the mechanism by which ego integrity is assured. Some current research and clinical applications of the life review concept were described.

The final topic discussed in the survey of psychodynamic issues in the dying process of older persons was depression. Briefly the chapter considered the interrelationships between physical illness, depression, and death.

All of the psychological issues of death and dying have relevance to providing care for the dying older person. In the discussion of specific issues of care, the importance of communication with the older person, and the messages transmitted verbally and nonverbally in that process, were emphasized. Some indications of how to interpret behavioral cues of a dying elder were suggested.

Dying is more than a medical or psychiatric issue. Much contemporary discussion of death focuses on the ethical dimensions of the topic. The final section of this chapter was devoted to an exploration of the ethical aspects of the process of dying.

If one were to ask almost any health care professional who cares for a dying older person, "What is the major goal of your program of care?" the answer would probably be: "death with dignity." This slogan has become a catchword in many discussions of death and dying. Death with dignity implies holistic and responsive care. In contemporary clinical practice, these objectives are not easily met.

Death with dignity is also suggestive to some of *euthanasia*. The meanings of this term are as varied as the people who express positions about it. The principal meaning describes a quiet and painless death. Another meaning focuses on the means for procuring a tranquil death. A third definition stresses the acts that bring about such a death. This third definition is what many people understand by the term *mercy killing*.

A three-tiered set of distinctions classifies euthanasia as voluntary and involuntary, active and passive, direct and indirect. These distinctions clarify certain issues in the ethical debate surrounding euthanasia. The Living Will has been conceived in response to the question of voluntary, passive, and indirect euthanasia.

The American Medical Association's statement on euthanasia underscores the ethical problems encountered by practicing physicians. What are a physician's duties and responsibilities in maintaining life? How are these responsibilities reconciled with a person's right to die with dignity? How are the costs and benefits of prolonged terminal care assessed? The chapter reviewed these important issues.

While public acceptance of euthanasia has continued to grow over the past 30 years, the cohort of older persons may be less accepting of euthanasia than their younger counterparts. This may stem from the fear in some older persons that active and direct euthanasia may be simply a form of gerontocide. Attitudes of older persons toward euthanasia may also be tied to the quality of life they have experienced, and not specifically to the effects of aging.

Epilogue:
The Health Care
Professional,
Death, and Dying

In an essay entitled "Our attitude towards death," Sigmund Freud (1957) urged his readers to let go of their denials of death. He reasoned that a sober recognition of the brevity of a human life has a unique way of enriching that very life. He said:

> Would it not be better to give death the place in actuality and in our thoughts which properly belong to it, and to yield a little more prominence to that unconscious attitude toward death which we have hitherto so carefully repressed?. . . We remember the old saying: *Si vis pacem, para bellum*. If you desire peace, prepare for war. It would be timely thus to paraphrase it: *Si vis vitam, para mortem*. If you would endure life, be prepared for death.

Freud's simple insight is profoundly true. Often the things that concern us the most deeply are the very things we talk about the least. Death certainly figures prominently among these topics.

Elizabeth Kubler-Ross, in person and through her popular book *On death and dying* (1969), has helped people to understand and begin to discuss death and dying in an open and productive way. What was once taboo has now become the object of intensive professional and lay research and discourse. Although death is achieving legitimacy in the arena of popular debate, the stigma associated with death has not been erased. Rollo May's description of death in *Love and will*, published the same year as Kubler-Ross's bench mark work, reflects the way many still feel about the subject: "Death is obscene, unmentionable, pornographic; death is a nasty mistake. Death is not to be talked of in front of children, nor talked about at all if we can help it" (May, 1969).

Uneasy feelings about death are probably more universally shared than any others. Avoidance is a defense people naturally employ to minimize the anxieties experienced when they encounter dying persons or death itself. For some people, the topic of death or personal involvement with dying persons and their families seems to threaten their own emotional well-being.

Nurses, physicians, and other health care professionals are not immune from negative feelings and reactions in relation to death. Socialization processes in contemporary culture do not adequately prepare people for encounters with death in the human life cycle. American society does everything possible to shelter and protect individuals from the signs, symbols, and experiences of death. Death itself is disguised and mourning rituals are devalued and trivialized. Grieving is considered a private affair: public expressions of grief are discouraged.

The practice of clinical medicine and nursing reinforces these cultural attitudes. Even professional education and experiential learning may not succeed in countering the cultural bias against death. Education may fail to help health care professionals themselves learn to accept the reality and thereby thwart their attempts to assist dying persons.

Many medical schools recognize the benefits of a course in clinical thanatology, but relatively few schools in the United States have made such a course an integral part of their curricula. As a result, the majority of graduates of medical schools have limited formal education about death and dying; what little exposure there is to these topics comes from brief discussions in clinical courses. Some physicians maintain that this is evidence of an imbalance in professional medical education. Moreover, when the topic of death is actually discussed in these courses, emphasis usually falls on the biophysical aspects of dying, while its psychosocial dimensions are often excluded. A professor at the Harvard Medical School has noted: "Physicians have been taught how to pronounce the patient dead, but not how to ease the psychological distress of dying" (Hackett, 1976).

In institutions where thanatology courses are offered, they often turn out to be undersubscribed electives. To make matters worse, poor enrollment figures often result in the outright cancellation of the courses. Faculty who teach such courses, generally conducted as clinical seminars, have commented that students who elect and participate in them are frequently highly motivated and naturally oriented to a more humanistic approach to patient care. These faculty acknowledge that they often fail to reach students who could benefit most from an encounter with the issues explored.

Nursing schools have been generally more successful in achieving an integration of thanatology into their curricula. In her extensive workshops and lectures for health care professionals during the past 15 years, Kubler-Ross has noted that most of her participants are women and that a large majority of these are nurses. Most of the professional literature related to the psychosocial care of the dying is written by nurses. The dichotomy between nursing and medicine in this regard is striking.

Like most people, health care professionals will have difficulty both in discussing the topic of death and in relating to dying persons. One explanation for the ambivalent attitudes and behaviors of health care professionals toward death and the dying rests in this paradox: those who deal the most with death and dying people are professionally committed to the preservation of life. A nurse or a physician is one who heals and who must try to prevent death from happening. How do these same professionals learn to *accept* death and assist dying persons? In routine practice, professionals are nevertheless required to make some contact with dying persons and their families, even when others in the society have the luxury to deny and withdraw.

Analyzing the same paradox, traditional psychoanalytic theory has suggested that certain unconscious forces influence the choice of medicine as a personal life vocation. In the opinion of some psychoanalysts, medicine is considered a reaction formation to the unconscious fear of death that is acquired early in childhood. Medicine thus represents a way of waging war against this enemy, death. Physicians may also choose their areas of specialization as a way of protecting themselves from the fear of death, by selecting a practice not so closely associated with death as some. Although no specialty in clinical medicine is completely immune from encounters with death and dying persons, specialties such as pediatrics, gynecology, and psychiatry may be challenged less in this respect.

Most physicians and other health care professionals resist the implications of psychoanalytic theory, realizing that even if unconscious forces and the fear of death influenced their choice to enter the medical field, clinical medicine can sustain life but not defeat death.

The perceived *failure* of medicine to prevent death has generated considerable discussion among professionals. Some analytic commentators contend that it is precisely the inability of medicine to prevent death that explains certain modern developments within the practice of medicine. Although medicine is often defined as both the *art* and *science* of diagnosis, treatment of disease, and maintenance of health, to many people it describes a system of thought and practice that is strictly scientific, rational, mechanistic, and technological. Much has been written about the way in which medical practice has been dehumanized throughout history. Art has yielded to science; personal care and compassion have surrendered to objective technological sophistication. In like manner, death is scientifically attacked and humanly denied.

The striving for perfection in science and technology seems to correspond to a deemphasis on the human dimensions of medicine and hence to the dehumanization of the patients it is intended to serve. Because of its scientific concentration, medicine has also been fragmented into many different specializations. The specialized approach to the delivery of medical service diminishes or precludes significant interpersonal involvement between patient and physician and weakens the important psychosocial supports that should be a part of comprehensive care. Science, technology, and specialization have been achieved at a very high human cost.

The popular image of the medical profession is another symptom of the basic difficulty. A profession that was once considered to be among the most prestigious no longer commands universal respect and esteem. Patients distrust their physicians; physicians are unwilling to make a personal investment in their patients' well-being. On the other hand, many people still cherish an image of the ideal physician as a caring, listening and consoling person who is always available and who is ever ready to make the patient feel better. While this portrait may seem romantic, it shows the premium people place on human and interpersonal qualities in medical care. It also informs the expectations many people have of the family doctor. Fortunately, the renaissance of interest in the family practice of medicine may help to restore some of the respect for the profession of medicine that has been eroding during the past 30 years.

The expectations of what medical professionals can accomplish and the conditions in which they often must work have been similarly problematic. The contemporary practice of medicine is seriously compromised by the herculean demands made on physicians, nurses, and other allied health professionals. The volume of work required of these persons, coupled with the urgency, gravity, and intensity of the demands of medical intervention, seriously affect their ability to manage equally well all the important dimensions of effective patient care. Providing medical care is an emotionally complex task. The profession places great strain on its members in terms of personal investment, effort, and energy as well as commitment of time.

These pressures affect not only professionals but patients as well. Nowhere are iatrogenic stresses more apparent than in their effect on persons with life-threatening or terminal illnesses. A patient's serious illness challenges the health care team's abilities as healers. No less significantly, it places the professional in a position wherein he or she must encounter the fact of personal death.

The realization that human life is temporary can have positive as well as negative consequences, however. Positively, the encounters with death can underscore the inherent meanings of life and catalyze a personal integration of personal mortality into one's personality and outlook. Negatively, the confrontation with death can make a person fearful and anxious and excite a variety of unhelpful reactions.

When this confrontation with death is not accepted or not dealt with effectively by a patient, nurses and physicians become especially vulnerable to feelings of inadequacy, anger, guilt, helplessness, and frustration as they attempt to care for a terminally ill person. Professional competence and personal effort are not lacking; feelings—often unconscious and unexpressed—are the source of the difficulty. The negative consequences of frequent and prolonged encounters with dying persons may engage a variety of psychological defenses that shield the doctor or nurse from disquieting feelings. One common manifestation of such a defense is the subtle retreat behind a facade of formality. The professional resorts to the use of technical jargon in conversations with or about a patient and gradually withdraws from significant emotional contact with the patient.

A dying person described this phenomenon in vivid language. This 46-year-old mother of four, in the terminal stages of Hodgkin's disease, talked about her perceptions of the attending physician.

Whenever he comes to see me he has a real sadness on his face, yet he tries so hard not to let it show. His responses are so evasive. No matter what question I ask him, he retorts, "Oh, you really don't want to know all that." Whenever I succeed in cornering him on an issue, he overwhelms me with medical language that I can't possibly understand.

I know that he is terribly disappointed that all his efforts don't seem to be working. He has tried everything, and I'm grateful for what he has done. My husband told me that he put the question to him directly: "How much longer has Anne to live?" He got very disturbed and told Gerry not to be so pessimistic. "She's going to lick this thing and she needs all the help you can give her." While Gerry and I would both like to believe that, we both know that I am dying. Dr. Hayes knows it better than we do, but he doesn't seem comfortable admitting it.

This makes it very hard on us, because we are not able to speak openly and freely with him. It always seems like we are playing roles in a play. I've noticed that he spends less time with me when he comes in to examine me. His attempts to encourage me and cheer me up actually make me more anxious and upset. I don't know how to tell him all these things I feel.

This verbatim account highlights the ways in which a physician's discomfort with death adversely affects the quality of interaction with a dying person. The relationship comes to be characterized by well-meaning but dishonest communication on both sides. A physician's realization that medical objectives cannot be reached sometimes sets in motion a chain of negative reactions that can seriously compromise the quality of terminal care. Underlying many of these negative results are unresolved attitudes and feelings about death.

Another symptom pointing to the same problem is some patients' belief that they will suffer poorer medical and nursing attention if they make reference to their dying. A patient's need and desire to talk honestly about the approach of his or her death can be very distressing to some professionals who provide terminal care. A late adolescent dying of Ewing's sarcoma shared this experience.

Everybody here tries very hard to cheer me up. But I'm not getting better. I've noticed that the nurses and doctors really don't like to think that one of the kids here is going to die.

They (the hospital staff members) want you to believe that you are going to get better. I used to believe that, but now I know that I am going to die. I'm afraid sometimes, and other times I am not. But whenever I mention that I think I am going to die to one of the nurses, she makes some joke, or passes if off. They are constantly telling me that I shouldn't give up on life.

Do you think I'm giving up on life?. . . If you keep a cheery disposition and keep quiet about dying, then everyone is great. They talk with you and make you feel like everything's fine. But if you say anything about dying, they avoid you like the plague. I guess the message is pretty clear: keep your mouth shut about dying and just die.

This confession of a dying teenager is a poignant one. The bitterness and frustration she feels is evident in her choice of language and expression. As a long-term cancer patient with multiple hospital admissions during the course of her disease, she has been socialized to institutional expectations. The hospital has been successful in getting its message across. It is a place where people come to be restored to health; it is not a place where people come to die. The social structure of the hospital has reinforced this message. In realistic terms, the patient has received it and realizes that her physical and emotional care may be compromised if she speaks openly of her impending death. To state it bluntly, the denial of death ensures better care. Yet the same patient resents this message and wishes it were different. This interview took place in a very prestigious hospital renowned for cancer research and treatment. It is evidence that the competence of professionals in the treatment of disease is no insurance that they can meet the human needs of their dying patients.

Self-awareness in the health care professional is an indispensable component in efforts to provide competent care. To know and understand one's fears and feelings about death make it possible to deal more constructively with dying persons. To deny these feelings may lead to a routinization of care that may communicate callousness or indifference to patients and their families. Especially when they are unidentified, preexisting feelings about death can color interactions with dying patients and their families. Training and experience do not always temper these ambivalent or negative attitudes. If the dying person stimulates latent fears and feelings, the professional may become angry or frustrated with the patient or begin to withdraw from personal involvement, taking refuge in a mantle of objective clinical diagnoses and prescription. Not only will negative feelings and reactions intensify the level of a professional's anxiety, frustration, and fatigue, but they may contribute to "burnout"—a state of physical and emotional depletion that can cause some people to leave the helping professions.

Loss of valuable and skilled persons from the health care professions is troubling and unnecessary. Although it is not always easy to help persons in the health professions to come to terms with their latent fears and feelings about death, the effort to do so often brings very satisfactory results. Kubler-Ross frequently alludes to the problems she has encountered in her seminars with hospital staff persons and medical and nursing students who exhibit a natural tendency to intellectualize their feelings and to seek solutions in traditional retreats.

A psychologist (Schreibaum, 1975) writes of his experiences in trying to gain access to an oncology department in a general hospital for purposes of research. The reaction of the chief medical officer in that department reveals some of the difficulties that can be encountered in efforts to facilitate discussion of nonmedical issues related to the care of terminally ill persons.

Professor R. read the letter [of introduction and recommendation] attentively, looked me over thoughtfully and enquired, "Are the honorable doctors who signed this letter Ph.D.'s or M.D.'s?" I answered that they were Ph.D.'s. Professor R. continued to examine me with his piercing gaze and stated rather than asked, "So what have you to look for on this subject? Have psychologists ever seen a dying patient? What do they know about cancer?" I tried to explain that the knowledge psychologists have is not medical, but is connected with the understanding of human beings, their needs, their feelings, their relations with other people. Just as medical doctors can help in the medical field, psychologists can help in handling the mental problems which develop in the sick person.

Professor R., with unshakable conviction, declared on the contrary: "The cancer patient has no mental problems. His problems are not Freudian. All his problems lie in the domain of medicine. The patients are in pain. What preoccupies them is not in a domain where psychologists can help. Here there is nothing constructive, and psychologists can help only when there is something constructive. To be a cancer patient who is dying, or who is afraid of dying, is to exist in a different world. It is difficult, sad and dry as this table. (Then with clenched fist he banged on the table.) We are not dealing here with the romanticism of psychologists. There is nothing for you to look for here. A dying patient lives in a world which those who are well cannot enter. The only person who can help is his doctor." (Schreibaum, 1975, pp. 266–267)

The psychologist reporting this interview noted that this respected oncologist, despite his brusque approach, was completely dedicated to his patients and his work. However, one wonders about the success he may have in assisting some of his patients to prepare for death.

Fears and ambivalent feelings are often a function of one's discomfort with death. This discomfort unfortunately affects efforts to care for dying persons. It has been the experience of many who have offered death education courses to allied health professionals and students that discomfort with the topic of death is broadly shared among them. For this reason, an approach that combines didactic and experiential methods provides a safe vehicle by which insight and feelings can be processed. The dynamic interplay between instruction and experience gradually reduces the level of discomfort with the subject of death and consequently with dying persons as well.

Professionals who have facilitated learning experiences of this sort often report that participants found the course or seminar to be personally significant. It has been this author's own personal experience that many professionals recognize the importance of the subject of death, despite the biases they may have or the resistance they feel. There is a genuine desire on their part to learn more about it. How often the chorus played: "We never had anything like this in medical school or nursing school." The process of learning about death and dying, once engaged, is met with high motivation. Students willingly seek to acquire the knowledge and skills that will enable them to support persons who are dying, as well as their families.

In a collegial setting, professionals gradually begin to share with others some of their fears and feelings. It is not uncommon that physicians and nurses will admit that they tend to favor caring for a patient they can cure over a patient who is going to die. It is interesting to hear these professionals acknowledge their resistance to being involved with a patient whom they could not cure. A discussion of *cure* versus *care* invariably surfaces among them. It is only when the issue of *caring* for the dying person becomes the focus of conversation that the cutting edge of growth becomes apparent.

Some professionals will admit that when it was evident that they could no longer do anything to cure a disease, they could sense themselves withdrawing from the patient, but few have ever attempted to process these feelings. The psychological literature on this issue reveals that deep down the physician or nurse feels that he or she has *failed*.

The following vignette exemplifies the feeling of failure some professionals experience when their best efforts to maintain life prove unsuccessful. The case in question involved a 66-year-old man who had recently retired and with his wife moved to Florida. During the summer they had returned for a 2-week visit to their former town. While dining with his sister-in-law's family, Mr. Fitzpatrick suffered an apparent heart attack and was brought by ambulance to the emergency room of a community hospital.

The activity in the emergency room was frantic. The seriousness of his condition was apparent. Mr. Fitzpatrick was in coronary arrest. The entire resuscitation team was jammed into the small treatment area; more than a dozen professionals were involved in a complex series of medical and surgical interventions.

Since no staff member was free to leave the treatment area to speak with Mrs. Fitzpatrick and her sister, who were nervously sitting in the waiting room, I went out to provide some information and support to them. Although there was little to report, they appreciated the opportunity to talk with someone who was directly involved with Donald Fitzpatrick. They were consoled to know that everything possible was being done for him.

When I returned to the treatment area, a number of the team working on Fitzpatrick had already departed. Now there were about four people continuing to attend the dying man. Despite the fact that they were successful in reestablishing minimal cardiac functioning, his arterial blood pressure was dangerously weak.

As chaplain, I was invited to administer the sacrament of the sick. Recognizing the reality for what it was, I began to read the prayers for the dying as the remaining physicians and nurses continued their interventions. I noticed a perceptible discomfort among these people as the prayers were recited. One by one they began to withdraw from the treatment cubicle until there was but one physician and myself remaining.

When the cardiac monitor reflected no electrical activity, the remaining doctor said: "Father, there's nothing more I can do for him. Will you come with me to inform his family?" As I accompanied him the short distance from the treatment area to the waiting room, I could sense his fatigue and his quiet disappointment.

As we approached the family members, Mrs. Fitzpatrick rushed toward us. "How is my Donald?" she asked. The doctor replied: "We were not able to help him this time. He has been sent upstairs [that is, to the hospital morgue]." Mrs. Fitzpatrick responded: "What do you mean, Doctor? Can I see him?" "Your husband is dead; I'm sorry—we did all we could for him." Mrs. Fitzpatrick asked no further questions, but threw her arms around my neck and began to sob deeply.

This story highlights two issues, professional withdrawal as a person draws nearer to death and the discomfort in acknowledging the efforts to *cure* have been unsuccessful. In this case, this experienced senior physician was extremely awkward in communicating with the family of the deceased; he found it very difficult to say: "Your husband has died." The choice of words—"We were not able to help him this time"—gives some indication of how the physician was feeling about the recent death of this patient. His discomfort appeared to be tied to his own lack of success in rescuing the patient.

I have personally observed many professionals who are similarly uncomfortable in the presence of a dying person. If there is nothing more they can do for the patient, they tend to rationalize reasons to leave. If they do visit, some of these physicians and nurses become victims of what might be termed the "stethoscope syndrome." Armed with this instrument, they approach the dying person. Monitoring respiratory, cardiac, pleural, or intestinal sounds provides a way of attempting care when cure is impossible. This medical activity seems to legitimize contact. Without the stethoscope, the professional might find it exceedingly difficult to relate in a human and caring way to the *person* who is dying.

In seminars with professionals and students, the questions are often raised: "How do you learn to accept death? Where do you find the courage to support a patient who is facing death?" The answers of many professionals are the same: they learn to accept death through experience and derive courage from the dying persons whom they serve. The many cases reported in this book enriched the author's own understanding of death and have been a source of inspiration and encouragement. Dying persons have a unique ability to teach those who attempt to care for them in their final days.

In addition, the support that one receives from colleagues, both social and professional, is important. The way a profession defines itself is crucial to the way it carries out its work. If the health sciences neglect the importance of personal and psychosocial attitudes toward death and dying persons, then effective care of the dying will continue to be seriously compromised. Peers may make it possible to talk about the meaning of experiences of death. In many hospitals today, particularly among nurses, regular groups are established in which personal experiences can be shared and processed. Psychologists and social workers have frequently been invited to facilitate these staff groups. Evaluative reports that have been published describe the benefits that participants derive from such experiences. Not only do they have preventive value in mitigating factors contributing to burnout, but they have a positive effect of helping staff to become more comfortable with their own feelings about death and the care of dying persons. Quality staff support, provided in this manner and through a variety of other in-service programs, can do much for the individual professional and greatly enhance the ways staff relate to dying patients and their families.

The health care professions have a serious obligation to dying persons at each stage of the human life cycle. To be able to extend care in ways that promote dignity and that preserve a sense of identity, self-worth, and self-respect requires coming to terms with the issue of personal mortality. This humanistic objective is one of the greatest challenges to society. The common task of medical science is to reorient a profession that has been weaned from dealing with death and nurtured on death-defying, death-denying philosophies and technologies. Health professionals must accept and care for those who are dying as conscientiously as they have traditionally sought to restore the diseased and injured to wholeness of life.

Bibliography

CHAPTER ONE: STILLBIRTH AND PERINATAL DEATH

Adolf, A. & Patt, R. (1980). Neonatal death: The family is the patient. *Journal of Family Practice, 10*(10), 317–321.

Alexy, W.D. (1982). Dimensions of psychological counseling that facilitate the grieving process of bereaved parents. *Journal of Counseling Psychology, 29*, 498–507.

Benfield, D.G., Lieb, S.A., & Vollman, J.H. (1978). Grief responses of parents to neonatal death and parent participation in deciding care. *Pediatrics, 62*(2), 171–177.

Bourne, S. (1968). The psychological effects of stillbirth on women and their doctors. *Journal of the Royal College of General Practitioners, 16*, 103–112.

Bourne, S. (1983). Psychological impact of stillbirth. *Practitioner, 227*(1375), 53–60.

Bullock, M. (1981). The grief-relief process: Coping with the life and death of physically and mentally disabled children. *Orthopedic Clinics of North America, 12*(1), 193–200.

Cain, A. & Cain, B. (1964). On replacing a child. *Journal of the American Academy of Child Psychiatry, 3*, 443–455.

Campbell, A.G. (1979). Deciding the care of severely malformed or dying infants. *Journal of Medical Ethics, 5*(2), 65–67.

Chase, T.M. (1980). Perinatal death: Initiating positive family grief. *Journal of the Medical Association of the State of Alabama, 50*(1), 26–27.

Chernus, L.A. (1982). Marital treatment following early infant death. *Clinical Social Work Journal, 10*(1), 28–38.

Clyman, R.I., Green, C., Mikkelsen, C., Rowe, J. & Ataide, L. (1979). Do parents utilize physician follow-up after death of their newborn? *Pediatrics, 64*(5), 665–667.

Clyman, R.I., Green, C., Rowe, J., Mikkelsen, C. & Ataide, L. (1980). Issues concerning parents after the death of their newborn. *Critical Care Medicine, 8*(4), 215–218.

Cohen, L., Zilkha, S., Middleton, J., & O'Donohue, N. (1978). Perinatal mortality: Assisting parental affirmation. *American Journal of Orthopsychiatry, 48*(4), 727–731.

Craig, Y. (1977). The bereavement of parents and their search for meaning. *British Journal of Social Work, 7*(1), 41–54.

Crout, T.K. (1980). Caring for the mother of a stillborn baby. *Nursing (Horsham), 10*(4), 70–73.

Cullberg, J. (1972). Mental reactions of women to perinatal death. In N. Morris (ed.), *Psychosomatic Medicine in Obstetrics and Gynecology*. Basel: Karger.

David, C.J. (1975). Grief, mourning and pathological mourning. *Primary Care*, 2, 81– 92.

Drotar, D. (1976). Consultation in the intensive care nursery. *International Journal of Psychiatry in Medicine*, 7(1), 69–81.

Drotar, D. & Irvin, N. (1979). Disturbed maternal bereavement following infant death. *Child: Care, Health and Development*, 5(4), 239–247.

Elliott, B.A. & Hein, H.A. (1978). Neonatal death: Reflections for physicians. *Pediatrics*, 62(1), 96–99.

Elliott, B.A. (1978). Neonatal death: Reflections for parents. *Pediatrics*, 62(1), 100– 102.

Estok, P.J. & Lehman, A. (1983). Perinatal death: Grief support for families. *Birth: Issues in Perinatal Care and Education*, 10(1), 17–25.

Forrest, G.C., Standish, E. & Baum, J.D. (1982). Support after perinatal death: A study of support and counseling after perinatal bereavement. *British Medical Journal*, 285(6353), 1475–1479.

Furlong, R.M. & Hobbins, J.C. (1983). Grief in the perinatal period. *Obstetrics and Gynecology*, 61(4), 497–500.

Furman, E.P. (1976). Comment on J. Kennell and M. Klaus "Caring for the parents of an infant who dies." In M. Klaus & J. Kennell (Eds.), *Maternal-infant bonding*. St. Louis: C.V. Mosby.

Furman, E.P. (1978). The death of a newborn: Care of the parents. *Birth and the Family Journal*, 5(4), 214–218.

Grief and stillbirth. (1977). (Editorial). *British Medical Journal*, 1(6054), 126.

Haller, J.A. (1978). Newborns with major congenital malformations: Can the anguish of decisions regarding management be shared? *AORN Journal*, 27(6), 1070–1075.

Harman, W.V. (1981). Death of my baby. *British Medical Journal*, 282, 35–37.

Harrington, V. (1982). Bereavement and childbirth: Look, listen, support. *Nursing Mirror* (England), 154(2), 21–28.

Helmrath, T.A. & Steinitz, E.M. (1978). Death of an infant: Parental grieving and the failure of social support. *Journal of Family Practice*, 6(4), 785–790.

Help for parents after stillbirth. (1978). (Letter). *British Medical Journal*, 1(6106), 172– 173.

Hemphill, M. & Freeman, J.M. (1977). Ethical aspects of care of the newborn with serious neurological disease. *Clinics in Perinatology*, 4(1), 201–209 (27 ref.).

Hildebrand, W.L. & Schreiner, R.L. (1980). Helping parents cope with perinatal death. *American Family Physician*, 22(5), 121–125.

Jolly, H. (1976). Family reactions to stillbirth. *Proceedings of the Royal Society of Medicine*, 69(11), 835–837.

Jolly, H. (1977). Loss of a baby. *Australian Nurses Journal*, 7(4), 40–41.

Jolly, H. (1983). Parental bereavement in the perinatal period *European Journal of Obstetrics and Gynecology*, 15(4–6), 233–237.

Kellner, K.R., Best, E., Chesborough, S., Donnelly, W. & Green, M. (1981). Perinatal mortality counseling program for families who experience a stillbirth. *Death Education*, 5(1), 29–35.

Kennell, J.H., Slyter, H. & Klaus, M.H. (1970). The mourning response of parents to the death of a newborn infant. *New England Journal of Medicine*, 283, 344–349.

Kirkley-Best, E. & Kellner, K.R. (1982). The forgotten grief: A review of the psychology of stillbirth. *American Journal of Orthopsychiatry*, 52(3), 420–429.

Klaus, M.H. & Kennell, J. (1976). Caring for the parents of a stillborn or an infant who dies. In Klaus, M.H. & Kennell, J. (eds.) *Parent-Infant Bonding*, 209–239. St. Louis: C.V. Mosby.

Knapp, R.J., & Peppers, L.G. (1979). Doctor-patient relationships in fetal/infant death encounters. *Journal of Medical Education, 54*(10), 755–780.

Kovalesky, A. (1978). Encounters with grief: That night in the neonatal nursery. *American Journal of Nursing, 78*(3), 414–416.

Kowalski, K. & Osborn, M.R. (1977). Helping mothers of stillborn infants to grieve. *Maternal-Child Nursing Journal, 2*(1), 29–32.

Krein, N. (1979). Sudden infant death syndrome: Acute loss and grief reactions. *Clinical Pediatrics, 18*, 414–423.

Kulkarni, P., et al. (1978). Postneonatal infant mortality in infants admitted to a neonatal intensive care unit. *Pediatrics, 62*(2), 178–183.

Kushner, L. (1979). Infant death and the childbirth educator. *Maternal-Child Nursing Journal, 4*(4), 231–233.

Lake, M., Knippel, R.A., Murphy, J. & Johnson, T.M. (1983). The role of a grief support team following stillbirth. *American Journal of Obstetrics and Gynecology, 146*(8), 877–881.

LaRoche, C., et al. (1982). Grief reactions to perinatal death: An exploratory study. *Psychosomatics, 23*(5), 510–511, 514, 516–518.

Lewis, E. (1976). Points of view. The management of stillbirth: Coping with an unreality. *Lancet, 2*(7896), 619–620.

Lewis, E. (1979a). Mourning by the family after a stillbirth or neonatal death. *Archives of Diseases in Childhood, 54*(4), 303–306.

Lewis, E. (1979b). Inhibition of mourning by pregnancy: Psychopathology and management. *British Medical Journal, 2*(6181), 27–28.

Lewis, E. (1983). Stillbirth: Psychological consequences and strategies of management. In A. Miunsky, E.A. Friedman & L. Cluck (eds.), *Advances in Perinatal Medicine*: Vol. 3, 205–245. New York: Plenum Publishing Corporation.

Lewis, E. & Page, A. (1978). Failure to mourn a stillbirth: An overlooked catastrophe. *British Journal of Medical Psychology, 51*(3), 237–241.

Lewis, M.S., Gottesman, D. & Gutstein, S. (1979). The course and duration of crisis. *Journal of Consulting and Clinical Psychology, 47*(1), 128–134.

Limerick, L. (1979). Counselling parents who have lost an infant. *Journal of the Royal College of Physicians of London, 13*(4), 242–245.

Lockwood, S. (1983). Parental reactions to stillbirth. *Australian Family Physician, 12*(4), 234–235.

Lovell, A. (1983). Some questions of identity: Late miscarriage, stillbirth and perinatal loss. *Social Science and Medicine, 17*(11), 755–761.

Lovell, A. (1983). Women's reactions to late miscarriage, stillbirth and perinatal death. *Health Visitor, 56*(9), 325–327.

Mahan, C.K., Perez, R.H., Ratliff, M. & Schreiner, R.L. (1980). Neonatal death: Parental evaluation of the NICU experience. *Issues in Comprehensive Pediatric Nursing, 5*(5–6), 279–292.

Mahan, C.K. & Schreiner, R.L. (1981). Management of perinatal death: Role of the social worker in the ICU. *Social Work in Health Care, 6*(3), 69–76.

Meyer, R. & Lewis, E. (1979). The impact of a stillbirth on a marriage. *Journal of Family Therapy, 1*, 361–369.

Middleton, J. (1979). The perinatal bereavement crisis. Michele and James. *Journal of Nurse-Midwifery*, 19–21.

Morgan, J.H. & Goering, R. (1978). Caring for parents who have lost an infant. *Journal of Religion and Health, 17*(4), 290–298.

Morris, D. (1976). Parental reactions to perinatal death. *Proceedings of the Royal Society of Medicine, 69*(11), 837–838.

Orfirer, A.P. (1970). Loss of sexual function in the male. In B. Schoenberg *et al.* (eds.), *Loss and grief: Psychological management in medical practice* (156–177). New York: Columbia University Press.

O'Donohue, N. (1978). Perinatal bereavement: The role of the health care professional. *QRB. Quality Review Bulletin, 4*(9), 30–32.

O'Donohue, N. (1979). The perinatal bereavement crisis. Facilitating the grief process. *Journal of Nurse-Midwifery, 24*(5), 16–19.

Parrish, S. (1980). Letting go. *Canadian Nurse, 76*(3), 34–37.

Peppers, L.G. & Knapp, R.J. (1980). *Motherhood and mourning*. New York: Praeger.

Peppers, L.G. & Knapp, R.J. (1980). Maternal reactions to involuntary fetal/infant death. *Psychiatry, 43*(2), 155–159.

Phipps, S. (1981). Mourning response and intervention in stillbirth: An alternative genetic counseling approach. *Social Biology, 28*(1–2), 1–13.

Poznanski, E.O. (1972). The "replacement child": A saga of unresolved parental grief. *Journal of Pediatrics, 81*, 1190–1193.

Quirk, T.R. (1979). The perinatal bereavement crisis. Crisis theory, grief theory, and related psychosocial factors: The framework for intervention. *Journal of Nurse-Midwifery, 24*(5), 13–16.

Rabin, A.T. (1965). Motivation for parenthood. *Journal of Projective Techniques of Personality Assessment, 29*, 405–411.

Reid, R. (1977). Spina bifida: The fate of the untreated. *Hastings Center Report, 7*(4), 16–19.

Rowe, J., Clyman, R., Green, C., Mikkelson, C., Haight, J. & Ataide, L. (1978). Follow-up families who experience a perinatal death. *Pediatrics, 62*(2), 166–170.

Sahu, S. (1981). Coping with perinatal death. *Journal of Reproductive Medicine, 26*(3), 129–132.

Savage, W. (1978). Perinatal loss and the medical team. *Midwife, Health Visitor, and Community Nurse, 14*(9), 292–295.

Saylor, D.E. (1978). Nursing response to mothers of stillborn infants. *JOGN Nursing, 6*(4), 39–42.

Scupholme, A. (1978). Who helps? Coping with the unexpected outcomes of pregnancy. *JOGN Nursing, 7*(4), 36–39.

Seibel, M. & Graves, W.L. (1980). The psychological implications of spontaneous abortions. *Reproductive Medicine, 24*, 161–165.

Seitz, P.M. & Warrick, L.H. (1974). Perinatal death: The grieving mother. *American Journal of Nursing, 74*(11), 2028–2033.

Shaw, C.T. (1983). Grief over fetal loss. *Family Practice Recertification, 5*, 129–145.

Shokeir, M. (1979). Managing the family of the abnormal newborn. In B.D. Hall (ed.), *Proceedings of the 1978 Birth Defects Conference*. New York: National Foundation–March of Dimes.

Silverman, W.A. (1981). Mismatched attitudes about neonatal death. *Hastings Center Report, 11*(6), 12–16.

Slade, C.I., Reidl, C.J. & Mangurten, H.H. (1977). Working with parents of high-risk newborns. *JOGN Nursing, 6*(2), 21–26.

Speck, P. (1978). Easing the pain and grief of still-birth. *Nursing Mirror, 146*(22), 38–41.

Stack, J.M. (1980). Spontaneous abortion and grieving. *American Family Physician, 21,* 99–102.

Stringham, J.G., Riley, J.H. & Ross, A. (1982). Silent birth: Mourning a stillborn baby. *Social Work, 27*(4), 322–327.

Support for parents experiencing perinatal loss. (1983). *Canadian Medical Association Journal, 129*(4), 335–339.

Thomas, J.V. (1980). A validation of a grief scale used with parents of critically ill infants. *Dissertation Abstracts International, 41*(1–B), 335–336.

Todres, I.D., Krane, D., Howell, M.C., *et al.* (1977). Pediatricians' attitudes affecting decision making in defective newborns. *Pediatrics, 60*(2), 197–201.

Whitfield, J.M., *et al.* (1982). The application of hospice concepts to neonatal care. *American Journal of Diseases of Children, 136*(5), 421–424.

Wilson, A.L. & Soule, D.J. (1981). The role of self-help groups in working with parents of a stillborn baby. *Death Education, 5*(2), 175–186.

Winnicott, D.W. (1958). Primary maternal preoccupation. In *Collected Papers.* London: Tavistock.

Wolff, J.R., Nielson, P.E. & Schiller, P. (1970). The emotional reaction to a stillbirth. *American Journal of Obstetrics and Gynecology, 108*(1), 73–77.

Yu, V.Y., Jamieson, J. & Astbury, J. (1981). Parent's reactions to unrestricted parental contact with infants in the intensive care nursery. *Medical Journal of Australia, 1*(6), 294–296.

CHAPTER TWO: SUDDEN INFANT DEATH SYNDROME

American Academy of Pediatrics. (1978). Task force on prolonged apnea. *Pediatrics, 61,* 651–652.

Bakke, K. & Dougherty, J. (1981). Sudden infant death syndrome and infant apnea: Current questions, clinical management and research directions. *Issues in Comprehensive Pediatric Nursing, 5*(2), 77–88.

Beal, S.M. (1979). Sudden infant death syndrome. *Australian Family Physician, 8*(12), 1279–1283.

Beckwith, J.B. (1973). The sudden infant death syndrome. *Current Problems in Pediatrics, 3,* (1).

Beckwith, J.B. (1977). The sudden infant death syndrome. *Public Health Service,* 8–16.

Bergman, A.B. (1976). Sudden Infant Death Syndrome: An approach to management. *Primary Care, 3,* 1–8.

Bergman, A.B., Ray, C.G. & Pomeroy, M.A. (1972). Studies of the Sudden Infant Death Syndrome in Kings County, Washington. *Pediatrics, 49*(6), 860.

Black, D. (1978). The bereaved child. *Journal of Child Psychology Psychiatry, 19,* 287–292.

Bluglass, K. (1981). Psychological aspects of the sudden infant death syndrome ("cot death"). *Journal of Child Psychology and Psychiatry, 22*(4), 411–421.

Brooks, J.G. (1982). Apnea of infancy and sudden infant death syndrome. *American Journal of Diseases of Children, 136*(11), 1012–1023.

Brown, A. (1978). A case study in family systems consultations for community health nurses working with Sudden Infant Death (SIDS) families. *Family Therapy, 5*(3), 233–244.

Camfield, P., Camfield, C., Bagnell, P. & Rees, E. (1982). Infant apnea syndrome: A prospective evaluation of etiologies. *Clinical Pediatrics, 21*(11), 684–687.

Cepeda, M.L. (1981). Sudden infant death syndrome: Helping bereaved parents talk with children. *Southern Medical Journal, 74*(1), 9–10.

Chernus, L.A. (1982). Marital treatment following early infant death. *Clinical Social Work Journal, 10*(1), 28–38.

Colton, R.H. & Steinschneider, A. (1981). The cry characteristics of an infant who died of the Sudden Infant Death Syndrome. *Journal of Speech and Hearing Disorders, 46*(4), 359–363.

Cornwell, J., Nurcombe, B. & Stevens, L. (1977). Family response to loss of a child by sudden infant death syndrome. *Medical Journal of Australia,* 656–658.

Crawshaw, L. (1978). The sudden infant death syndrome: A psychological consideration. *Smith College Studies in Social Work, 48*(2), 132–170.

DeFrain, J.D. & Ernst, L. (1978). The psychological effects of sudden infant death syndrome on surviving family members. *Journal of Family Practice, 6*(5), 985–989.

DeFrain, J.D., Taylor, J. & Ernst, L. (1982). *Coping with sudden infant death.* Lexington, Mass.: D.C. Heath Company (Lexington Books).

Emery, J.L. (1972). Welfare of families of children found unexpectedly dead ("cot death"). *British Medical Journal, 2,* 612–615.

Emery, J.L. & Dinsdale, F. (1978). Structure of periadrenal brown fat in childhood in both expected and cot deaths. *Archives of the Diseases of Childhood, 53, 154.*

Franciosi, R.A. (1983). Evolution of SIDS diagnosis. *Minnesota Medicine, 66*(7), 411–413.

Freud, S. (1957). Mourning and melancholia. In *Standard edition of the complete psychological works of Sigmund Freud, 14,* 237–260. London: Hogarth Press. (Original work published in 1917.)

Froggatt, P., Lynas, M.A. & MacKenzie, G. (1971). Epidemiology of sudden unexpected death in infants ("cot death") in northern Ireland. *British Journal of Preventive Social Medicine, 25,* 119–134.

Golub, H.L. & Corwin, M.J. (1982). Infant cry: A clue to diagnosis. *Pediatrics, 69*(2), 197–201.

Greenough, W.T. (1975). Experiential modification of the developing brain. *American Scientist, 63,* 37–46.

Greenough, W.T., Wolkmar, F.R. & Fleischman, T.B. (1976). Environmental effects on brain connectivity and behavior. In D.I. Mostofsky (ed.), *Behavior control and modification of physiological activity,* 220–245. Englewood Cliffs, N.J.: Prentice-Hall.

Guilleminault, C., Souquet, M., Ariagno, R.L., Korobkin, R. & Simmons, F.B. (1984). Five cases of near-miss sudden infant death syndrome and development of obstructive sleep apnea syndrome. *Pediatrics, 73*(1), 71–78.

Guntheroth, W.G. (1970). Some physiologic considerations in sudden infant death syndrome. In A.B. Bergman, J.B. Beckwith and C.G. Ray (eds.), *Sudden Infant Death Syndrome,* 181. Seattle: University of Washington Press.

Guntheroth, W.G. (1973). The significance of pulmonary petechiae in crib death. *Pediatrics, 52,* 601–603.

Guntheroth, W.G., Kawabori, I., Breazeale, D.G., *et al.* (1980). The role of respiratory infection in intrathoracic petechiae. *American Journal of the Diseases of Childhood, 134,* 364–366.

Harper, R.M. *et al.* (1981). Periodicity of sleep states is altered in infants at risk for the Sudden Infant Death Syndrome. *Science, 213*(4511), 1030–1032.

Hawkins, D.G. (1980). Enigma in swaddling clothes: Sudden infant death. *Health and Social Work, 5*(4), 21–27.

Heinen, B.N. (1983). Etiology of sudden infant death. *Journal of Family Practice, 16*(1), 22–23.

Hoppenbrouwers, T., Hodgman, J.E., Harper, R.M. & Sterman, M.B. (1982). Temporal distribution of sleep states, somatic activity and autonomic activity during the first half year of life. *Sleep, 5*(2), 131–144.

Johnson, M.P. & Hufbauer, K. (1982). Sudden Infant Death Syndrome as a medical research problem since 1945. *Social Problems, 30*(1), 65–81.

Katona, Peter G. & Egbert, J.R. (1978). Heart rate and respiratory rate differences between preterm and full-term infants during quiet sleep: Possible implications for SIDS. *Pediatrics, 62*(1), 91–95.

Kraus, J.F. & Borkani, N.O. (1972). Post-neonatal sudden, unexpected death in California: A cohort study. *American Journal of Epidemiology, 95,* 497.

Krein, N. (1979). Sudden infant death syndrome: Acute loss and grief reactions. *Clinical Pediatrics, 18,* 414–423.

Kulkarni, P. *et al.* (1978). Postneonatal infant mortality in infants admitted to a neonatal intensive care unit. *Pediatrics, 62* (2).

Lewak, N. *et al.* (1979). Sudden infant death syndrome risk factors: prospective data reviewed. *Clinical Pediatrics, 18*(7), 404–411.

Lewis, S. (1981). Some psychological consequences of bereavement by sudden infant death syndrome. *Health Visitor, 54,* 322–325.

Limerick, S. (1981). The role of the Foundation for the Study of Infant Deaths. *Medical Science and Law, 21*(2), 143–144.

Lipsitt, L.P. (1979). Infants at risk: Perinatal and neonatal factors. *International Journal of Behavioral Development, 2*(1), 23–42.

Lipsitt, L.P., Sturner, W.Q. & Burke, P. (1979). Perinatal indicators and subsequent crib death. *Infant Behavior and Development, 2*(4), 325–328.

Lipsitt, L. P. *et al.* (1981). Perinatal indicators of Sudden Infant Death Syndrome: A study of 34 Rhode Island cases. *Journal of Applied Developmental Psychology, 2*(1), 79–88.

Lowman, J. (1979). Grief intervention and sudden infant death syndrome. *American Journal of Community Psychology, 7*(6), 665–677.

Mandell, F., McAnulty, E. & Reece, R. (1980). Observations of paternal response to sudden unanticipated infant death. *Pediatrics, 65,* 221–225.

Mandell, F., Wolfe, L.C. (1975). Sudden infant death syndrome and subsequent pregnancy. *Pediatrics, 56,* 774–776.

Markusen, E., Owen, G., Fulton, R. & Bendiksen, R. (1977). SIDS: The survivor as victim. *OMEGA: Journal of Death & Dying, 8*(4), 277–284.

May, H.J. & Breme, F.L. (1983). SIDS Family Adjustment Scale: A method of assessing family adjustment to Sudden Infant Death Syndrome. *OMEGA: Journal of Death and Dying, 13*(1), 59–74.

McCoy, K.S. (1981). Sudden infant death syndrome. *Arizona Medicine, 38*(6), 432–435.

Meier, C.A. (1973). Sudden infant death syndrome: Death without apparent cause. *Life-Threatening Behavior, 3*(4),298–304.

Naeye, R.L. (1976). Brain-stem and adrenal abnormalities in the sudden infant death syndrome. *American Journal of Clinical Pathology, 66*, 526.

Naeye, R.L. (1980). Sudden infant death. *Scientific American, 242*(4), 56–62.

Naeye, R.L., Fisher, R., Ryser, M. *et al.* (1976). Carotid body in the sudden infant death syndrome. *Science, 191*, 567.

Nikolaisen, S. (1981). The impact of sudden infant death on the family: Nursing intervention. *Topics in Clinical Nursing, 3*(3), 45–53.

Pasquis, P., Tardif, C. & Nouvet, G. (1983). Reflux gastro-oesphagien et affections respiratoires. *Bulletin European Physiopathologie Respiratoire, 19*(6), 645–658.

Peterson, D.R., Chinn, N.M. & Fisher, L.D. (1972). Sudden and unexpected death in infants: Incidence in two climactically dissimilar metropolitan communities. *American Journal of Epidemiology, 95*, 95–98.

Pierson, P.S. *et al.* (1972). Sudden deaths in infants born to methadone-maintained addicts. *Journal of the American Medical Association, 220*(13), 1733–1734.

Read, D.J., Jeffery, H.W. & Rahilly, P. (1982). Sudden infant death syndrome and suspected "near-miss": An overview for clinicians. *Medical Journal of Australia, 1*(2), 82–87.

Rubin, S. (1977). Bereavement and vulnerability: A study of mothers of sudden infant death syndrome children. *Dissertation Abstracts International, 38*(4–B), 1902–1903.

Rubin, S. (1982). Persisting effects of loss: A model of mourning. *Series in Clinical and Community Psychology: Stress and Anxiety, 8*, 275–282.

Shaddy, R.E. & McIntire, M.S. (1982). Sudden infant death syndrome: A review for primary care physicians. *Nebraska Medical Journal*, 74–79.

Smialek, Z. (1978). Observations on immediate reactions of families to sudden infant death. *Pediatrics, 62*(2), 160–165.

Steinmarc, P.L. (1979). When a young child dies: The interactionist approach to the crisis of sudden infant death syndrome and its case management. *Dissertation Abstracts International, 40*(2–A), 1111.

Steinschneider, A. (1972). Prolonged apnea and the sudden infant death syndrome: Clinical and laboratory observations. *Pediatrics, 50*(4), 646–654.

Stevenson, K.M. (1981). Parental utilization and perceptions of helpful social networks following a sudden infant death. *Dissertation Abstracts International, 41*(11–A), 4841.

Stockard, J.L. (1982). Brainstem auditory evoked potentials in adult and infant sleep apnea syndromes, including sudden infant death syndrome and near-miss for sudden infant death. *Annals of the New York Academy of Sciences, 388*, 443–465.

Takashima, S., Armstrong, D. & Becker, L.E. (1978). Cerebral white matter lesions in sudden infant death syndrome. *Pediatrics, 62*(2), 155–159.

Valdes-Dapena, M.A. (1967). Sudden and unexpected death in infancy: A review of the world literature 1954–1966. *Pediatrics, 39*, 123–135.

Valdes-Dapena, M.A. (1970). Progress in sudden infant death research, 1963–1969. In A.B. Bergman, J.B. Beckwith & C.G. Ray (eds.), *Sudden Infant Death Syndrome*, 3. Seattle: University of Washington Press.

Valdes-Dapena, M.A. (1977). Sudden unexplained infant death, 1970 through 1975: An evolution in understanding. *Pathology Annual, 12*, 117.

Valdes-Dapena, M.A. (1980). Sudden infant death syndrome: A review of medical literature 1974–1979. *Pediatrics, 66,* 597–613.

Weinstein, S.E. (1978). Sudden infant death syndrome: Impact on families and a direction for change. *American Journal of Psychiatry, 135*(7), 831–834.

Weissbluth, M. (1981). Infantile colic and near-miss sudden infant death. *Medical Hypotheses, 7*(9), 1193–1199.

Weitzman, E.D. (1981). Sleep and its disorders. *Annual Review of Neuroscience, 4,* 381–417.

Werne, J. (1942). Postmortem evidence of acute infection in unexpected death in infancy. *American Journal of Pathology and Bacteriology, 18,* 759.

Werne, J. & Garrow, I. (1947). Sudden death of infants allegedly due to mechanical suffocation. *American Journal of Public Health, 37,* 675.

Werne, J. & Garrow, I. (1953). Pathologic findings in infants dying immediately after violence contrasted with those after sudden apparently unexplained death. *American Journal of Pathology, 29,* 833.

Williams, A. (1981). SIDS: A pathologist's diagnosis. *Pathology, 13*(3), 405–407.

Williams, M.L. (1981). Sibling reaction to cot death. *The Medical Journal of Australia, 2,* 227–231.

Williams, R.A. & Nikolaisen, S.M. (1982). Sudden Infant Death Syndrome: Parents' perceptions and responses to the loss of their infant. *Research in Nursing and Health, 5*(2), 55–61.

Williams, W.V., Lee, J. & Polak, P.R. (1976). Crisis intervention: Effects of crisis intervention on family survivors of sudden death situations. *Community Mental Health Journal, 12*(2), 128–136.

Young, P.C. (1981). Another aspect of the SIDS problem [letter]. *Pediatrics, 68*(1), 143–144.

CHAPTER THREE: CHILDHOOD BEREAVEMENT

Balk, D. (1983). The effects of sibling death on teenagers. *Journal of School Health, 53*(1), 14–18.

Becker, D. & Margolin, F. (1967). How surviving parents handled their young children's adaptation to the crisis of loss. *American Journal of Orthopsychiatry, 37*(4), 753–757.

Bendiksen, R. & Fulton, R. (1975). Death and the child: An anterospective test of the childhood bereavement and later behavior disorder hypothesis. *Omega, 6,* 45–59.

Berlinsky, E.B. & Biller, H.B. (1982). *Parental death and psychological development.* Lexington, Mass.: D.C. Heath, Lexington Books.

Birk, A. (1966). The bereaved child. *Mental Health, 25*(4), 9–11.

Birtchnell, J. (1969a). Parent death in relation to age and parental age at birth in psychiatric patients and general population controls. *British Journal of Preventive and Social Medicine, 23,* 244.

Birtchnell, J. (1969b). The possible consequences of early parent death. *British Journal of Medical Psychology, 42*(1), 1–12.

Birtchnell, J. (1970a). Early parent death and mental illness. *British Journal of Psychiatry, 116,* 281–288.

Birtchnell, J. (1970b). Recent parent death and mental illness. *British Journal of Psychiatry, 116,* 289–297.

Birtchnell, J. (1970c). Depression in relation to early and recent parent death. *British Journal of Psychiatry, 116,* 299–306.

Birtchnell, J. (1970d). The relation between attempted suicide, depression and parent death. *British Journal of Psychiatry, 116,* 307–313.

Birtchnell, J. (1971). Case register study of bereavement. *Proceedings of the Royal Society of Medicine, 64,* 279–282.

Birtchnell, J. (1972a). Early parent death and psychiatric diagnosis. *Social Psychiatry, 7,* 202–210.

Birtchnell, J. (1972b). The inter-relationship between social class, early parent death and mental illness. *Psychological Medicine, 2,* 166–175.

Birtchnell, J. (1974). Is there a scientifically acceptable alternative to the epidemiological study of familial factors in mental illness? *Social Science and Medicine, 8,* 335–350.

Birtchnell, J. (1975). The personality characteristics of early bereaved psychiatric patients. *Social Psychiatry, 10,* 97–103.

Birtchnell, J. (1978). Early parent death and the clinical scales of the MMPI. *British Journal of Psychiatry, 132,* 574–579.

Birtchnell, J. (1981). In search of correspondences between age at psychiatric breakdown and parental age at death—"anniversary reactions". *British Journal of Medical Psychology, 54*(pt. 2), 111–120.

Black, C.P. (1979). Young children's understandings about death as perceived by parents, teachers, and a recorder. *Dissertation Abstracts International, 40*(1–B), 157.

Bluebond-Langner, M. (1978). *The private world of dying children.* New Jersey: Princeton University Press.

Blum, H.P. (1983). The psychoanalytic process and analytic inference: A clinical study of a lie and loss. *International Journal of Psychoanalysis, 64,* 17–33.

Bowlby, J. (1960). Grief and mourning in infancy and early childhood. In *Psychoanalytic Study of the Child, 15.* New York: International Universities Press.

Bowlby, J. (1969). *Attachment and loss: Attachment* (Vol. 1). New York: Basic Books.

Bowlby, J. (1973). *Attachment and loss: Separation: Anxiety and anger* (Vol. 2). New York: Basic Books.

Bowlby, J. (1980). *Attachment and loss: Loss, sadness and depression* (Vol. 3). New York: Basic Books.

Brent, D.A. (1983). A death in the family: The pediatrician's role. *Pediatrics, 72*(5), 645–651.

Cain, A.C. & Fast, I. (1966). Children's disturbed reactions to parent suicide. *American Journal of Orthopsychiatry, 36,* 874–885.

Cairns, N.U., Clark, G.M., Smith, S.D. & Lansky, S.B. (1979). Adaptation of siblings to childhood malignancy. *Journal of Pediatrics, 95*(3), 484–487.

Codden, P. (1977). The meaning of death for parents and the child. *Maternal-Child Nursing Journal, 6*(1), 9–16.

Dietrich, D.R. (1979). Psychopathology and death fear: A quasi-experimental investigation of the relationship between psychopathology and death fear and fantasies as psychological sequelae in young adults who experienced the death of a parent during childhood or adolescence. *Dissertation Abstracts International, 40*(2–B), 910–911.

Feinberg, D. (1970). Preventive therapy with siblings of a dying child. *Journal of the American Academy of Child Psychiatry, 9*(4), 644–668.

Freud, S. (1957). Mourning and melancholia. In *Standard edition of the complete psychological works of Sigmund Freud, 14,* 237–260. London: Hogarth Press. (Original work published in 1917.)

Furman, E. (1974). *A child's parent dies: Studies in childhood bereavement.* New Haven: Yale University Press.

Furman, R.A. (1970). The child's reaction to death in the family. In B. Schoenberg, A.C. Carr, D. Peretz & A.H. Kutscher (eds.), *Loss and grief: Psychological management in medical practice.* New York: Columbia University Press.

Gardner, R.A. (1977a). Children's guilt reactions to parental death: Psychodynamics and therapeutic management. *Hiroshima Forum for Psychology, 4,* 45–50.

Gardner, R.A. (1977b). Author's reply to the comments. *Hiroshima Forum for Psychology, 4,* 55–57.

Gogan, J.L. & Slavin, L.A. (1981). Interviews with brothers and sisters. In G.P. Koocher & J.E. O'Malley (eds.), *The Damocles syndrome: Psychological consequences of surviving childhood cancer.* New York: McGraw-Hill.

Hagin, R.A. & Corwin, C.G. (1974). Bereaved children. *Journal of Clinical Child Psychology, 3*(2), 39–40.

Johnson, P.A. (1982). After a child's parent has died. *Child Psychiatry and Human Development, 12*(3), 160–170.

Kane, B. (1979). Children's concepts of death. *Journal of General Psychology, 134,* 141–153.

Kohut, H. (1971). *Analysis of the self.* New York: International Universities Press.

Koocher, G.P. (1973). Childhood, death, and cognitive development. *Developmental Psychology, 9*(3), 369–375.

Krueger, D.W. (1983). Childhood parent loss: Developmental impact and adult psychopathology. *American Journal of Psychotherapy, 37*(4), 582–592.

Lebovici, S. (1974). Observations on children who have witnessed the violent death of one of their parents: A contribution to the study of traumatization. *International Review of Psychoanalysis, 1*(1–2), 117–123.

Long, K. A. (1983). The experience of repeated and traumatic loss among Crow Indian children: Response patterns and intervention strategies. *American Journal of Orthopsychiatry, 53*(1), 116–126.

Mitchell, N.L. & Schulman, K.R. (1981). The child and the fear of death. *Journal of the National Medical Association, 73*(10), 963–967.

Nagaraja, J. (1977). Child's reaction to death. *Child Psychiatry Quarterly, 10*(2), 24–28.

Nagera, H. (1970). Children's reactions to the death of important objects: A developmental approach. *Psychoanalytic Study of the Child, 25,* 360–400.

Nagy, M.H. (1948). The child's theories concerning death. *Genetic Psychology, 73,* 3–27.

Ney, P.G. & Barry, J.E. (1983). Children who survive. *New Zealand Medical Journal, 96*(726), 127–129.

Nixon, J. & Pearn, J. (1977). Emotional sequelae of parents and siblings following the drowning or near-drowning of a child. *Australian & New Zealand Journal of Psychiatry, 11*(4), 262–268.

Palgi, P. (1983). Reflections on some creative modes of confrontation with the phenomenon of death. *International Journal of Social Psychiatry, 29*(1), 29–37.

Palombo, J. (1981). Parent loss and childhood bereavement: Some theoretical considerations. *Clinical Social Work Journal, 9*(1), 3–33.

Persson-Goran. (1980). Relation between early parent death and life event ratings among 70-year-olds: A test of a sensitization theory. *ACTA Psychiatrica Scandinavica*, 62(4), 392–397.

Piaget, J. (1929). *The child's conception of the world*. London: Kegan Paul.

Plank, E.N. & Plank, R. (1978). Children and death. In A. J. Solnit (ed.), *Psychoanalytic study of the child*. New Haven: Yale University Press.

Pollock, G.H. (1972). Bertha Pappenheim's pathological mourning: Possible effects of childhood sibling loss. *Journal of the American Psychoanalytic Association*, 20(3), 476–493.

Raphael, B. (1982). The young child and the death of a parent. In C.M. Parkes & J. Stevenson-Hinde (eds.), *The place of attachment in human behavior*. New York: Basic Books, 1982.

Raphael, B., Field, J. & Kvelde, H. (1980). Childhood bereavement: A prospective study as a possible prelude to future preventive intervention. In E.J. Anthony & C. Chiland (eds.), *Preventive psychiatry in an age of transition* (Yearbook of the International Association for Child and Adolescent Psychiatry and Allied Professions, Vol. 6). New York: Wiley.

Rheingold, J. (1967). *The mother, anxiety and death*. Boston: Little, Brown.

Rosenheim, E. & Ichilov, Y. (1979). Short-term preventive therapy with children of fatally-ill parents. *Israel Annals of Psychiatry & Related Disciplines*, 17(1), 67–73.

Rosenthal, P.A. (1980). Short-term family therapy and pathological grief resolution with children and adolescents. *Family Process*, 19, 151–159.

Rosen, H. & Cohen, H.L. (1981). Children's reactions to sibling loss. *Clinical Social Work Journal*, 9(3), 211–219.

Salladay, S.A. & Royal, M.E. (1981). Children and death: Guidelines for grief work. *Child Psychiatry & Human Development*, 11(4), 203–212.

Salzberger, R.C. (1975). Death: Beliefs, activities and reactions of the bereaved: Some psychological and anthropological observations. *Human Context*, 7(1), 103–116.

Small, G.W. & Nicholi, A.M., Jr. (1982). Mass hysteria among school-children: Early loss as a predisposing factor. *Archives of General Psychiatry* (U.S.), 39(6), 721–724.

Tallmer, F. & Tallmer, J. (1974). Factors influencing children's concepts of death. *Journal of Clinical Child Psychology*, 3(2), 17–19.

Taylor, D.A. (1984). Views of death from sufferers of early loss. *Omega*, 14, 77–82.

Tennant, C. & Bebbington, P. & Hurry, J. (1980). Parental death in childhood and risk of adult depressive disorders: A review. *Psychological Medicine*, 10(2), 289–299.

Tousley, M.M. (1982). The use of family therapy in terminal illness and death. *Journal of Psychosocial Nursing Mental Health Services*, 20(1), 17–22.

Wessel, M.A. & McCullough, W.B. (1982). Bereavement—An etiologic factor in peptic ulcer in childhood and adolescence? *Journal of Adolescent Health Care*, 2(4), 287–288.

White, E., Elsom, B.F. & Prawat, R.S. (1978). Children's conceptions of death. *Child Development*, 49(2), 307–310.

Wolfenstein, M. (1966). How is mourning possible? *Psychoanalytic Study of the Child*, 21, 93–123.

Zilboorg, G. (1943). Fear of death. *Psychoanalytic Quarterly*, 12, 465–475.

CHAPTER FOUR: CHILDHOOD AND ADOLESCENT CANCER

Adams, D.W. (1979). *Childhood malignancy: The psychosocial care of the child and his family.* Springfield, Ill.: Charles C. Thomas.

Adams, M.A. (1976). A hospital play program: Helping children with serious illness. *American Journal of Orthopsychiatry, 46*(3), 416 – 424.

Adams, M.A. (1978). Medical progress: Helping the parents of children with malignancy. *Journal of Pediatrics, 93*(5), 734 –738.

Alexy, W.D. (1982). Dimensions of psychological counseling that facilitate the grieving process of bereaved parents. *Journal of Counseling Psychology, 29*, 498–507.

American Cancer Society (1983). *Cancer facts and figures, 1983.* New York: American Cancer Society, Inc.

Bigner, S.H. & Johnson, W.W. (1984). The diagnostic challenge of tumors manifested initially by the shedding of cells into cerebrospinal fluid. *Acta Cytologica, 28*(1), 29–36.

Binger, C.M., Ablin, A.R., Feuerstein, R.C., Kushner, J.H., Zoger, S., & Mikkelsen, C. (1969). Childhood leukemia: Emotional impact on patient and family. *New England Journal of Medicine, 280*, 414 – 418.

Bruneau, J.P. (1981). Psychological aspects of nursing care of the dying leukemic child. *SOINS, 26*(15–16), 79–87.

Brunnquell, D. & Hall, M.D. (1982). Issues in the psychological care of pediatric oncology patients. *American Journal of Orthopsychiatry, 52*(1), 32– 44.

Bryant, E.H. (1978). Teacher in crisis: A classmate is dying. *Elementary School Journal, 78*(4), 233–241.

Burns, W.J. & Zweig, A.R. (1980). Self-concepts of chronically ill children. *Journal of Genetic Psychology, 137*(2), 179–190.

Carella, A.M., Santini, G., Frassoni, F., Giordano, D., Congiu, A., Nati, S., Risso, M., Cerri, R., Occhini, D., Damasio, E. *et al.* (1983). Il trapianto di midollo osseo autologo senza criopreservazione dopo megadosi di chemioterapia oncolitica. [Autologous bone marrow transplantation without cryopreservation after megadoses of oncolytic chemotherapy.] *Haematologica, 68*(5), 620 – 637.

Chapman, J.A. & Goodall, J. (1980). Helping a child to live whilst dying. *Lancet, 1*(8171), 753–756.

Ch'ien, L.T., Aur, R.J.A., Stagner, S., Cavallo, K., Wood, A., Goff, J., Pitner, S., Hutsu, H.O., Seifert, M.J. & Simone, J.V. (1980). Long term neurological implications of Somnolence Syndrome in children with acute lymphocytic leukemia. *Annals of Neurology, 8*(3), 273–277.

Coddington, M.N. (1976). A mother struggles to cope with her child's deteriorating illness. *Maternal-Child Nursing Journal, 5*(1), 39– 44.

Cotter, J.M. & Schwartz, A.D. (1978). Psychological and social support of the patient and family. *Major Problems in Clinical Pediatrics, 18*, 120 –127.

Craig, Y. (1977). The bereavement of parents and their search for meaning. *British Journal of Social Work, 7*, 41–54.

Dash, J. (1980). Hypnosis for symptom amelioration. In J. Kellerman (Ed.), *Psychological aspects of childhood cancer.* Springfield, Ill.: Charles C. Thomas, Publisher.

Death, the child and his family. (1980). *Nursing Times, 76*(10), suppl. 4 – 6.

Drotar, D. (1977). Family oriented intervention with the dying adolescent. *Journal of Pediatric Psychology, 2*, 68–71.

Easson, W.M. (1970). *The dying child: The management of the child or adolescent who is dying.* Springfield, Ill.: Charles C. Thomas.

Eiser, C. (1978). Intellectual abilities among survivors of childhood leukemia as a function of CNS irradiation. *Archives of the Diseases of Childhood, 53,* 391–395.

Eiser, C. (1979). Psychological development of the child with leukemia: A review. *Journal of Behavioral Medicine, 2*(2), 141–157.

Eiser, C. (1980). How leukemia affects a child's schooling. *British Journal of Social and Clinical Psychology, 19*(4), 365–368.

Eiser, C. & Landsdown, R. (1977). A retrospective study of intellectual development in children treated for acute lymphoblastic leukemia. *Archives of the Diseases of Childhood, 52*(7), 525–529.

Farkas, A. (1974). Research on families of terminally ill children: Problems and rewards. *Journal of Clinical Child Psychology, 3*(2), 41–43.

Farrell, F. & Hutter, J.J., Jr. (1980). Living until death: Adolescents with cancer. *Health and Social Work, 5*(4), 35–38.

Fife, B.L. (1980). Childhood cancer is a family crisis: A review. *Journal of Psychiatric Nursing, 18*(10), 29–34.

Flaherty, M. (1978). Use of control by an eleven-year-old with a neoplastic disease. *Maternal-Child Nursing Journal, 7*(2), 61–72.

Fochtman, D. (1979). How adolescents live with leukemia. *Cancer Nursing, 2*(1), 27–31.

Foster, D.J., O'Malley, J.E. & Koocher, G.P. (1981). The parent interviews. In G.P. Koocher & J.E. O'Malley (eds.), *The Damocles syndrome: Psychosocial consequences of surviving childhood cancer.* New York: McGraw-Hill.

Freeman, J.E., Johnston, P.G.B. & Voke, J.M. (1973). Somnolence after prophylactic cranial irradiation in children with acute lymphoblastic leukemia. *British Medical Journal, 4,* 523.

Frydman, M.I. (1980). Perception of illness severity and psychiatric symptoms in parents of chronically ill children. *Journal of Psychosomatic Research, 24*(6), 361–369.

Furth, G.M. (1974). Impromptu paintings by terminally ill, hospitalized and healthy children: What can we learn from them? *Dissertation Abstracts International, 34*(8–A, Pt. 1), 4739–4740.

Geist, R.A. (1979). Onset of chronic illness in children and adolescents: Psychotherapeutic and consultative intervention. *American Journal of Orthopsychiatry, 49,* 4–23.

George, S.L., Aur, R.J.A., Maurer, A.M. & Simone, J.V.A. (1979). A reappraisal of stopping therapy in childhood leukemia. *New England Journal of Medicine, 303,* 269–273.

Gilpin, B.L. (1980). The intercorrelation of amount of interaction and coping response in mothers of children with leukemia. *Dissertation Abstracts International, 40*(10–B), 5000.

Gogan, J.L. et al. (1979). Pediatric cancer survival and marriage: Issues affecting adult adjustment. *American Journal of Orthopsychiatry, 19*(3), 423–430.

Gogan, J.L., O'Malley, J.E. & Foster, D.J. (1977). Treating the pediatric cancer patient: A review. *Journal of Pediatric Psychology, 2*(2), 42–48.

Gogan, J.L., et al. (1977). Impact of childhood cancer on siblings. *Health Social Work, 2,* 42–57.

Goodell, A.S. (1979). Perceptions of nurses toward parent participation on pediatric oncology units. *Cancer Nursing, 2*(1), 38– 46.

Goodell, A.S. (1980). Responses of nurses to the stresses of caring for pediatric oncology patients. *Issues in Comprehensive Pediatric Nursing, 4*(1), 2– 6.

Grave, G.D. & Pless, I.B. (eds). (1974). *Chronic childhood illness: Assessment and outcome* (Fogarty International Center Series on the Teaching of Preventive Medicine, Vol. 3). DHEW Publication No. (NIH) 76–877. Washington, D.C.: U.S. Government Printing Office.

Green-Epner, C.S. (1976). The dying child. In R.E. Caughill (ed.), *The dying patient: A supportive approach.* Boston: Little, Brown.

Guimond, J. (1974). We knew our child was dying. *American Journal of Nursing, 74*(2), 248–249.

Hanefeld, F. & Riehm, H. (1980). Therapy of acute lymphoblastic leukemia in childhood: Effects on the nervous system. *Neuropaediatrie, 11*(1), 3–16.

Healey, J.M. (1980). The death of Chad Green. *Connecticut Medicine, 44*(2), 117.

Hinton, P.E. (1980). How a ten-year-old girl faced her death. *Journal of Child Psychotherapy, 6,* 107–116.

Hirsch, J.F., Reiner, D., Czernichow, P. *et al.* (1979). Medulloblastoma in childhood: Survival and functional results. *Acta Neurochirurgica, 48*(1–2), 1–15.

Hodges, D.M. (1981). Using art and poetry with terminally ill children in the hospital. *Arts in Psychotherapy, 8*(1), 55–59.

Holdsworth, C. & Whitmore, K. (1974). A study of children with epilepsy attending ordinary schools: Their seizure patterns, progress and behavior in school. *Developmental Medicine and Child Neurology, 16,* 746–758.

Iles, J.P. (1979). Children with cancer: Healthy siblings' perceptions during the illness experience. *Cancer Nursing, 2*(5), 371–377.

Jampolsky, G.G. (1980). The future is now. *Journal of Clinical Child Psychology, 9*(2), 182–184.

Johnson, F.L., Rudolph, L.A. & Hartmann, J.R. (1979). Helping the family coping with childhood cancer. *Psychosomatics, 20*(4), 241, 245–247, 251.

Kagen, B. (1976). Use of denial in adolescents with bone cancer. *Health and Social Work, 1,* 71–87.

Kagen-Goodheart, L. (1977). Reentry: Living with childhood cancer. *American Journal of Orthopsychiatry, 47*(4), 651– 658.

Kalnins, I.V., Churchill, M.P. & Terry, G.E. (1980). Concurrent stresses in families with a leukemic child. *Journal of Pediatric Psychology, 5*(1), 81–92.

Karon, M. (1975). Acute leukemia in childhood. In H.F. Conn (ed.), *Current therapy, 1975.* Philadelphia: W.B. Saunders.

Katz, E.R. (1980). Illness impact and social reintegration. In J. Kellerman (ed.), *Psychological aspects of childhood cancer.* Springfield, Ill.: Charles C. Thomas, Publisher.

Katz, E.R. (1981). Beta-endorphin and acute behavioral distress in children with leukemia. *Dissertation Abstracts International, 41*(7–B), 2764–2765.

Katz, E.R., Kellerman, J. & Siegel, S.E. (1980). Behavioral distress in children with cancer undergoing medical procedures: Developmental considerations. *Journal of Consulting & Clinical Psychology, 48*(3), 356–365.

Kellerman, J. (1979). Single case study: Behavioral treatment of night terrors in a child with acute leukemia. *Journal of Nervous & Mental Disease, 167*(3), 182–185.

Kellerman, J. (1980). *Psychological aspects of childhood cancer.* Springfield, Ill.: Charles C. Thomas, Publisher.

Koocher, G.P. (1980). Initial consultation with the pediatric cancer patient. In J. Kellerman (ed.), *Psychological aspects of childhood cancer,* 231–237. Springfield, Ill.: Charles C. Thomas, Publisher.

Koocher, G.P. & O'Malley, J.E. (1981). *The Damocles syndrome: Psychosocial consequences of surviving childhood cancer.* New York: McGraw-Hill.

Koocher, G.P. & Sallan, S.E. (1978). Psychological issues in pediatric oncology. In P.R. Magrab (ed.), *Psychological management of pediatric problems.* College Park, Md.: College Park Press.

Koocher, G.P., Sourkes, B. & Keane, W. (1979). Pediatric oncology consultations: A generalizable model for medical settings. *Professional Psychology, 10,* 467–474.

Kornfeld, M.S. & Siegel, I.M. (1979). Parental group therapy in the management of a fatal childhood disease. *Health and Social Work, 4*(3), 99–118.

Krueger, A., Gyllenskold, K., Pehrsson, G. & Sjolin, S. (1981). Parent reactions to childhood malignant diseases: Experiences in Sweden. *Journal of Pediatric Hematology/Oncology, 3*(3), 233–238.

Lacasse, C.M. (1975). A dying adolescent. *American Journal of Nursing, 75*(3), 433–434.

Lamb, M.A. & Woods, N.F. (1981). Sexuality and the cancer patient. *Cancer Nursing, 4*(2), 137–144.

Lansky, S.B. (1978). Childhood cancer: Parental discord and divorce. *Pediatrics, 62*(2), 184–188.

Lanksy, S.B., Cairns, N.U., Clark, G.M., Lowman, J.T., Miller, L. & Trueworthy, R.C. (1979). Childhood cancer: Non-medical costs of the illness. *Cancer, 43,* 403–408.

Lansky, S.B., Cairns, N.U., Hassanein, R., Wehr, J. & Lowman, J.T. (1978). Childhood cancer: Parental discord and divorce. *Pediatrics, 62,* 184–188.

Lansky, S.B., Cairns, N.U. & Zwartjes, W. (1983). School attendance among children with cancer: A report from two centers. *Journal of Psychosocial Oncology, 1,* 75–82.

Lansky, S.B., Lowman, J.T., Vats, T. & Grulay, J. (1975). School phobias in children with malignant neoplasms. *American Journal of Diseases of Children, 129,* 42–46.

Lenarsky, C. & Feig, S.A. (1983). Bone marrow transplantation for children with cancer. *Pediatric Annals, 12*(6), 428–436.

Lewis, S. & Armstrong, S.H. (1977). Children with terminal illness: A selected review. *International Journal of Psychiatry in Medicine, 8*(1), 73–82.

Lindemann, E. (1944). Symptomatology and management of acute grief. *American Journal of Psychiatry, 101,* 141–148.

Margolies, C. & McCredie, K.B. (1983). *Understanding leukemia.* N.Y.: Charles Scribner & Sons.

Martinson, I.M. et al. (1978). Home care for children dying of cancer. *Pediatrics, 62*(1), 106–113.

Miller, J.A. (1980). Hypnosis in a boy with leukemia. *American Journal of Clinical Hypnosis, 22*(4), 231–235.

Moss, H.A. & Nannis, E.D. (1980). Psychological effects of central nervous system treatment of children with acute lymphocyctic leukemia. In J. Kellerman (ed.), *Psychological aspects of childhood cancer,* 171–183. Springfield, Ill.: Charles C. Thomas, Publisher.

Nir, Y. & Maslin, B. (1982). Liaison psychiatry in childhood cancer: A systems approach. *Psychiatric Clinics of North America, 5*(2), 379–386.

Nitschke, R., Wunder, S., Sexauer, C.L. & Humphrey, G.B. (1977). The final-stage conference: The patient's decision on research drugs in pediatric oncology. *Journal of Pediatric Psychology, 2*(2), 58–64.

Nordmark-Lindberg, I. & Lindberg, T. (1977). A child's experience of imminent death. *Acta Paediatrica Scandinavica, 68*(5), 645–648.

Oury, N. (1981). Quelques reflexions a propos des enfants atteints de leucose et de leurs parents. [Some observations on children with leucoses and their parents (author's translation).] *Neuropsychiatrie de l'Enfance et de Adolescence* (Paris), *29*(7), 337–342.

O'Malley, J.E. & Koocher, G.P. (1979). Psychological consultation to a pediatric oncology unit: Obstacles to effective intervention. *Journal of Pediatric Psychology, 2*(2), 54–57.

O'Malley, J.E., Koocher, G., Foster, D. & Slavin, L. (1979). Psychiatric sequelae of surviving childhood cancer. *American Journal of Orthopsychiatry, 49*(4), 608–616.

Peck, B. (1979). Effects of childhood cancer on long-term survivors and their families. *British Medical Journal, 1*, 1327–1329.

Peck, V. (1980). Childhood cancer: Death—the final relief. *Nursing Mirror, 151*(9), xxxii-xxxiv.

Pfefferbaum, B. & Lucas, R.H. (1979). Management of acute psychologic problems in pediatric oncology. *General Hospital Psychiatry, 1*(3), 214–219.

Plumb, M.M. & Holland, J. (1974). Cancer in adolescents: The symptom is the thing. In B. Schoenberg, A.C. Carr, A.H. Kutscher, D. Peretz & I. Goldberg (eds.), *Anticipatory grief.* New York: Columbia University Press.

Powazek, M., Goff, J.R., Scheving, J. & Paulson, M.A. (1978). Emotional reactions of children to isolation in a cancer hospital. *Journal of Pediatrics, 92*(5), 834–837.

Powers, M.A. (1977). The benefits of anticipatory grief for the parents of dying children. *American Journal of Family Therapy, 5*(2), 48–53.

Ross, J.W. (1979). Coping with childhood cancer: Group intervention as an aid to parents in crisis. *Social Work in Health Care, 4*(4), 381–391.

Ross, J.W. (1980). Childhood cancer: The parents, the patients, the professionals. *Issues in Comprehensive Pediatric Nursing, 4*(1), 7–16.

Ross, T. (1981). Compassionate friends: When time doesn't heal all . . . *Nursing Mirror, 153*(11), 24.

Sacerdote, P. (1970). Theory and practice of pain control in malignancy and other protracted or recurring painful illnesses. *International Journal of Clinical Experimental Hypnosis, 3*, 160.

Sachs, M.B. (1980). Helping the child with cancer go back to school. *Journal of School Health, 50*(6), 328–331.

Sallan, S.E. & Weinstein, H.J. (1980). Management of acute lymphoblastic and acute myeloblastic leukemia in childhood. *Pediatrician, 9*(2), 56–67.

Schnell, R. (1974). Helping parents cope with the dying child with a genetic disorder. *Journal of Clinical Child Psychology, 3*(2), 34–35.

Shephard, C.S. (1975). The effect of group counseling on death anxiety in children with cancer. *Dissertation Abstracts International, 36*(5–A), 2723–2724.

Sogn, D.L. (1980). The child with a life-threatening illness: An analysis of the impact of experience on the awareness of personal mortality. *Dissertation Abstracts International, 40*(8–A), 4765–4766.

Soni, S.S., Marten, G.W., Patner, S.E., Duenas, D.A. & Powazek, M. (1975). Effects of central nervous system irradiation on neuropsychologic functioning of children with acute lymphoblastic leukemia. *New England Journal of Medicine, 293,* 113–118.

Spinetta, J.J. (1972). Death anxiety in leukemic children. *Dissertation Abstracts International, 33*(4–B), 1807–1808.

Spinetta, J.J. (1974). The dying child's awareness of death: A review. *Psychological Bulletin, 81,* 256–260.

Spinetta, J.J. (1977). Adjustment in children with cancer. *Journal of Pediatric Psychology, 2*(2), 49–51.

Spinetta, J.J. (1978). Communication patterns in families dealing with life-threatening illness. In O.J.Z. Sahler (ed.), *The child and death.* St. Louis: C.V. Mosby.

Spinetta, J.J. (1980). Disease-related communication: How to tell. In J. Kellerman (ed.), *Psychological aspects of childhood cancer.* Springfield, Ill.: Charles C. Curran.

Spinetta, J.J. (1981). Adjustment and adaptation in children with cancer: A three-year study. In J.J. Spinetta & P. Deasy-Spinetta (eds.), *Living with childhood cancer.* St. Louis: C.V. Mosby.

Spinetta, J.J. & Deasy-Spinetta, P. (1981). *Living with childhood cancer.* St. Louis: C.V. Mosby.

Spinetta, J.J. & Maloney, L.J. (1975). Death anxiety in the outpatient leukemic child. *Pediatrics, 56,* 1034–1037.

Spinetta, J.J. & Maloney, L.J. (1978). The child with cancer: Patterns of communication and denial. *Journal of Consulting & Clinical Psychology, 46*(6), 1540–1541.

Spinetta, J.J., Rigler, D. & Karon, M. (1974). Personal space as a measure of a dying child's sense of isolation. *Journal of Consulting and Clinical Psychology, 42*(6), 751–756.

Spinetta, J.J., Swarner, J.A. & Sheposh, J.P. (1981). Effective parental coping following the death of a child from cancer. *Journal of Pediatric Psychology* (U.S.), 6(3), 251–263.

Spruce, W. E. (1983). Bone marrow transplantation. *American Journal of Pediatric Hematology and Oncology, 5*(3), 287–294.

Taylor, C.I., DeAntonio, M., Draffin, N.C. & Morgan, S.K. (1978). A group experience for parents of children with malignancy. *Journal of the South Carolina Medical Association, 74*(6), 290–292.

Taylor, M.M. & Williams, H.A. (1980). Use of therapeutic play in the ambulatory pediatric hematology clinic. *Cancer Nursing, 3*(6), 433–437.

Tietz, W., McSherry, L. & Britt, B. (1977). Family sequelae after a child's death due to cancer. *American Journal of Psychotherapy, 31*(3), 417–425.

Tiller, J.W., Ekert, H. & Richards, W.S. (1977). Family reactions in childhood lymphoblastic leukimia in remission. *Australian Paediatric Journal, 13*(3), 176–181.

Videka-Sherman, L. (1982). Coping with the death of a child: A study over time. *American Journal of Orthopsychiatry, 52,* 688–698.

When your child dies . . . The compassionate friends. (1980). *Lamp,* 41–43.

Wilbur, J. (1979). Sexual development and body image in the teenager with cancer. *Frontiers of Radiation Therapy and Oncology, 14,* 108–114.

Williams, H.A., Rivara, F.P. & Rothenberg, M.B. (1981). The child is dying: Who helps the family? *MCN,* 6, 261–265.

Willis, D.J. (1974). The families of terminally ill children: Symptomatology and management. *Journal of Clinical Child Psychology, 3*(2), 32—33.

Wright, L. (1974). An emotional support program for parents of dying children. *Journal of Clinical Child Psychology, 3*(2), 37—38.

Zeltzer, L.K. (1980) The adolescent with cancer. In J. Kellerman (ed.), *Psychological aspects of childhood cancer.* Springfield, Ill.: Charles C. Thomas.

CHAPTER FIVE: SUICIDE IN ADOLESCENCE AND YOUNG ADULTHOOD

Abraham, K. (1968). Notes on the psychoanalytical investigation and treatment of manic-depressive insanity and allied conditions. In W. Gaylin (Ed.), *The Meaning of Despair,* 26—49. New York: Science House, Inc. (Originally published in 1927.)

American Psychiatric Association. (1980). *The diagnostic and statistical manual of mental diseases.* Third edition. Washington, D.C.: American Psychiatric Association.

Bancroft, J. & Hawton, K. (1983). Why people take overdoses: A study of psychiatrists' judgments. *British Journal of Medical Psychology, 56*(2), 197—204.

Boyer, L.B. (1975). Meanings of a bizarre suicidal attempt by an adolescent. *Adolescent Psychiatry, 4,* 371—381.

Bunney, W.E., Fawcett, J.A., Davis, J.M. & Gifford, S. (1969). Further evaluation of urinary 17—hydroxycorticosteroids in suicidal patients. *Archives of General Psychiatry, 21,* 138—150.

Bunney, W.E. & Fawcett, J.A. (1965). Possibility of a biochemical test for suicidal potential. *Archives of General Psychiatry, 13,* 232—239.

Caine, E. (1978). Two contemporary tragedies: Adolescent suicide/adolescent alcoholism. *Journal of the National Association of Private Psychiatric Hospitals, 9*(3), 4—11.

Carlson, G.A. (1981). Phenomenology of adolescent depression. In S. C. Feinstein *et al.* (eds.), *Adolescent Psychiatry.* Chicago: University of Chicago Press.

Carmack, B.J. (1983). Suspect a suicide? Don't be afraid to act. *RN, 46*(4), 43—45, 90.

Catryn, L., McKnew, D.H. & Bunney, W.E. (1980). Diagnosis of depression in children: A reassessment. *American Journal of Psychiatry, 137,* 22—25.

Charry, D. (1983). The borderline personality. *American Family Physician, 27*(1), 195—202.

Cohen-Sandler, R., Berman, A.L. & King, R.A. (1982a). A follow-up study of hospitalized suicidal children. *Journal of the American Academy of Child Psychiatry, 21*(4), 398—403.

Cohen-Sandler, R., Berman, A.L. & King, R.A. (1982b). Life stress and symptomatology: Determinants of suicidal behavior in children. *Journal of the American Academy of Child Psychiatry, 21*(2), 178—186.

Cohen-Sandler, R. & Berman, A.L. (1980). Diagnosis and treatment of childhood depression and self-destructive behavior. *Journal of Family Practice, 11*(1), 51—58.

Coppen, A. (1972). Indoleamines and affective disorders. *Journal of Psychiatric Research, 9,* 163, 171.

Cotman, C.W. & McGaugh, J.L. (1980). *Behavioral neuroscience.* New York: Academic Press.

Crumley, F.E. (1982). The adolescent suicide attempt: A cardinal symptom of a serious psychiatric disorder. *American Journal of Psychotherapy, 36*(2), 158–165.

Danto, B.L. (1980). A case of female autoerotic death. *American Journal of Forensic Medicine & Pathology, 1*(2), 117–121.

Davidson, F., Choquet, M., Etienne, M. & Taleghani, M. (1972). Contribution a l'etude du suicide des adolescents. [Suicide among adolescents: A medical-social report of 139 who attempted suicide.] *Hygiene Mentale, 61*(1), 1–32.

DenHouter, K.V. (1981). To silence one's self: A brief analysis of the literature on adolescent suicide. *Child Welfare, 60*(1), 2–10.

Dublin, L.I. (1963). *Suicide: A sociological and statistical study.* New York: Ronald Press.

Eth, S. (1983). Adolescent separation-individuation and the court. *Bulletin of the American Academy of Psychiatry and the Law, 11*(3), 231–238.

Evans, D.L. (1982). Explaining suicide among the young: An analytical review of the literature. *Journal of Psychosocial Nursing and Mental Health Services, 20*(8), 9–16.

Feifel, H. & Nagy, V.T. (1980). Death orientation and life-threatening behavior. *Journal of Abnormal Psychology, 89*(1), 38–45.

Frederick, C.J. (1978). Current trends in suicidal behavior in the United States. *American Journal of Psychotherapy, 32*, 172–200.

Freud, S. (1957). Mourning and melancholia. In *Standard edition of the complete psychological works of Sigmund Freud, 14*, 237–260. London: Hogarth Press. (Original work published in 1917.)

Garfinkel, B. D. & Golombek, H. (1974). Suicide and depression in childhood and adolescence. *Canadian Medical Association Journal, 110*, 1278–1281.

Garfinkel, H., Froese, A. & Hood, J. (1982). Suicide attempts in children and adolescents. *American Journal of Psychiatry, 139*, 1257–1261.

Glaser, K. (1978). The treatment of depressed and suicidal adolescents. *American Journal of Psychotherapy, 32*(2), 252–269.

Glaser, K. (1981). Psychopathologic patterns in depressed adolescents. *American Journal of Psychotherapy, 35*, 368–382.

Greuling, J.W. & DeBlassie, R.R. (1980). Adolescent suicide. *Adolescence, 15*(59), 589–601.

Hendrin, H. (1982). *Suicide in America.* New York: W.W. Norton.

Herzog, D.B. & Rathbun, J.M. (1982). Childhood depression: Developmental considerations. *American Journal of Diseases in Children, 136*(2), 115–120.

Hirsch, S.R., Walsh, C. & Draper, R. (1982). Parasuicide: A review of treatment interventions. *Journal of Affective Disorders, 4*(4), 299–311.

Hodgman, C.H. (1983). Current issues in adolescent psychiatry. *Hospital and Community Psychiatry, 34*(6), 514–521.

Hollinger, P.C. (1978). Adolescent suicide: An epidemiological study of recent trends. *American Journal of Psychiatry, 135*, 754.

Hollinger, P.C. & Offer, D. (1981). Perspectives on suicide in adolescence. In R. Simmons (ed.), *Research in Community and Mental Health.* Greenwich, Conn.: JAI Press.

Ishii, K. (1981). Adolescent self-destructive behavior and crisis intervention in Japan. *Suicide and Life-Threatening Behavior, 11*(1), 51–61.

Kaizuka, T. (1977). Can guilt feelings be a key concept in understanding Japanese children's social behavior? Comments on Dr. Gardner's paper. *Hiroshima Forum for Psychology, 4*, 51–54.

Keidel, G.C. (1983). Adolescent suicide. *Nursing Clinics of North America*, *18*(2), 323–332.

Kovacs, M. & Beck, A.T. (1977). An empirical approach toward definition of childhood depression. In J. Schulterbrandt & A. Raskin (eds.), *Depression in childhood: diagnosis, treatment and conceptual models*, 20–23. New York: Raven Press.

LaGrand, L.E. (1981). Loss reactions of college students: A descriptive analysis. *Death Education*, *5*, 235–248.

Lerner, H. (1983). An object representation approach to psychostructural change: A clinical illustration. *Journal of Personality Assessment*, *47*(3), 314–323.

Lesse, S. (1981). Hypochondriacal and psychosomatic disorders masking depression in adolescents. *American Journal of Psychotherapy*, *35*, 356–365.

Levy, B. & Hanson, E. (1969). Failure of the urinary test for suicidal potential. *Archives of General Psychiatry*, *20*, 415–418.

Marcelli, D. (1978). Les tentatives de suicide de l'enfant: aspects statistiques et epidemiologiques. [Suicidal attempts of the child: Statistical and general epidemiological aspects.] *ACTA Paedopsychiatrica*, *43*(5–6), 213–221.

Maris, R.W. (1981). *Pathways to suicide: A survey of self-destructive behaviors*. Baltimore: Johns Hopkins University Press.

Markush, R.E. & Bartolucci, A.A. (1984). Firearms and suicide in the United States. *American Journal of Public Health*, *74*(2), 123–127.

McGuire, D.J. & Ely, M. (1984). Childhood suicide. *Child Welfare*, *63*(1), 17–26.

McKenry, P.C., Tishler, C.L. & Kelley, C. (1982). Adolescent suicide: A comparison of attempters and non-attempters in an emergency room population. *Clinical Pediatrics*, *21*(5), 266–270.

Mehr, M., Zeltzer, L.K. & Robinson, R. (1981). Continued self-destructive behaviors in adolescent suicide attemptors. *Journal of Adolescent Health Care*, *1*(4), 269–274.

Miller, D. (1981). Adolescent suicide: Etiology and treatment. *Adolescent Psychiatry* (U.S.), *9*, 327–342.

Mintz. R.S. (1970). Prevalence of persons in the city of Los Angeles who have attempted suicide: A pilot study. *Bulletin of Suicidology*, *7*, 9–16.

Mouren, M.C. & Soulayrol, R. (1978). La depression chez l'enfant: aspects cliniques et psychopathologiques. [Depression in the child: Clinical and psychopathological aspects.] *Annales Medico-Psychologiques*, *136*(10), 1147–1165.

Ostroff, R., Giller, E. *et al.* (1982). Neuroendocrine risk factors of suicidal behavior. *American Journal of Psychiatry*, *139*, 1323–1325.

Patel, A.R., Roy, M. & Wilson, G.M. (1972). Self-poisoning and alcohol. *Lancet*, *2*, 1099–1102.

Pattison, E.M. & Kahan, J. (1983). The deliberate self-harm syndrome. *American Journal of Psychiatry*, *140*(7), 867–872.

Petzel, S.V. & Cline, D.W. (1978). Adolescent suicide: Epidemiological and biological aspects. *Adolescent Psychiatry*, *6*, 239–266.

Petzel, S.V. & Riddle, M. (1981). Adolescent suicide: Psychosocial and cognitive aspects. *Adolescent Psychiatry*, *9*, 343–398.

Pfeffer, C.R. (1981a). The family system of suicidal children. *American Journal of Psychotherapy*, *35*, 330–341.

Pfeffer, C.R. (1981b). Suicidal behavior of children: A review with implications for research and practice. *American Journal of Psychiatry*, *138*(2), 154–159.

Puig-Antich, J. *et al.* (1979). Plasma levels of imipramine and desmethylimpramine and clinical response in prepubertal major depressive disorder. *Journal of the American Academy of Child Psychiatry*, *18*, 616–627.

Remschmidt, H. & Schwab, T. (1978). Attempted suicide in children and young people. *Acta Paedopsychiatrica, 43*(5–6), 197–208.

Reynolds, D.K. & Nelson, F.L. (1981). Personality, life situation, and life expectancy. *Suicide and Life-Threatening Behavior, 11*(2), 99–110.

Richman, J. (1978). Symbiosis, empathy, suicidal behavior and the family. *Suicide and Life-threatening Behavior, 8,* 139–149.

Robbins, D. & Conroy, R. C. (1983). A cluster of adolescent suicide attempts: Is suicide contagious? *Journal of Adolescent Health Care, 3*(4), 253–255.

Rosenthal, M. J. (1981). Sexual differences in the suicidal behavior of young people. In S. C. Feinstein (ed.), *Adolescent Psychiatry*. Chicago: University of Chicago Press.

Rudestam, K.E. & Imbroll, D. (1983). Societal reactions to a child's death by suicide. *Journal of Consulting and Clinical Psychology, 7,* 97–113.

Seiden, R.H. (1969). Suicide among youth. *Public Health Service Publication*, No. 1971, 1–60.

Seiden. R.H. (1981). Mellowing with age: Factors influencing the nonwhite suicide rate. *International Journal of Aging and Human Development, 13*(4), 265–284.

Stack, S. (1982). Suicide: A decade review of the sociological literature. *Deviant Behavior, 4*(1), 41–66.

Struve, F.A., Klein, D.F. & Saraf, K.R. (1972). Electroencephalographic correlates of suicide. *Archives of General Psychiatry, 27,* 363–365.

Suter, B. (1976). Suicide and women. In B. B. Wolman & H. H. Krauss (eds.), *Between survival and suicide*. New York: Gardner Press.

Tishler, C.L., McKenry, P.C. & Morgan, K.C. (1981). Adolescent suicide attempts: Some significant factors. *Suicide and Life-threatening Behavior, 11,* 31.

Tishler, C.L. & McKenry, P.C. (1982). Parental negative-self and adolescent suicide attempts. *Journal of the American Academy of Child Psychiatry, 21,* 404–408.

Toolan, J.M. (1962a). Suicide and suicidal attempts in children and adolescents. *American Journal of Psychiatry, 118,* 719–724.

Toolan, J.M. (1962b). Depression in children and adolescents. *American Journal of Orthopsychiatry, 32,* 404–415.

Toolan, J.M. (1975). Suicide in children and adolescents. *American Journal of Psychotherapy, 29,* 339–344.

Toolan, J.M. (1978). Therapy of depressed and suicidal children. *American Journal of Psychotherapy, 32,* 243–251.

Toolan, J.M. (1981). Depression and suicide in children: An overview. *American Journal of Psychiatry, 35*(3), 311–322.

Walker, B.A. & Mehr, M. (1983). Adolescent suicide—a family crisis: A model for effective intervention by family therapists. *Adolescence, 18*(70), 285–292.

Weisman, M.M. (1974). The epidemiology of suicide attempts, 1960–1971. *The American Journal of Psychotherapy, 32,* 243–251.

Wilkins, J., Robert, M., Barker, M. & Frappier, J.Y. (1983). Les tentatives de suicide chez les adolescents: Revue de 93 dossiers. [Attempted suicide among adolescents: A review of 93 case reports.] *Union des Medecins Canadiens, 112*(8), 682–684.

Wolfgang, M.E. (1959). Suicide by means of victim-precipitated homicide. *Journal of Clinical and Experimental Psychopathology, 20,* 335–349.

CHAPTER SIX: CATASTROPHIC LIFE-THREATENING
EVENTS IN ADULTHOOD

Allyn, P. & Bartlett, R. (1981). Management of the burn patient. In D.A. Zschoche (ed.), *Comprehensive review of critical care*. St. Louis: C.V. Mosby.

Alonzo, A.A. (1975). Illness behavior during acute episodes of coronary heart disease. *Dissertation Abstracts International, 36*(3–A), 1842–1843.

Appels, A. (1980). Psychological prodromata of myocardial infarction and sudden death. *Psychotherapy and Psychosomatics, 34*(2–3), 187–195.

Arndt, H.C.M. & Gruber, M. (1977). Helping families cope with acute and anticipatory grief. In. E.R. Prichard, J. Collard, B.A. Orcutt, A.H. Kutscher, I. Seeland & N. Lefkowitz (eds.), *Social work with the dying patient and family*. New York: Columbia University Press.

Artz, C.P., Moncreif, J.A. & Pruitt, B.A. (eds.) (1979). *Burns: A team approach*. Philadelphia: W.B. Saunders.

Barton, D. (1977). The family of the dying person. In D. Barton (ed.), *Dying and death: A clinical guide for caregivers*. Baltimore: Williams & Wilkins.

Beales, J.G. (1983). Factors influencing the expectation of pain among patients in a children's burns unit. *Burns Including Thermal Injuries, 9*(3), 187–192.

Bernstein, N.R. (1976a). *Emotional care of the facially burned and disfigured*. Boston: Little, Brown.

Bernstein, N.R. (1976b). Medical tragedies in facial burn disfigurement. *Psychiatric Annals, 6*(10), 475–483.

Bernstein, N.R. (1983). Child psychiatry and burn care. *Journal of the American Academy of Child Psychiatry, 22*(2), 202–204.

Binik, Y.M., Theriault, G. & Shustack, B. (1977). Sudden death in the laboratory rat: Cardiac function, sensory and experimental factors in swimming deaths. *Psychosomatic Medicine, 39*, 82–92.

Blades, B.C., Jones, C. & Munster, A.M. (1979). Quality of life after major burns. *Journal of Trauma, 19*(8), 556–558

Burns, A.C. & Steger, H.G. (1983). Intervention strategies for victims of work-related burn injuries. *Occupational Health Nursing, 31*(7), 29–31, 44.

Byrne, D.G. (1982a). Psychological responses to illness and outcome after survived myocardial infarction: A long-term follow-up. *Journal of Psychosomatic Research, 26*(2), 105–112.

Byrne, D.G. (1982b). Illness behavior and psychosocial outcome after a heart attack. *British Journal of Clinical Psychology, 21*(2), 145–146.

Byrne, D.G. & Whyte, H.M. (1984). State and trait anxiety correlates of illness behavior in survivors of myocardial infarction. *International Journal of Psychiatry in Medicine, 13*(1), 1–9.

Byrne, D.G., Whyte, H.M. & Butler, K.L. (1981). Illness behaviour and outcome following survived myocardial infarction: A prospective study. *Journal of Psychosomatic Research, 25*(2), 97–107.

Byrne. D.G. (1981). Type A behavior, life-events and myocardial infarction: Independent or related risk factors? *British Journal of Medical Psychology, 54*(4), 371–377.

Cahners, S.S. (1978). Group meetings for families of burned children. *Health and Social Work, 3*(3), 165–172.

Cahners, S.S. (1979). A strong hospital-school liaison: A necessity for good rehabilitation planning for disfigured children. *Scandinavian Journal of Plastic and Reconstructive Surgery* (Supplementum), *13*(1), 167–168.

Cahners, S.S. & Bernstein, N.R. (1979). Rehabilitating families with burned children. *Scandinavian Journal of Plastic & Reconstructive Surgery* (Supplementum), *13*(1), 173–175.

Caplan, G. (1964). *Principles of Preventive Psychiatry*. New York: Basic Books.

Clarke, A.M. (1980). Thermal injuries: The care of the whole child. *Journal of Trauma, 20*(10), 823–829.

Cope, O. & Long, R.T. (1961). Emotional problems of burned children. *New England Journal of Medicine, 264*, 22.

Cottington, E.M., Matthews, K.A., Talbott, E. & Kuller, L.H. (1980). Environmental events preceding sudden death in women. *Psychosomatic Medicine, 42*(6), 567–574.

Croog, S.H., Kosolowsky, M. & Levine, S. (1976). Personality self-perceptions of male heart attack patients and their wives: Issues of congruence and "coronary personality." *Perceptual and Motor Skills, 43*(3), 927–937.

Davidson, G.P. (1981). Sudden death: Bereavement sequelae and interventions. *New Zealand Medical Journal, 94*, 265–267.

Davidson, T.N., Bowden, M.L., Tholen, D., James, M.H. & Feller, I. (1981). Social support and post-burn adjustment. *Archives of Physical Medicine and Rehabilitation, 62*(6), 274–278.

Derogatis, L.R. & King, K.M. (1981). The coital coronary: A reassessment of the concept. *Archives of Sexual Behavior, 10*(4), 325–335.

DeSilva, R.A. (1982). Central nervous system risk factors for sudden cardiac death. *Annals of the New York Academy of Science, 382*, 143–161.

DeSilva, R.A. & Lown, B. (1978). Ventricular premature beats, stress and sudden death. *Psychosomatics, 19*, 649–659.

Dimsdale, J.E. (1977). Emotional causes of sudden death. *American Journal of Psychiatry, 134*(12), 1361–1366.

Earle, E.M. (1979). The psychological effects of mutilating surgery in children and adolescents. *Psychoanalytical Study of the Child, 34*, 527–546.

Elliott, C.H. & Olson, R.A. (1983). The management of children's distress in response to painful medical treatment for burn injuries. *Behavioral Respiratory Therapy, 21*(6), 675–683.

Engel, G.L. (1968). A life setting conducive to illness, the giving-up–given-up complex. *Annals of Internal Medicine, 69*, 293–300.

Engel, G. L. (1971). Sudden and rapid death during psychological stress: Folklore or folk wisdom? *Annals of Internal Medicine, 74*, 771–782.

Epperson, M.M. (1977). Families in sudden crisis: Process and intervention in a critical care center. *Social Work in Health Care, 2*(3), 265–273.

Frances, A. & Perry, S.W. (1983). Burn victim faces impending divorce, potential job loss. *Hospital and Community Psychiatry, 34*(6), 499–500, 502.

Friedman, G., Vry, H.K., Klatsky, A.L. & Siegelaub, A.B. (1974). A psychological questionnaire predictive of myocardial infarction. *Psychosomatic Medicine, 36*, 327–343.

Friedman, M. & Rosenman, R.H. (1974). *Type A behavior and your heart*. Greenwich, Conn.: Fawcett.

Friedman, S.B., Glasgow, L.A. & Ader, R. (1969). Psychosocial factors modifying host resistance to experimental infections. *Annals of the New York Academy of Sciences, 164,* 381–393.

Friedman, S.B., Glasgow, L.A. & Ader, R. (1970). Differential susceptibility to a viral agent in mice housed alone or in groups. *Psychosomatic Medicine, 32,* 285–299.

Garts, K. & Garland, S. (1983). Marital satisfaction of the post-rehabilitation burn patient. *Occupational Health Nursing, 31*(7), 35–37.

Gentry, W.D. & Williams, R.B. (eds.) (1979). *Psychological aspects of myocardial infarction and coronary care.* St. Louis, Mo.: C. V. Mosby.

Glass, D.C. (1977). *Behavior patterns, stress and coronary disease.* Hillsdale, N.J.: Lawrence Erlbaum Associates, Publishers.

Glinsky, J. (1983). When fears collide. *Canadian Journal of Psychiatric Nursing, 24*(4), 18–19.

Griffiths, W.J. (1960). Responses of wild and domestic rats to forced swimming. *Psychological Reports, 6,* 39–49.

Gulledge. A.D. (1979). Psychological aftermaths of myocardial infarction. In W.D. Gentry & R.B. Williams (eds.), *Psychological aspects of myocardial infarction and coronary care.* St. Louis, Mo: C.V. Mosby.

Hackett, T.P. & Cassem, N.H. (1979). Psychological intervention in myocardial infarction. In W.D. Gentry & R.B. Williams (eds.), *psychological aspects of myocardial infarction and coronary care.* St. Louis, Mo: C.V. Mosby.

Hamera, E.K. (1978). Positive and negative effects of life-threatening illness. *Dissertation Abstracts International, 38*(7–B), 3469–3470.

Hamera, E.K. & Shontz, F.C. (1978). Perceived positive and negative effects of life-threatening illness. *Journal of Psychosomatic Research, 22*(5), 419–424.

Hellerstein, H.K. & Friedman, E.H. (1969). Sexual activity and the post coronary patient. *Medical Aspects of Human Sexuality, 3,* 70–96.

Hellerstein, H.K. & Friedman, E.H. (1978). Managing the sexual fears of cardiac patients. *Sexual Medicine Today, 2,* 12–14.

Henry, J.P. (1975). The induction of acute and chronic cardiovascular disease in animals by psychosocial stimulation. *International Journal of Psychiatry in Medicine, 6*(1–2), 147–158.

Hughes, C.W. & Lynch, J.J. (1978). A reconsideration of psychological precursors of sudden death in infrahuman animals. *American Psychologist, 33*(5), 419–429.

Hughes, C.W. & Preskorn, S.H. (1980). Considerations of physiologic mechanisms in animal models of "sudden death." *OMEGA: Journal of Death and Dying, 11*(2), 113–118.

Imbus, S.H. & Zawacki, B.E. (1977). Autonomy for burned patients when survival is unprecedented. *New England Journal of Medicine, 197,* 308.

Jayne, D. (1979). The burn survivor's point of view. *Journal of Trauma, 19*(11 Supp.), 920–921.

Jenkins, C.D. (1979). The coronary-prone personality. In W.D. Gentry & R.B. Williams (eds.), *Psychological aspects of myocardial infarction and coronary care.* St. Louis, Mo: C. V. Mosby.

Kavanagh, C. (1983a). Alternative approach to burned children. *American Journal of Psychiatry, 140*(2), 268–269.

Kavanagh, C. (1983b). Psychological intervention with the severely burned child: Report of an experimental comparison of two approaches and their effects on psychological sequelae. *Journal of the American Academy of Child Psychiatry, 22*(2), 145–156.

Kiely, W.F. & Procci, W.R. (1981). Psychiatric aspects of critical care. In D. A. Zschoche (ed.), *Comprehensive review of critical care*. St. Louis, Mo: C. V. Mosby.

Lebovits, B., Lichter, E. & Moses, V.K. (1975). Personality correlates of coronary heart disease: A re-examination of the MMPI data. *Social Science and Medicine, 9*, 207–219.

Levinson, P. (1972). On sudden death. *Psychiatry* (Washington, D.C.), *35*(2), 160–173.

Lown, B., DeSilva, R.A., Reich, P. & Murawski, B.J. (1980). Psychophysiologic factors in sudden cardiac death. *American Journal of Psychiatry, 137*(11), 1325–1335.

Lynch, J.J. (1977). *The broken heart: The medical consequences of loneliness*. New York: Basic Books.

Lynch, J.J., Paskewitz, D.A., Gimbel, K.S. & Thomas, S.A. (1977). Psychological aspects of cardiac arrhythmia. *American Heart Journal, 93*, 645–657.

Lynch, J.J., Thomas, S.A., Mills. M. *et al*. (1974). The effects of human contact in coronary care patients. *Journal of Nervous and Mental Disease, 158*, 88–99.

Lynch, J.J. & Katcher, A.H. (1974). Human handling and sudden death in laboratory rats. *Journal of Nervous and Mental Disease, 159*, 362–365.

Mann, J.K. & Oakes, A.R. (eds.). (1980). *Critical care nursing of the multi-injured patient*. Philadelphia: W.B. Saunders Company.

Marvin, J.A. (1983). Crisis management for patients/families experiencing acute physiological crisis (burn/trauma). *Washington State Journal of Nursing, 54*(2), 8–11.

Marvin, J.A. (1983). Planning home care for burn patients. *Nursing, 13*(8), 65–67.

May, S.R. & DeClement, F.A. (1983). Effects of early hypnosis on the cardiovascular and renal physiology of burn patients. *Burns Including Thermal Injuries, 9*(4), 257–266.

McCrady, V.L. & Kahn, A.M. (1980). Life or death for burn patients? (Editorial). *Journal of Trauma, 20*(4), 356–357.

McNaughton, M.W. (1978). Heart rate and blood pressure response to stair climbing and sexual activity. *Circulation, 57*, 215.

Meerloo, J.A.M. (1962). The reflex of surrender and capitulation. *Psychiatry, Neurology and Neuropsychology, 65*, 225–232.

Meislin, H.W. (ed.). (1980). *Priorities in multiple trauma*. Germantown, Md: Aspen Systems Corporation.

Mendelsohn, I. E. (1983). Liaison psychiatry and the burn center. *Psychosomatics, 24*(3), 235–243.

Merz, B. (1983). Hypnosis for burn patients: Healing body and spirit. *Journal of the American Medical Association, 249*(3), 321–323.

Miller, D.H. & Borer, J.S. (1982). Exercise testing early after myocardial infarction: Risks and benefits. *American Journal of Medicine, 72*(3), 427–438.

Modestin, J., Krapf, R. & Boker, W. (1981). A fatality during haloperidol treatment: Mechanism of sudden death. *American Journal of Psychiatry, 138*(12), 1616–1617.

Moonilal, J.M. (1982). Trauma centers: A new dimension for hospital social work. *Social Work in Health Care. 7*(4), 15–25.

Moos, R.H. & Tsu, V.D. (1977). The crisis of physical illness: An overview. In R.H. Moos (ed.), *Coping with physical illness*. New York: Plenum.

Murray, K.H. (1983). Burn recovery: Transition to full employment. *Occupational Health Nursing, 31*(2), 35–36, 47.

Nemec, E.D., Mansfield, L. & Kennedy, J.D. (1976). Heart rate and blood pressure responses during sexual activity in normal males. *American Heart Journal, 92,* 274–277.

Nishimura, N. & Hiranuma, N. (1982). Respiratory changes after major burn injury. *Critical Care Medicine, 10*(1), 25–28.

Noyes, R. & Kletti, R. (1976). Depersonalization in the face of life-threatening danger: A description. *Psychiatry, 39*(1), 19–27.

Olton, D.S. & Noonberg, A.R. (1980). *Biofeedback: Clinical applications in behavioral medicine.* Englewood Cliffs, N.J.: Prentice-Hall, Inc.

Paffenbarger, R.S. & Hale, W.E. (1975). Work activity and coronary heart mortality. *New England Journal of Medicine, 292*(11), 545–550.

Parkes, C.M. & Brown, R.J. (1972). Health after bereavement: A controlled study of young Boston widows and widowers. *Psychosomatic Medicine, 34*(5), 449–461.

Perry, R.R., Buffler, P.A. & Sanderson, L.M. (1982). A research model for the study of rehabilitation among adult burn injury patients. *Rehabilitation Literature, 43*(3–4), 77–81.

Plattner, P.B. & Ripley, H.S. (1982). The fatally burned suicidal patient. *Crisis, 3*(2), 88–94.

Price, T. & Bergen, B.J. (1977). The relationship to death as a source of stress for nurses on a coronary care unit. *OMEGA: Journal of Death and Dying, 8*(3), 229–238.

Rainsford, G.L. & Schuman, S.H. (1981). The family in crisis. A case study of overwhelming illness and stress. *Journal of the American Medical Association, 246*(1), 60–63.

Ravenscroft, K. (1982). The burn unit. *Psychiatric Clinics of North America, 5*(2), 419–432.

Richter, C.P. (1957). On the phenomenon of sudden death in animals and man. *Psychosomatic Medicine, 19,* 190–198.

Roi, L.D., Flora, J.D., Davis, T.M., Cornell, R.G. & Feller, I. (1981). A severity grading chart for the burned patient. *Annals of Emergency Medicine, 10*(3), 161–163.

Roi, L.D., Flora, J.D., Davis, T.M. & Wolfe, R.A. (1983). Two new burn severity indices. *Journal of Trauma, 23*(12), 1023–1029.

Rosellini, R.A., Binik, Y.M. & Seligman, M.E.P. (1976). Sudden death in the laboratory rat. *Psychosomatic Medicine, 38,* 55–58.

Sanders, C.M. (1982). Effects of sudden versus chronic illness death on bereavement outcome. *Omega, 13,* 227–241.

Saul, L. (1966). Sudden death at impasse. *Psychoanalytical Forum, 1,* 88–89.

Sawyer, M.G., Minde, K. & Zuker, R. (1983). The burned child— scarred for life? A study of the psychosocial impact of a burn injury at different developmental stages. *Burns Including Thermal Injuries, 9*(3), 205–213.

Schmale, A. (1958). Relationship of separation to disease. *Psychosomatic Medicine, 20,* 259–277.

Schnaper, N. & Cowley, R.A. (1976). Overview: Psychiatric sequelae to multiple trauma. *American Journal of Psychiatry, 133*(8), 883–890.

Schotz, S. (1977). Myocardial infarction: A personal history. *Psychosomatics, 18*(4), 17–23.

Scully, J.H. & Hutcherson, R. (1983). Suicide by burning. *American Journal of Psychiatry, 140*(7), 905–906.

Seligman, M.E.P. (1975). *Helplessness: On depression, development and death.* San Francisco: Freeman.

Selye, H. (1956). *Stress of life*. New York: McGraw-Hill.

Shady, G.A. (1977). Death anxiety and AB therapeutic styles as factors in helping patients with different coping styles accept life-threatening illness. *Dissertation Abstracts International, 38*(2–B), 916–917.

Slater, H. & Gaisford, J.C. (1981). Burns in older patients. *Journal of the American Geriatrics Society, 29*(2), 74–76.

Solomon, J.R. (1981). Care and needs in a children's burn unit. *Progress in Pediatric Surgery, 14*, 19–32.

Stern, M. & Waisbren, B.A. (1976). A method by which burn units may compare their results with a baseline curve. *Surgery, Gynecology and Obstetrics, 142*, 230.

Stoddard, F.J. (1982). Coping with pain: A developmental approach to treatment of burned children. *American Journal of Psychiatry, 139*(6), 736–740.

Stoupel, E. (1982). Le stress, facteur declenchant ou reaction secondaire de l'infarctus du myocarde. [Stress: causative factor or secondary reaction to myocardial infarct.] *Revue de Medecine (Liege), 37*(1), 25–28.

St. Lawrence, J.S. & Drabman, R.S. (1983). Interruption of self-excoriation in a pediatric burn unit. *Journal of Pediatric Psychology, 8*(2), 155–159.

Theorell, T.G. (1982). Review of research on life events and cardiovascular illness. *Advances in Cardiology, 29*, 140–149.

Thomas, S.A. & Lynch, J.J. (1979). Human contact, coping and cardiac function in coronary patients. In W.D. Gentry & R.B. Williams (eds.), *Psychological aspects of myocardial infarction and coronary care*. St. Louis, Mo: C. V. Mosby.

Tobiason, J., Hiebert, J.H. & Edlich, R.F. (1982). Prediction of burn mortality. *Surgery, Gynecology and Obstetrics, 154*(5), 711–714.

Tringali, R. (1982). The role of the psychiatric nurse consultant on a burn unit. *Issues in Mental Health Nursing, 4*(1), 17–24.

Ueno, M. (1963). The so-called coition death. *Japanese Journal of Legal Medicine, 17*, 333–337.

Wasow, M. (1978). Human sexuality and serious illness. In C.A. Garfield (ed.), *Psychosocial care of the dying patient*. New York: McGraw-Hill.

Weinberg, N. & Miller, N.J. (1983). Burn care: A social work perspective. *Health Social Work, 8*(2), 97–106.

Wenger, N.K. (1981). Rehabilitation of the patient with myocardial infarction. *Primary Care, 8*(3), 491–507.

Williams, R.D. (1979). Physiological mechanisms underlying the association between psychosocial factors and coronary disease. In W.D. Gentry & R.B. Williams (eds.), *Pychological aspects of myocardial infarction and coronary care*. St. Louis, Mo: C. V. Mosby.

Williams, W.V., Lee, J. & Polak, P.R. (1976). Crisis intervention: Effects of crisis intervention on family survivors of sudden death situations. *Community Mental Health Journal, 12*(2), 128–136.

Williams, W.V. & Polak, P.R. (1979). Follow-up research in primary prevention: A model of adjustment in acute grief. *Journal of Clinical Psychology, 35*(1), 35–45.

Wise, T.N. (1983). Sexual dysfunction in the medically ill. *Psychosomatics, 24*(9), 787–801.

Zawacki, B.E., Azen, S.P., Imbus, S.H. & Chang, Y.T. (1979). Multifactorial probit analysis of mortality in burned patients. *Annals of Surgery, 189*(1), 1–5.

Zschoche, D.A. (ed.). (1981). *Comprehensive review of critical care*. St. Louis, Mo: C. V. Mosby.

CHAPTER SEVEN: CONJUGAL BEREAVEMENT

Abraham, K. (1969). A short study on the development of the libido. In *Selected papers on psychoanalysis*. London: Hogarth Press. (Originally published in 1927.)

Alrich, C.K. (1974). Some dynamics of anticipatory grief. In B. Schoenberg, D. Peretz & I. Goldberg (eds.), *Anticipatory grief*. New York: Columbia University Press.

Arens, D.A. (1983). Widowhood and well-being: An examination of sex differences within a causal model. *International Journal of Aging and Human Development, 15*(1), 27–40.

Arkin, A.M. (1981). Emotional care of the bereaved. In O.S. Margolis, H.C. Raether, A.H. Kutscher, J.B. Powers, I.B. Seeland, R. DeBellis & D.J. Cherico (eds.), *Acute grief: Counseling the bereaved*. New York: Columbia University Press.

Augspurger, R.E. (1978). Grief resolution among recent spouse-bereaved individuals. *Dissertation Abstracts International, 38*(9–A), 5534.

Ball, J.F. (1977). Widow's grief: The impact of age and mode of death. *OMEGA: Journal of Death and Dying, 7*(4), 307–333.

Benner, B.J. (1980). Cognitive changes during the grief process. *Dissertation Abstracts International, 40*,(11–B), 5397–5398.

Blanchard, C.G., Blanchard, E.B. & Becker, J.V. (1976). The young widow: Depressive symptomatology throughout the grief process. *Psychiatry, 39*(4), 394–399.

Bowlby, J. (1960). Grief and mourning in infancy and early childhood. *Psychoanalytic Study of the Child, 15*, 9–52.

Bowlby, J. (1973). *Separation: Anxiety and anger*, Vol. 2 of *Attachment and loss*. New York: Basic Books.

Carey, R.G. (1977). The widowed: A year later. *Journal of Counseling Psychology, 24*(2), 125–131.

Carey, R.G. (1979). Weathering widowhood: Problems and adjustments of the widowed during the first year. *Omega, 10*(2), 163–174.

Ciocco, A. (1940). On the mortality in husbands and wives. *Human Biology, 12*, 508–531.

Clayton, P.J. (1973). The clinical morbidity of the first year of bereavement: A review. *Comprehensive Psychiatry, 14*(2), 151–157.

Clayton, P.J. (1974). Mortality and morbidity in the first year of widowhood. *Archives of General Psychiatry, 30*, 747–750.

Clayton, P.J. (1979). The sequelae and nonsequelae of conjugal bereavement. *American Journal of Psychiatry, 136*(12), 1500–1534.

Clayton, P.J. (1982). Bereavement. In E. S. Paykel (ed.), *Handbook of affective disorders*. London: Churchill Livingstone.

Clayton, P.J., Halikas, J.A., Maurice, W.L. & Robins, E. (1973). Anticipatory grief and widowhood. *British Journal of Psychiatry, 122*, 47–51.

Clayton, P.J., Halikas, J.A. & Maurice, W.L. (1971). The bereavement of the widowed. *Diseases of the Nervous System, 32*, 597–604.

Clayton, P.J., Halikas, J.A. & Maurice, W.L. (1972). The depression of the widowed. *British Journal of Psychiatry, 120*, 71–78.

Clayton, P.J., Parilla, R.H. & Bieri, M.D. (1980). Bereavement research: Methodological problems in assessing the relationship between acuteness of death and the bereavement outcome. In J. Reiffel *et al.*, (eds.), *Psychosocial aspects of cardiovascular disease: The patient, the family and the staff*. New York: Columbia University Press.

Conroy, R.C. (1977). Widows and widowhood. *New York State Journal of Medicine*, *77*(3), 357–360.

Cox, P.R. & Ford, J.R. (1964). The mortality of widows shortly after widowhood. *Lancet*, *1*, 163–164.

Davidson, G. (1975). The waiting vulture syndrome. In B. Schoenberg, I. Gerber, A. Weiner, A.H. Kutscher, D. Peretz & A.C. Carr (eds.), *Bereavement: Its psychosocial aspects*. New York: Columbia University Press.

Demi, A.M. (1978). Adjustment to widowhood after a sudden death: Suicide and non-suicide survivors compared. *Dissertation Abstracts International*, *38*(12–B), 5847–5848.

Epstein, G., Weitz., Roback, H. & McKee, E. (1975). Research on bereavement: A selective and critical review. *Comprehensive Psychiatry*, *16*(6), 537–546.

Frankel, S. & Smith, D. (1982). Conjugal bereavement amongst the Huli people of Papua New Guinea. *British Journal of Psychiatry*, *141*, 302–305.

Franklin, H.J. (1979). The problem of grief among family members. *Dissertation Abstracts International*, *39*(8–B), 4028.

Freud, S. (1957a). Mourning and melancholia. In *Standard edition of the complete psychological works of Sigmund Freud*, *14*, 237–260. London: Hogarth Press. (Originally published in 1917.)

Freud, S. (1957b). On transcience. In *Standard edition of the complete psychological works of Sigmund Freud*, *14*, 305–307. London: Hogarth Press. (Originally published in 1916.)

Freud, S. (1957c). Premonitory dreams fulfilled. In *Standard edition of the complete psychological works of Sigmund Freud*, *5*, 623–625. London: Hogarth Press. (Originally published in 1899.)

Frost, N.R. & Clayton, P.J. (1977). Bereavement and psychiatric hospitalization. *Archives of General Psychiatry*, *34*, 1172–1175.

Fulton, R. & Gottesman, D.J. (1980). Anticipatory grief: A psychological concept reconsidered. *British Journal of Psychiatry*, *137*, 45–54.

Gallagher, D.E., Thompson, L.W. & Peterson, J.A. (1982). Psychosocial factors affecting adaptation to bereavement in the elderly. *International Journal of Aging and Human Development*, *14*(2), 79–95.

Gandour, M. (1978). Coping with grief as " 'bearing up' and 'bearing down' ": An exchange on James Agee's *A death in the family*. *Suicide and Life-Threatening Behavior*, *8(1)*, 60–64.

Gerber, I., Rusalem, R., Hannon, N., Battin, D. & Arkin, A. (1975). Anticipatory grief and aged widows and widowers. *Journal of Gerontology*, *30*(2), 225–229.

Golan, N. (1975). Wife to widow to woman. *Social Work*, *20*(5), 369–374.

Gorer, G. (1965). *Death, grief and mourning*. New York: Doubleday.

Greenblatt, M. (1978). The grieving spouse. *American Journal of Psychiatry*, *135*(1), 43–47.

Gullo, S.V. (1975). A study of selected psychological, psychosomatic, and somatic reactions in women anticipating the death of a husband. *Dissertation Abstracts International*, *35*(10–B), 5113–5114.

Hardt, D.V. (1979). An investigation of the stages of bereavement. *Omega*, *9*, 279–285.

Hays, D.R. (1978). Perceived needs for support of women who participate in a Red Cross Widows Program. *Dissertation Abstracts International*, *38*(7–B), 3129.

Heyman, D.K. & Gianturco, D.T. (1973). Long-term adaptation by the elderly to bereavement. *Journal of Gerontology*, *28*(3), 359–362.

Holmes, T. & Rahe, R. (1967). The social readjustment rating scale. *Journal of Psychosomatic Research, 11,* 213–218.

Horowitz, M.J., *et al.* (1980). Pathological grief and the activation of latent self-images. *American Journal of Psychiatry, 137*(10), 1157–1162.

Hudgens, R.W., Morrison, J.R. & Barchha, R.C. (1967). Life events and psychiatric illness. *British Journal of Psychiatry, 114,* 423–432.

Jacobs, S.C. & Ostfeld, A.M. (1980). The clinical management of grief. *Journal of the American Geriatrics Society, 28*(7), 331–335.

Jacobs, S. & Douglas, L. (1979). Grief: A mediating process between a loss and illness. *Comprehensive Psychiatry, 20*(2), 165–176.

Jacobs, S.C. & Ostfeld, A. (1977). An epidemiological review of the mortality of bereavement. *Psychosomatic Medicine, 39*(5), 344–357.

Jones, D. R. (1979). The grief therapy project: The effects of group therapy with bereaved surviving spouses on successful coping with grief. *Dissertation Abstracts International, 39*(12–B), 6121–6122.

Klein, M. (1940). Mourning and its relationship to manic-depressive states. *International Journal of Psychoanalysis, 21,* 125.

Klein, M. (1978). *Contributions to psychoanalysis.* London: Hogarth Press. (Originally published in 1940.)

Lewis, M.S., Gottesman, D. & Gutstein, S. (1979). The course and duration of crisis. *Journal of Consulting & Clinical Psychology, 47*(1), 128–134.

Lindemann, E. (1944). Symptomatology and management of acute grief. *American Journal of Psychiatry, 101,* 141–148.

Lopata, H.Z. (1972). *Widowhood in an American city.* Cambridge, Mass.: Schenkman.

Lopata, H.Z. (1973). Living through widowhood. *Psychology Today, 7*(2), 87–92.

Lopata, H.Z. (1975). On widowhood: Grief work and identity reconstruction. *Journal of Geriatric Psychiatry, 8*(1), 41–55.

MacMahon, B. & Pugh, T.F. (1965). Suicide in the widowed. *American Journal of Epidemiology, 81,* 23–31.

Maddison, D. & Viola, A. (1968). The health of widows in the year following bereavement. *Journal of Psychosomatic Research, 12,* 297–306.

Maddison, D. & Walker, W.L. (1967). Factors affecting the outcome of conjugal bereavement. *British Journal of Psychiatry, 113,* 1057–1067.

Maddison, D. & Walker, W.L. (1968). The relevance of conjugal bereavement for preventive psychiatry. *British Journal of Medical Psychology, 41,* 223–233.

Melson, S.J. & Rynearson, E.K. (1982). Unresolved bereavement: Medical reenactment of a loved one's terminal illness. *Postgraduate Medicine, 72*(1), 172–179.

Parkes, C.M. (1964). Effects of bereavement on physical and mental health: A study of the medical records of widows. *British Medical Journal, 2,* 274–279.

Parkes, C.M. (1970). The first year of bereavement: A longitudinal study of the reaction of London widows to the death of their husbands. *Psychiatry, 33,* 444–467.

Parkes, C.M. (1972). *Bereavement: Studies of grief in adult life.* N.Y.: International Universities Press, Inc..

Parkes, C.M. (1975). Determinants of outcome following bereavement. *OMEGA: Journal of Death and Dying, 6*(4), 303–323.

Parkes, C.M. (1981). Psychosocial care of the family after the patient's death. In O.S. Margolis, H.C. Raether, A.H. Kutscher, J.B. Powers, I.B. Seeland, R. DeBellis & D.J. Cherico (eds.), *Acute grief: Counseling the bereaved.* New York: Columbia University Press.

Parkes, C.M. (1981). Emotional involvement of the family during the period preceding death. In O.S. Margolis, H.C. Raether, A.H. Kutscher, J.B. Powers, I.B. Seeland, R. DeBellis & D.J. Cherico, (eds.), *Acute grief: Counseling the bereaved*. New York: Columbia University Press.

Parkes, C.M., Benjamin, B. & Fitzgerals, R.G. (1969). Broken heart: A statistical study of increased mortality among widowers. *British Medical Journal, 1*, 740.

Parkes, C.M. & Brown, R.J. (1972). Health after bereavement: A controlled study of young Boston widows and widowers. *Psychosomatic Medicine, 34*(5), 449–461.

Parkes, C.M. & Weiss, R.S. (1983). *Recovery from bereavement*. New York: Basic Books.

Paulay, D. (1977). Slow death: One survivor's experience. *OMEGA: Journal of Death and Dying, 8*(2), 173–179.

Paykel, E.S., Myers, J.K., Dienelt, M.N., Klerman, G.L., Lindenthal, J.J. & Pepper, M.P. (1969). Life events and depression: A controlled study. *Archives of General Psychiatry, 21*, 753–760.

Paykel, E.S., Prusoff, B.A. & Uhlenhuth, E.H. (1971). Scaling of life events. *Archives of General Psychiatry, 25*, 340–347.

Pincus, L. (1984). The process of mourning and grief. In E.S. Shneidman (ed.), *Death: Current perspectives*. Third edition. Palo Alto, Calif.: Mayfield Publishing Company.

Ramsay, R.W. (1977). Behavioural approaches to bereavement. *Behaviour Research and Therapy, 15*, 131–135.

Ramsay, R.W. (1979). Bereavement: A behavioral treatment of pathological grief. In P.O. Sjoden, S. Bates & W.S. Dockins (eds.), *Trends in behavior therapy*. New York: Academic Press.

Ramsay, R.W. & Happee, J.A. (1977). The stress of bereavement: Components and treatment. In C.D. Spielberger & I.G. Sarason (eds.), *Stress and anxiety*, Vol. 4. New York: Wiley.

Rando, T.A. (1984). *Grief, dying and death: Clinical interventions for caregivers*. Champaign, Ill.: Research Press.

Raphael, B. (1977). Preventive intervention with the recently bereaved. *Archives of General Psychiatry, 34*, 1450–1454.

Raphael, B. (1980). A psychiatric model for bereavement counseling. In B. Mark Scheonberg (ed.), *Bereavement counseling: A multidisciplinary handbook*. Westport, Conn.: Greenwood Press.

Raphael, B. (1983). *The anatomy of bereavement*. New York: Basic Books.

Rees, W.D. & Lutkins, S.G. (1967). Mortality of bereavement. *British Medical Journal, 4*, 13–16.

Rubin, S. (1981). A two-track model of bereavement: Theory and application in research. *American Journal of Orthopsychiatry, 51*(1), 101–109.

Saunders, J.M. (1980). A clinical study of widow bereavement involving various modes of death. *Dissertation Abstracts International, 40*(12–B, Pt. I), 5606.

Schultz, C.A. (1979). The dynamics of grief. *JEN, 5*(5), 26–30.

Silverman, P.R., MacKenzie, D., Pettipas, M. & Wilson, E. (eds.). (1975). *Helping each other in widowhood*. New York: Health Services Publishing Corporation.

Silverman, P.R. & Cooperband, A. (1975). On widowhood: Mutual help and the elderly widow. *Journal of Geriatric Psychiatry, 8*(1), 9–27.

Silverman, S.M. & Silverman, P.R. (1979). Parent-child communication in widowed families. *American Journal of Psychotherapy, 33*(3), 428–441.

Stedeford, A. (1981). Couples facing death. I—Psychological aspects. *British Medical Journal*, *283*(6298), 1033–1036.

Stroebe, M.S. & Stroebe, W. (1983). Who suffers more? Sex differences in health risks of the widowed. *Psychological Bulletin*, *93*(2), 279–301.

Stroebe, M.S., Stroebe, W., Gergen, K.J. & Gergen, M. (1981). The broken heart: Reality or myth? *OMEGA: Journal of Death and Dying*, *12*(2), 87–106.

Stubblefield, K.S. (1977). A preventive program for bereaved families. *Social Work in Health Care*, *2*(4), 379–389.

Vachon, M.L.S., Freedman, K., Formo, A., Rogers, J., Lyall, W.A.L. & Freeman, S.J.J. (1977). The final illness in cancer: The widow's perspective. *Canadian Medical Association Journal*, *117*(10), 1151–1154.

Vachon, M.L.S., Lyall, W.A.L., Rogers, J., Freedman-Letofsky, K. & Freeman, S.J.J. (1980). A controlled study of self-help intervention for widows. *American Journal of Psychiatry*, *137*(11), 1380–1384.

Vachon, M.L.S., Sheldon, A.R., Lancee, W.J., Lyall, W.A., Rogers, J. & Freeman, S. (1982). Correlates of enduring stress patterns following bereavement: Social network, life situation, and personality. *Psychological Medicine*, *12*, 783–788.

Valanis, B.G. & Yeaworth, R. (1982). Ratings of physical and mental health in the older bereaved. *Research in Nursing and Health*, *5*(3), 137–146.

Vogelsang, J.D. (1983). A psychological and faith approach to grief counseling. *Journal of Pastoral Care*, *37*(1), 22–27.

Winn, R.L. (1981). Retrospective evaluations of marital interaction and post bereavement adjustment in widowed individuals. *Dissertation Abstracts International*, *42*(5–B), 2105–2106.

Worden, J.W. (1982). *Grief counseling and grief therapy: A handbook for the mental health practitioner*. New York: Springer.

Young, M., Benjamin, B. & Wallis, C. (1963). The mortality of widowers. *Lancet*, *2*, 454–456.

CHAPTER EIGHT: PSYCHOLOGICAL ASPECTS OF CANCER

Adams, J. (1979). Mutual-help groups: Enhancing the coping ability of oncology clients. *Cancer Nursing*, *2*(2), 95–98.

Allen, A. (1981). Psychosocial factors in cancer. *American Family Physician*, *23*(2), 197–201.

Allport, G.W. (1937). *Personality: A psychological interpretation*. New York: Holt, Rinehart & Winston.

Anderson, J.L. (1979). A practical approach to teaching about communication with terminal cancer patients. *Journal of Medical Education*, *54*, 823–824.

Bahnson, C.B. (1980). Stress and cancer: The state of the art. *Psychosomatics*, *21*(12), 975–981.

Bateson, G., Jackson, D.D., Haley, J. & Weakland, J. (1956). Double-bind hypothesis of schizophrenia. *Behavioral Science*, *1*, 251–264.

Bean, G., Cooper, S., Alpert, R. & Kipnis, D. (1980). Coping mechanisms of cancer patients: A study of 33 patients receiving chemotherapy. *CA*, *30*(5), 256–259.

Beatty, L.F. (1978). *Still a lot of living: Coping with cancer*. New York: Macmillan.

Becker, H. (1979). Psychodynamic aspects of breast cancer: Differences in younger and older patients. *Psychotherapy and Psychosomatics*, *32*(1–4), 287–296.

Blumenfield, M., Levy, N.B. & Kaufman, D. (1978). The wish to be informed of a fatal illness. *Omega, 9*(4), 323–326.

Brehm, J.W. (1966). *A theory of psychological reactance.* New York: John Wiley.

Brewin, T.B. (1977). The cancer patient: Communication and morale. *British Medical Journal, 2*(6103), 1623–1627.

Burnet, M. (1957). Cancer—A biological approach. *British Medical Journal, 1,* 779–786; 841–847.

Burnet, M. (1971). *Genes, dreams and realities.* Aylesbury: Medical Technical Publishing Company.

Cahen, R. (1979). Cancer and depth psychology: Reflections and hypotheses. *Journal of Analytical Psychology, 24*(4), 343–347.

Campbell, T.W., VanGee, S.J., Brock, G. & Greenfield, G. (1980). Use of multiple family group for crisis intervention. *General Hospital Psychiatry, 2,* 95–99.

Cantor, R.C. (1978). *And a time to live.* N.Y.: Harper & Row.

Cantor, R.C. (1980). Self-esteem, sexuality and cancer-related stress. *Frontiers of Radiation Therapy and Oncology,* (14), 51–54.

Capone, M.A., *et al.* (1979). Crisis intervention: A functional model for hospitalized cancer patients. *American Journal of Orthopsychiatry, 49*(4), 598–607.

Dansak, D.A. & Selgas-Cordes, R. (1979). Cancer: Denial or suppression? *International Journal of Psychiatry in Medicine, 9*(3–4), 257–262.

Derogatis, L.R. & Kourlesis, S.M. (1981). An approach to evaluation of sexual problems in the cancer patient. *CA, 31*(1), 46–50.

Duszynski, K.R., Shaffer, J.W. & Thomas, C.B. (1981). Neoplasm and traumatic events in childhood: Are they related? *Archives of General Psychiatry, 38*(3), 327–331.

Farberow, N.L., Ganzler, S., Cutter, F. *et al.* (1971). An eight-year survey of hospital suicides. *Suicide and Life-Threatening Behavior, 1,* 184–202.

Farberow, N.L., McKelligott, W., Cohen, S. & Darbonne, A. (1966). Suicide among patients with cardiorespiratory illnesses. *Journal of the American Medical Association, 195,* 422–428.

Farberow, N.L., Shneidman, E.S. & Leonard, C.V. (1963). Suicide among general medical and surgical hospital patients with malignant neoplasms. *Medical Bulletin of the Veteran's Administration, 9*(2), 1–11.

Fay, M. (1983). *A mortal condition.* New York: Coward-McCann.

Ferlic, M., Goldman, A. & Kennedy, B.J. (1979). Group counseling in adult patients with advanced cancer. *Cancer, 43*(2), 760–766.

Fiore, N. (1979). Fighting cancer: One patient's perspective. *New England Journal of Medicine, 300*(6), 284–289.

Fitzpatrick, J.J., Donovan, M.J. & Johnston, R.L. (1980). Experience of time during the crisis of cancer. *Cancer Nursing, 3*(3), 191–194.

Forman, B.F. (1979). Cancer and suicide. *General Hospital Psychiatry, 1*(2), 108–114.

Freidenbergs, I., Gordon, W., Hibbard, M.R. & Diller, L (1980). Assessment and treatment of psychosocial problems of the cancer patient: A case study. *Cancer Nursing, 3*(2), 111–119.

Garusi, G.F. (1978). Psychological problems of the cancer patient. *Zeitschrift für Krebsforschung und Klinische Onkologie, 91,* 117–125.

Gazut, M. (1981). La mort de ma mere. *Soins infirmiers, 9,* 79–81.

Giacquinta, B. (1977). Helping families face the crisis of cancer. *American Journal of Nursing, 77*(10), 1585–1588.

Gottheil, E., McGurn, W.C. & Pollak, O. (1979). Awareness and disengagement in cancer patients. *American Journal of Psychiatry*, *136*(5), 632–636.

Greenberg, R.P. & Dattore, P.J. (1981). The relationship between dependency and the development of cancer. *Psychosomatic Studies*, *43*(1), 35–43.

Greene, W.A., Young, L.E. & Swisher, S.N. (1956). Psychological factors and reticuloendothelial disease: Observations on a group of women with lymphomas and leukemias. *Psychosomatic Medicine*, *18*, 284–303.

Greer, S. (1979). Psychological enquiry: A contribution to cancer research. *Psychological Medicine*, *9*(2), 81–89.

Grossarth-Maticek, R. (1980). Psychosocial predictors of cancer and internal diseases: An overview. *Psychotherapy and Psychosomatics*, *33*, 122–128.

Gussow, Z. & Tracy, G.S. (1976). The role of self-help clubs in adaptation to chronic illness and disability. *Social Science and Medicine*, *10*(7–8), 407–414.

Hanson, M.R., McKay, F.W. & Miller, R.W. (1980). Three-dimensional perspective of U.S. cancer mortality. *Lancet*, 246–247.

Hardy, R.E., Green, D.R., Jordan, H.W. & Hardy, G. (1980). Communication between cancer patients and physicians. *Southern Medical Journal*, *73*(6), 755–757.

Hardy, R.E., & Hardy, G. (1979). Patterns of communication to cancer patients: A descriptive analysis. *Journal of the Tennessee Medical Association*, *72*(9), 656–658.

Heim, E., Moser, A. & Adler, R. (1978). Defense mechanisms and coping behavior in terminal illness: An overview. *Psychotherapy and Psychosomatics*, *30*(1), 1–17.

Herzoff, N.E. (1979). A therapeutic group for cancer patients and their families. *Cancer Nursing*, *2*(6), 469–474.

Jacobs, T.J. & Charles, E. (1980). Life events and the occurrence of cancer in children. *Psychosomatic Medicine*, *42*(1), 11–24.

Jordan, H.W. (1979). Psychosocial aspects of cancer. *Journal of the Tennessee Medical Association*, *72*(1), 41–42.

Kay, E. (1979). Cancer: I faced the facts—in my own time. *Nursing Mirror*, *149*(17), 18–19.

Kaplan, D.M., Grobstein, R. & Smith, A. (1976). Predicting the impact of severe illness in families: A study of the variety of responses to fatal illness. *Health and Social Work*, *1*, 71–82.

Kelly, P.P. & Ashby, G.C. (1979). Group approaches for cancer patients: Establishing a group. *American Journal of Nursing*, *79*(5), 914–915.

Kennedy, B.J. & Lillehaugen, A. (1979). Patient recall of informed consent. *Medical and Pediatric Oncology*, *7*(2), 173–178.

Lamb, M.A. & Woods, N.F. (1981). Sexuality and the cancer patient. *Cancer Nursing*, *4*(2), 139–144.

Leiber, L., Plumb, M.M., Gerstenzang, M.L. & Holland, J. (1976). The communication of affection between cancer patients and their spouses. *Psychosomatic Medicine*, *38*, 379–389.

Leigh, H., Ungerer, J. & Percarpio, B. (1980). Denial and helplessness in cancer patients undergoing radiation therapy: Sex differences and implications for prognosis. *Cancer*, *45*(12), 3086–3089.

Lewis, M.S., Gottesman, D. & Gutstein, S. (1979). The course and duration of crisis. *Journal of Consulting and Clinical Psychology*, *47*(1), 128–134.

Lickiss, J.N. (1980). Psychological aspects of cancer. *The Medical Journal of Australia*, *1*, 297–302.

Longhofer, J. & Floersch, J.E. (1980). Dying or living?: The double bind. *Culture, Medicine and Psychiatry*, *4*, 119–136.

Louhivouri, K.A. & Hakama, M. (1979). Risk of suicide among cancer patients. *American Journal of Epidemiology, 109*(1), 59–65.

Love, R.R., Hayward, J. & Stone, H.L. (1980). Attitudes about cancer medicine among primary care residents and their teachers. *Journal of Medical Education, 55*(3), 211–212.

Marshall, J.R., Burnett, W. & Brassure, J. (1983). On precipitating factors: Cancer as a cause of suicide. *Suicide and Life-Threatening Behavior, 13*(1), 15–27.

Maxwell, M.B. (1980). Cancer and suicide. *Cancer Nursing, 3*(1), 33–38.

Meares, A. (1979). The psychologcial treatment of cancer. *Australian Family Physician, 8*, 801–805.

Meryman, R. (1980). *Hope: A loss survived*. Boston: Little, Brown.

Morrow, G.R., Chiarello, R.J. & Derogatis, L.R. (1978). A new scale for assessing patients' psychosocial adjustment to medical illness. *Psychological Medicine, 8*(4), 605–610.

Morrow, G.R., Gootnick, J. & Schmale, A. (1978). A simple technique for increasing cancer patient's knowledge of informed consent to treatment. *Cancer, 42*(2), 793–799.

Murray, J.B. (1980). Psychosomatic aspects of cancer: An overview. *Journal of Genetic Psychology, 136*(Second Half), 185–194.

Nordlicht, S. (1980). Psychiatric support during cancer treatment. *New York State Journal of Medicine, 80*(10), 1557–1559.

Novack, D.H., Plumer, R., Smith, R.L. *et al.* (1979). Changes in physicians' attitudes toward telling the cancer patient. *Journal of the American Medical Association, 241*(9), 897–900.

Oakley, A. (1979). Living in the present: A confrontation with cancer. *British Medical Journal, 1*, 861–862.

Oken, D. (1961). What to tell cancer patients: A study of medical attitudes. *Journal of the American Medical Association, 175*, 1120–1128.

Paget, J. (1870). *Surgical Pathology*. London: Longmans Green.

Peteet, J.R. (1979). Depression in cancer patients: An approach to differential diagnosis and treatment. *Journal of the American Medical Association, 241*(14), 1487–1489.

Peterson, L.G. & Popkin, M.K. (1980). Neuro-psychiatric effects of chemotherapeutic agents for cancer. *Psychosomatics, 21*(2), 141–153.

Popkin, M.K., Prem, K.A., Hall, R.C. *et al.* (1978). Single case study: A novel psychiatric adjunct to cancer therapy. *Journal of Nervous and Mental Disease, 166*(3), 217–218.

Rando, T.A. (1983). An investigation of grief and adaptation in parents whose children have died from cancer. *Journal of Pediatric Psychology, 8*(1), 3–20.

Reich, P. & Kelly, M.J. (1976). Suicide attempts by hospitalized medical and surgical patients. *New England Journal of Medicine, 294*, 298–301.

Richards, W.A. (1975). Counseling, peak experiences and the human encounter with death: An empirical study of the efficacy of DPT-assisted counseling in enhancing the quality of life of persons with terminal cancer and their closest family members. *Dissertation Abstracts International, 36*(3–A), 1314.

Ryan, M. (1979). Ethics and the patient with cancer. *British Medical Journal, 2*, 480–481.

Ryan, M.E. & Neuenshwander, B. (1977). Team approach to psychological management of patients with neoplastic disease. *Radiologic Technology, 49*(3), 285–289.

Sachtleben, C.R. (1978). The role of belief systems in cancer therapy. *The Delaware Medical Journal, 50*(2), 71–72.

Schain, W.S. (1979). Sexual functioning, self-esteem and cancer care. *Frontiers of Radiation Therapy and Oncology, 14*, 12–19.

Schain, W.S. (1980). Patients' rights in decision making: The case for personalism versus paternalism in health care. *Cancer, 46*, 1035–1041.

Schildkraut, J.J. (1965). The catecholamine hypothesis of affective disorders: A review of supporting evidence. *American Journal of Psychiatry, 122*, 509–522.

Schmale, A.H. & Iker, H. (1971). Hopelessness as a predictor of cervical cancer. *Social Science and Medicine, 5*, 95–100.

Seligman, M.E. (1975). *Helplessness: On depression, development and death*. San Francisco: W.H. Freeman.

Shanfield, S.B. (1980). On surviving cancer: Psychological considerations. *Comprehensive Psychiatry, 21*(2), 128–134.

Snow, H. (1893). *Cancer and the cancer process*. London: Churchill.

Spence, D. (1979, September). Somatopsychic signs of cervical cancer. Paper presented at the meeting of the 87th annual American Psychiatric Association. New York.

Tasman, A. (1982). Loss of self-cohesion in terminal illness. *Journal of the American Academy of Psychoanalysis, 10*(4), 515–526.

The cancer patient's view of chemotherapy. (1979). *Cancer Nursing, 2*(4), 283–286.

Thomas, C.B. & Duszynski, D.R. (1974). Closeness to parents and the family constellation in a prospective study of five disease states: Suicide, mental illness, malignant tumor, hypertension and coronary heart disease. *Johns Hopkins Medical Journal, 134*, 251–270.

Thomas, C.B. & Greenstreet, R.L. (1973). Physiobiological characteristics in youth as predictors of five disease states: Suicide, mental illness, hypertension, coronary heart disease and tumor. *Johns Hopkins Medical Journal, 132*, 16–43.

Todres, R. & Wojtuik, R. (1979). The cancer patient's view of chemotherapy. *Cancer Nursing, 2*(4), 283–286.

Trillin, A.S. (1981). Of dragons and garden peas: A cancer patient talks to doctors. *New England Journal of Medicine, 300*(12), 699–700.

Weisman, A.D. & Worden, J.W. (1975). Psychological analysis of cancer deaths. *OMEGA: Journal of Death and Dying, 6*(1), 61–75.

Weisman, A. D. (1979). *Coping with cancer*. New York: McGraw-Hill.

Welch, D.A. (1981). Waiting, worry, and the cancer experience. *Oncology Nursing Forum, 8*(2), 14–18.

Welsh, D.A. (1982). Anticipatory grief reactions in family members of adult patients. *Issues in Mental Health Nursing, 4*(2), 149–158.

Wellisch, D.K., *et al.* (1978). Management of family emotional stress: Family group therapy in a private oncology practice. *International Journal of Group Psychotherapy, 28*(2), 225–231.

West, D.E. (1977). Social adaptation patterns among cancer patients with facial disfigurements resulting from surgery. *Archives of Physical Medicine and Rehabilitation, 58*(11), 473–479.

Whitlock, F.A. & Siskind, M. (1979). Depression and cancer: A follow-up study. *Psychological Medicine, 9*(4), 747–752.

Whitman, H.H., Gustafson, J.P. & Coleman, F.W. (1979). Group approaches for cancer patients: Leaders and members. *American Journal of Nursing, 79*(5), 910–913.

Wicklund, D. (1974). *Freedom and reactance.* (1974). Potomac, Md: Lawrence Erlbaum Associates.

Wood, P.E., Milligan, M., Christ, D. *et al.* (1978). Group counseling for cancer patients in a community hospital. *Psychosomatics, 19*(9), 555−557, 561.

Worden, J.W. & Weisman, A.D. (1980). Do cancer patients really want counseling?
General Hospital Psychiatry, 2(2), 100−103.

Wortman, C. B. & Brehm, J. W. (1975). Responses to uncontrollable outcomes: An
integration of reactance theory and the learned helplessness model. In L. Berkowitz
(ed.), *Advances in experimental social psychology,* Vol. 8. New York: Academic
Press.

CHAPTER NINE: HOSPICE TERMINAL CARE

Aiken, L.H. & Marx, M.M. (1982). Hospices: Perspectives on the public policy debate. *American Psychologist, 37*(11), 1271−1279.

Amenta-Madalon, M. & Weiner, A.W. (1981a). Death anxiety and purpose in life in
hospice workers. *Psychological Reports, 49*(3), 920.

Amenta-Madalon, M. & Weiner, A.W. (1981b). Death anxiety and general anxiety in
hospice workers. *Psychological Reports, 49*(3), 962.

Baines, M. (ed.) (1984). Drug control of common symptoms. Unpublished pamphlet
for the physicians of Saint Christopher's Hospice, Sydenham, England.

Barber, J. & Gitelson, J. (1980). Cancer pain: Psychological management using hypnosis. *Cancer Journal for Clinicians, 30*(3), 130−136.

Bass, D.M. (1983). Response bias in studying hospice clients' needs. *OMEGA: Journal
of Death and Dying, 13*(4), 305−318.

Bayer, R., Callahan, D., Fletcher, J., Hodgson, T., Jennings, B., Monsees, D., Siev-
erts, S. & Veatch, R. (1983). The care of the terminally ill: Morality and economics.
New England Journal of Medicine, 309(24), 1490−1494.

Benoliel, J.Q. & Crowley, D.M. (1974). The patient in pain: New concepts. *Proceedings of the National Conference on Cancer Nursing.* New York: American Cancer
Society.

Bertman, S.L. (1980). Lingering terminal illness and the family: Insights from literature.
Family Process, 19, 341−348.

Bertman, S.L., Greene, H. & Wyatt, C.A. (1982). Humanistic health care education
in a hospice/palliative care setting. *Death Education, 5*(4), 391− 408.

Bichekas, G. (1980). Life style analysis of hospice home care nurses. *Dissertation
Abstracts International, 41*(3−B), 1157.

Bitensky, R. (1979). Death: The psychotherapeutic cure for cancer. *Journal of Health
Politics, Policy & Law, 4*(1), 5−10.

Bonica, J.J. & Ventafridda, V. (eds.) (1979). *Advances in pain research and therapy,*
Vol. 2. New York: Raven Press.

Brann, J. (1983). Hospice home care—A pilot project in West Australia. *Australian
Nurses Journal, 13*(1), 47− 49.

Buckingham, R.W. (1983). Hospice care in the United States: The process begins.
OMEGA: Journal of Death and Dying, 13(2), 159−171.

Butler, R.N. (1979). The need for quality hospice care. *Quality Review Bulletin, 5*(5),
2−7.

Butterfield-Picard, H. & Magno, J.B. (1982). Hospice the adjective, not the noun: The future of a national priority. *American Psychologist, 37*(11), 1254–1259.

Cameron, J. & Parkes, C.M. (1983). Terminal care: Evaluation of effects on surviving family of care before and after bereavement. *Postgraduate Medicine Journal, 59*(688), 73–78.

Carey, R.G. & Posavac, E.J. (1979). Holistic care in a cancer care center. *Nursing Research, 28*(4), 213–216.

Clouet, A.M. (1981). Etre vieux a l'hospice. [Being old in a hospice.] *Soins, 26*(23–24), 75–80.

Cohen, K.P. (1979). Hospice: Prescription for terminal care. Germantown, Md: Aspen Systems Corporation.

Cohen, M.M. & Wellisch, D.K. (1978). Living in limbo: Psychosocial intervention in families with a cancer patient. *American Journal of Psychotherapy, 32*(4), 561–571.

Corbett, T.L. & Hai, D.M. (1979). Searching for euthanatos: The hospice alternative. *Hospital Progress, 60*(3), 38–41, 76.

Corr, C.A. & Corr, D.M. (eds.) (1983). *Hospice care: Principles and practice.* New York: Springer.

Creek, L.V. (1982). A homecare hospice profile: Description, evaluation, and cost analysis. *Journal of Family Practice, 14*(1), 53–58.

Dawson, E.E. (1981). The hospice: An educational-service model providing counseling opportunities and indirect benefits for older widows. *Death Education, 5*(2), 107–119.

Doka, K.J. (1983). The spiritual needs of the dying patient. *Newsletter of the Forum for Death Education and Counseling, 6,* 2–3.

Donovan, M., Burns, D., Daley, M., Dietz, K., Faut, M., Gardenhire, J., Ivantic, E., McGuire, L., Steinweg, C., Wangler, N., Wright, Z. & Yuska, C. (1981). Pain and symptom management (Facilitator Manual). In U.S. Department of Health and Human Services, *Hospice education program for nurses* (Publication No. HRA 81–27). Washington, D.C.: U.S. Government Printing Office.

Doyle, D. (1982a). Nerve blocks in advanced cancer. *Practitioner, 226*(1365), 539, 541–544.

Doyle, D. (1982b). Hospice: An education center for professionals *Death Education, 6*(3), 213–226.

Eastman, M. (1978). "Feelings are facts in this house." Hospice care for those with no cure. *American Pharmacy, 18*(12), 18–22.

Edelstyn, G.A., MacRae, K.D. & MacDonald, F.M. (1979). Improvement in life quality in cancer patients undergoing chemotherapy. *Clinical Oncology, 5,* 43–49.

Ferszt, G. & Houck, P.D. (1983). Integration of the community health nurse in a hospital-based hospice program. *Oncology Nursing Forum, 10*(3), 36–39.

Garfield, C.A., Larson, D.G. & Schuldberg, D. (1982). Mental health training and the hospice community: A national survey. *Death Education, 6*(3), 189–204.

Garner, J. (1976). Palliative care: It's the quality of life remaining that matters. *Canadian Medical Association Journal, 115*(2), 179–180.

Gibbs, H.W. & Achterberg, L.J. (1978). Spiritual values and death anxiety: Implications for counseling with terminal cancer patients. *Journal of Counseling Psychology, 25*(6), 563–569.

Glassman, S.M. & Popkin, B.H. (1980). Cancer audit: How the quality of care improves the quality of life. *Cancer Nursing, 3*(5), 379–383.

Gotay, C.C. (1983). Models of terminal care: A review of the research literature. *Clinical Investigations in Medicine, 6*(3), 131–141.

Gray-Toft, R. (1980). Effectiveness of a counseling support program for hospice nurses. *Journal of Counseling Psychology, 27*(4), 346–454.

Greco, F.A. & Hande, K.R. (1979). The clinical pharmacology and use of antineoplastic drugs. *Journal of the Tennessee Medical Association, 79*(1), 23–33.

Greer, D.S. (1983). Hospice: Lessons for geriatricians. *Journal of the American Geriatrics Society, 31*(2), 67–70.

Hamilton, M.P. & Reid, H.F. (eds.) (1980). *A Hospice handbook.* Grand Rapids, Mich.: William B. Eerdmans Publishing Company.

Hinton, J. (1979). Comparison of places and policies for terminal care. *Lancet, 1*(8106), 29–32.

Jarolim, D.R. (1983). Hospice care without hospice. *Journal of the Oklahoma State Medical Association, 76*(4), 87–89.

Jenkins, G.J. (1981). Stress and coping of hospice nurses. *Dissertation Abstracts International, 42*(6–B), 2600–2601.

Kassakian, M.G., Bailey, L.R., Rinker, M., Stewart, C.A. & Yates, J.W. (1979). The cost and quality of dying: A comparison of home and hospital. *Nurse Practitioner, 4*(1), 18–23.

Klagsbrun, S.C. (1982). Ethics in hospice care. *American Psychologist, 37*(11), 1263–1265.

Koff, T.H. (1980). *Hospice: A caring community.* Cambridge, Mass.: Winthrop.

Kraisman-Amit, U. (1977). The nature of change in a fatally ill individual. *Dissertation Abstracts International, 37*(12–B, pt. 1), 6406.

Krant, M.J. & Johnston, L. (1977). Family members' perceptions of communications in late stage cancer. *International Journal of Psychiatry in Medicine, 8*(2), 203–216.

Kuhl, S. (1983). Sharing: Hospice isn't just a place. *Nursing, 13*(9), 112.

Lamerton, R.C. (1979). Cancer patients dying at home: The last 24 hours. *Practitioner, 223*(1338), 813–817.

Lattanzi, M.E. (1982). Hospice bereavement services: Creating networks of support. *Family and Community Health, 5*(3), 54–63.

Lipman, A.G. (1979). Drug therapy of chronic pain. *The Journal of Continuing Education in Hospital and Clinical Pharmacy, 1,* 11–20.

Liss-Levinson, W.S. (1982). Reality perspectives for psychological services in a hospice program. *American Psychologist, 37*(11), 1266–1270.

MacElveen-Hoehn, P. & McIntosh, E.G. (1981). The hospice movement: Growing pains and promises. *Topics in Clinical Nursing, 3*(3), 29–38.

Markel, W.M. & Sinon, V.B. (1978). The hospice concept. *CA, 28*(4), 225–237.

McPhail, C. (1981). Nursing care study: Dying with dignity. *Nursing Times, 77*(42), 1792–1793.

McPhee, M.S., Arcand, R. & MacDonald, R.N. (1979). Taking the stigma out of hospice care: Flexible approaches for the terminally ill. *Canadian Medical Association Journal, 120*(10), 1284–1288.

Meichenbaum, D. & Turk, D. (1976). The cognitive-behavioral management of anxiety, anger, and pain. In P.O. Davidson (ed.), *The behavioral management of anxiety, depression, and pain.* New York: Brunner/Mazel.

Melzack, R. & Wall, P.D. (1983). The challenge of pain. New York: Basic Books.

Mor, V. & Birnbaum, H. (1983). Medicare legislation for hospice care: Implications of national hospice study data. *Health Affairs, 2*(2), 80–90.

Mount, B.M., Melzack, R. & MacKinnon, K.J. (1978). The management of intractable pain in patients with advanced malignant disease. *The Journal of Urology, 120,* 720–725.

Mudd, P. (1982). High ideals and hard cases: The evolution of a hospice. *The Hastings Center Report, 12*(2), 11–14.

Naiman, R. (1981). Characteristics associated with the extent of home or institutional care obtained by terminally ill cancer patients. *Dissertation Abstracts International, 41*(9–B), 3582–3583.

National Hospice Organization. (1981). Standards of a hospice program of care. Arlington, Va.

Noyes, R., Jr. (1981). Treatment of cancer pain. *Psychosomatic Medicine, 43*(1), 57–70.

Pannier, E.A. (1980). The hospice care giver: A qualitative study. *Dissertation Abstracts International, 41*(6 –A), 2456–2457.

Parkes, C.M. (1979). Terminal care: Evaluation of in-patient service at St. Christopher's Hospice. Part I. Views of surviving spouse on effects of the service on the patient. *Postgraduate Medical Journal, 55*(646), 517–522.

Parkes, C.M. (1981). Evaluation of a bereavement service. *Journal of Preventive Psychiatry, 1*(2), 179–188.

Pestello, F.P. & Bass, D.M. (1983). Goal impediments in two hospice programs. *Nursing Health Care, 4*(7), 397–399.

Peterson, L.G. & Popkin, M.K. (1980). Neuro-psychiatric effects of chemotherapeutic agents for cancer. *Psychosomatics, 21*(2), 141–153.

Rizzo, R.F. (1978). Hospice: Comprehensive terminal care. *New York State Journal of Medicine, 78*(12), 1902–1910.

Rossman, P. (1977). *Hospice: Creating new models of care for the terminally ill.* New York: Association Press.

Ryder, C.F. & Ross, D.M. (1977). Terminal care: Issues and alternatives. *Public Health Reports, 92*(1), 20–29.

Ryndes, T. & Brown, R.S. (1981). Care of the dying: Issues in pain management: Part I. *Minnesota Medicine, 64*(12), 774–775.

Ryndes, T. & Brown, R.S. (1982). Care of the dying: Issues in pain management: Part II. *Minnesota Medicine, 65*(3), 185–188.

Saunders, C.M. (1963). Management of intractable pain. *Proceedings of the Royal Society of Medicine, 191*(3), 195–197.

Saunders, C.M. (1966). Terminal patient care. *Geriatrics, 21*(12), 70–74.

Saunders, C.M. (1975). Terminal care. In K.D. Bagshawe (ed.), *Medical oncology: Medical aspects of malignant disease.* Oxford: Blackwell Scientific Publications.

Saunders, C.M. (1976). Care of the dying: The last achievement. *Nursing Times, 72*(32), 1247–1249.

Saunders, C.M. (1977). Palliative care for the terminally ill [letter]. *Canadian Medical Association Journal, 117*(1), 15.

Saunders, C.M. (1978a). Hospice care. *American Journal of Medicine, 65*(5), 726–728.

Saunders, C.M. (ed.) (1978b). *The management of terminal disease.* London: Edward Arnold.

Saunders, C.M. (1979). The nature and management of terminal pain and the hospice concept. In J.J. Bonica & V. Ventafridda (eds.), *Advances in pain research and therapy,* Vol. 2, 635–651. New York: Raven Press.

Saunders, C.M. & Baines, M. (1983). *Living with dying: The management of terminal disease*. Oxford: Oxford University Press.

Simpson, J. & Doyle, D. (1981). Protracted dying: A challenge to the caring team. *Nursing Times*, *77*(41), 1752−1754.

Stoddard, S. (1978). *The hospice movement*. Briarcliff Manor, N.Y.: Stein & Day.

Sweetser, C.J. (1979). Integrated care: The hospital-based hospice. *QRB. Quality Review Bulletin*, *5*(5), 18−21.

Tehan, C. (1982). Hospice in an existing home care agency. *Family and Community Health*, *5*(3), 11−20.

Theado, G.C. & Scarry, K.D. (1983). Networking community services: Politics of hospice development. *Nursing Health Care*, *4*(10), 568−572.

Tigges, K.N. & Sherman, L.M. (1983). The treatment of the hospice patient: From occupational history to occupational role. *American Journal of Occupational Therapy*, *37*(4), 235−238.

Twycross, R.G. (1974). Clinical experience with diamorphine in advanced malignant pain. *International Journal of Clinical Pharmacology*, *9*, 184−198.

Twycross, R.G. (1977). Choice of strong analgesic in terminal cancer: Diamorphine or morphine? *Pain*, *3*, 93−104.

Twycross, R.G. (1978a). The assessment of pain in advanced cancer. *Journal of Medical Ethics*, *4*, 112−116.

Twycross, R.G. (1978b). The target is a pain-free patient. *Nursing Mirror*, *147*(24), 38−39.

Twycross, R.G. (1978c). Relief of pain. In C.M. Saunders (ed.) *The management of terminal disease*, 65−92. London: Edward Arnold.

Twycross, R.G. (1979). Overview of analgesia. In J.J. Bonica & V. Ventafridda (eds.), *Advances in pain research and therapy*, Vol. 2, 617−633. New York: Raven Press.

Twycross, R.G. (1980a). Hospice care: Redressing the balance in medicine. *Journal of the Royal Society of Medicine*, *73*, 475−481.

Twycross, R.G. (1980b). Incidence and assessment of pain in terminal cancer. In R.G. Twycross & V. Ventafridda (eds.), *The continuing care of terminal cancer patients*, 65−74. Oxford: Pergamon Press.

Twycross, R.G. (1981). Rehabilitation in terminal cancer patients. *International Rehabilitation Medicine*, *3*(3), 135−144.

Vere, D.W. (1980). The hospital as a place of pain. *Journal of Medical Ethics*, *6*, 117−119.

Walsh, T.D. & Cheater, F.M. (1983). Use of morphine for cancer pain. *The Pharmaceutical Journal*, October, 1983, 525−527.

Ward, B.J. (1978). Hospice home care program. *Nursing Outlook*, *26*(10), 646−649.

Weisman, A.D. (1982). Special attention for the terminally ill. *Physician and Patient*, *1*, 28−34.

Weisman, A.D. & Sobel, H.J. (1979). Coping with cancer through self-instruction: A hypothesis. *Journal of Human Stress*, *5*, 3−8.

Wilson, B.P., Blosse, R.W., Tucker, J.L. & Spector, K.K. (1983). Hospice care: Perspectives on a Blue Cross Plan's community pilot program. *Inquiry*, *20*(4), 322−327.

Woodson, R. (1978). Hospice care in terminal illness. In C.A. Garfield (ed.), *Psychosocial care of the dying patient*. New York: McGraw-Hill.

Wright-St.Clair, R.E. (1983). Terminal care. *New Zealand Medical Journal*, *96*(724), 49−50.

Zimmerman, J.M. (1979). Experience with a hospice-care program for the terminally ill. *Annals of Surgery, 189*(6), 683–690.

CHAPTER TEN: THE ELDERLY AND DEATH

Abramson, R. (1975). A dying patient: The question of euthanasia. *International Journal of Psychiatry in Medicine, 6*(3), 431–454.

Averill, J.R. & Wisocki, P.A. (1981). Some observations on behavioral approaches to the treatment of grief among the elderly. In H.J. Sobel (ed.), *Behavior therapy in terminal care: A humanistic approach.* Cambridge, Mass.: Ballinger.

Bandman, E.L. & Bandman, B. (1979). The nurse's role in protecting the patient's right to live or die. *Advances in Nursing Science, 1*(3), 21–35.

Baron, C.H. (1981). Termination of life support systems in the elderly—Discussion: To die before the gods please: Legal issues surrounding euthanasia and the elderly. *Journal of Geriatric Psychiatry, 14*(1), 45–70.

Brace, S.M. (1978). A psychological study of the aged in the last stages of terminal illness. *Dissertation Abstracts International, 38*(8–A), 4671.

Bromberg, S. & Cassel, C.K. (1983). Suicide in the elderly: The limits of paternalism. *Journal of the American Geriatrics Society, 31*(11), 698–703.

Bumagin, V.E. & Hirn, K.F. (1982). Observations on changing relationships for older married women. *American Journal of Psychoanalysis, 42*(2), 133–142.

Butler, R.N. (1974). Successful aging and the role of the life review. *Journal of the American Geriatric Society, 22*, 529–535.

Butler, R.N. & Lewis, M.I. (1973). *Aging and mental health.* St. Louis, Mo.: C.V. Mosby.

Cape, E.A. (1979). "Going downhill" responses to terminality in a population of institutionalized aged ill. *Dissertation Abstracts International, 41*(2–A), 1107.

Cartwright, A. (1982). The role of the general practitioner in helping the elderly widowed. *Journal of the Royal College of General Practitioners, 32*(237), 215–227.

Cassem, N.H. (1981). Termination of life support systems in the elderly: Clinical issues. *Journal of Geriatric Psychiatry, 14*(1), 13–21.

Champlin, L. (1983). Early retirement: A catalyst for health problems? *Geriatrics, 38*(7), 106–109.

Chappell, N.L. (1975). Awareness of death in the disengagement theory: A conceptualization and an empirical investigation. *OMEGA: Journal of Death and Dying, 6*(4), 325–343.

Chisolm, S. (1981). Emotional stages of dying. *Michigan Nurse,* 8–9.

Cumming, E. & Henry, W.E. (1961). *Growing old: The process of disengagement.* N.Y.: Basic Books, Inc.

Deak, E.J. & Smith, W.J. (1979). Inflation and the elderly. *Aging, 299–300,* 3–9. [Department of Health, Education, and Welfare Publication No. (OHD/AoA) 79–20949]

Devins, G.M. (1979). Death anxiety and voluntary passive euthanasia: Influences of proximity to death and experiences with death in important other persons. *Journal of Consulting and Clinical Psychology, 47*(2), 301–309.

Devins, G.M. (1981). Contributions of health and demographic status to death anxiety and attitudes toward voluntary passive euthanasia. *OMEGA: Journal of Death and Dying, 11*(4), 293–302.

Engel, G.L. (1971). Sudden and rapid death during psychological stress: Folklore or folkwisdom? *Annals of Internal Medicine, 74,* 771–782.

Esberger, K. (1980). Dying and the aged. *Journal of Gerontology, 6*(1), 11–15.

Farquhar, C.M. (1980). Attitudes and beliefs concerning life and death of elderly persons. *New Zealand Medical Journal, 92*(665), 107–110.

Ficarra, B.J. (1978). The aged, the dying, the dead: Medical-legal considerations. *Psychosomatics, 19*(1), 41–45.

Fulmer, T.T. (1981). Termination of life support systems in the elderly—Discussion: The registered nurse's role. *Journal of Geriatric Psychiatry, 14*(1), 23–30.

Fulton, R., Gottesman, D.J. & Owen, G.M. (1982). Loss, social change, and the prospect of mourning. *Death Education, 6*(2), 137–153.

Gallagher, D., Thompson, L. & Peterson, J. (1982). Psychological factors affecting adaptation to bereavement in the elderly. *International Journal of Aging and Human Development, 14*(2), 79–95.

Gates, M.S. & Mayer, G.G. (1978). Are you too sure of your stand on the right to die? *R.N. Magazine, 41*(12), 76–82.

Gerber, I., Rusalem, R., Hannon, N., Battin, D. & Arkin, A. (1975). Anticipatory grief and aged widows and widowers. *Journal of Gerontology, 30*(2), 225–229.

Glaser, B.G. & Strauss, A.L. (1965). *Awareness of dying.* Chicago, Ill.: Aldine.

Greene, R.R. (1982). Life review: A technique for clarifying family roles in adulthood. *Clinical Gerontologist, 1*(2), 59–67.

Group for the Advancement of Psychiatry. (1973). The right to die: Decision and decision makers. *GAP Report, 8*(12), 667–751.

Hart, E.J. (1979). The effects of death anxiety and mode of "case study presentation on shifts of attitude toward euthanasia." *OMEGA: Journal of Death and Dying, 9*(3), 239–244.

Herst, L.D. (1983). Emergency psychiatry for the elderly. *Psychiatric Clinics of North America, 6*(2), 271–280.

Heyman, D.K. & Gianturco, D.T. (1973). Long-term adaptation by the elderly to bereavement. *Journal of Gerontology, 28*(3), 359–362.

Horan, D.J. (1978). Euthanasia and brain death: Ethical and legal considerations. *Annals of the New York Academy of Sciences, 315,* 363–375.

Hunter, R.C. (1980). Euthanasia: A paper for discussion by psychiatrists. *Canadian Journal of Psychiatry, 25*(5), 439–445.

Jaretski, A. (1976). Death with dignity: Passive euthanasia. Guide to physicians dealing with dying patients. *New York State Journal of Medicine, 76*(4), 539–543.

Jensen, G.D. (1980). Expectation of death: Case reports with implications for medical and psychiatric care. *Psychotherapy and Psychosomatics, 33,* 198–204.

Johnson, D., Fitch, S.D., Alston, J.P. & McIntosh, W.A. (1980). Acceptance of conditional suicide and euthanasia among adult Americans. *Suicide and Life-Threatening Behavior, 10*(3), 157–166.

Kalish, R. (1972). Of social values and the dying: A defense of disengagement. *Family Coordinator, 21*(1), 81–94.

Kearl, M.C. & Harris, R. (1982). Individualism and the emerging "modern" ideology of death. *OMEGA: Journal of Death and Dying, 12*(3), 269–280.

Keith, P.M. (1979). Life changes and perceptions of life and death among older men and women. *Journal of Gerontology, 34*(6), 870–878.

Kleemeier, R.W. (1962). Intellectual changes in the senium. *Proceedings of the American Statistical Association, 1,* 290–295.

Klerman, G.L. & Izen, J.E. (1977). The effects of bereavement and grief on physical health and general well-being. *Advances in Psychosomatic Medicine, 9,* 63–68.

Kimsey, L.R., Roberts, J.L. & Logan, D.L. (1972). Death, dying and denial in the aged. *American Journal of Psychiatry, 129*(2), 161–166.

Krant, M.J., Doster, N.J. & Ploof, S. (1980). Isolation in the aged: Individual dynamics, community and family involvement. *Journal of Geriatric Psychiatry, 13*(1), 53–61.

Kubler-Ross, E. (1969). *On death and dying.* New York: Macmillan.

Kuhnert, S. (1981). Selbstmord in Heimen. [Suicide in homes for the aged.] *Zeitschrift für Gerontologie, 14*(6), 501–507.

Kurlychek, R.T. (1976). Level of belief in afterlife and four categories of fear of death in a sample of 60+-year olds. *Psychological Reports, 38*(1), 228.

Kurlychek, R.T. & Trepper, T.S. (1982). Accuracy of perception of attitude: An intergenerational investigation. *Perceptual and Motor Skills, 54*(1), 271–274.

Ladd, J. (ed.) (1979). *Ethical issues relating to life and death.* New York: Oxford University Press.

Lauter, H. & Meyer, J.E. (1982). Mercy killing without consent: Historical comments on a controversial issue. *Acta Psychiatrica Scandinavica, 65*(2), 134–141.

Leering, C., Hilhorst, H.W. & Verhoef, M.J. (1979). Some remarks on the wish to die at life's end. *Aktuelle Gerontologie, 9*(6), 289–296.

Levinson, A.R. (1981). Termination of life support systems in the elderly: Ethical issues. *Journal of Geriatric Psychiatry, 14*(1), 71–85.

Maizler, J.S., Solomon, J.R. & Almquist, E. (1983). Psychogenic mortality syndrome: Choosing to die by the institutionalized elderly. *Death Education, 6*(4), 353–364.

Mandella, F. (1981). Morte naturale e longevità come progetto utopico della medicina. [Natural death and longevity as an ideal goal of clinical medicine.] *Minerva Medica* (Torino), *72*(32), 2123–2127.

Marshall, V.W. (1975). Age and awareness of finitude in developmental gerontology. *OMEGA: Journal of Death and Dying, 6*(2), 113–129.

McIntosh, J.L. & Santos, J.F. (1981). Suicide among minority elderly: A preliminary investigation. *Suicide and Life-Threatening Behavior, 11*(3), 151–166.

McIntosh, J.L., Hubbard, R.W. & Santos, J.F. (1981). Suicide among the elderly: A review of issues with case studies. *Journal of Gerontological Social Work, 4*(1), 63–74.

McMahon, M. & Miller, P. (1980). Behavioral cues in the dying process and nursing implications. *Journal of Gerontological Nursing, 6*(1), 16–20.

McMordie, W.R. (1981). The phenomenon of withdrawal in relation to the aging process: A developmental perspective. *Social Behavior and Personality, 9*(1), 71–79.

Meier, D.E. & Cassel, C.K. (1983). Euthanasia in old age: A case study and ethical analysis. *Journal of the American Geriatrics Society, 31*(5), 294–298.

Moss, D. (1980). Transient paranoia and the "gift" in terminal illness. *British Journal of Medical Psychology, 53*(2), 155–159.

Nagi, M., Pugh, M.D. & Lazerine, N.G. (1977). Attitudes of Catholic and Protestant clergy toward euthanasia. *OMEGA: Journal of Death and Dying, 8*(2), 153–164.

Neugarten, B. & Havighurst, R.J. (1969). Disengagement reconsidered in a cross national context. In R.J. Havighurst, J.M.A. Munnichs, B. Neugarten & H. Thomas (eds.), *Adjustments to retirement: A cross national study.* Assen, The Netherlands: Von Gorcum.

Noyes, R., Jochimsen, P.R. & Travis, T.A. (1977). The changing attitudes of physicians toward prolonging life. *Journal of the American Geriatric Society, 25*(10), 470–474.

Ouslander, J.G. (1982). Physical illness and depression in the elderly. *Journal of the American Geriatrics Society, 30*(9), 593–599.

Palmore, E. (1969). The effects of aging on activities and attitudes. *Gerontologist, 8,* 259–263.

Palmore, E. (1975). *The honorable elders: A cross cultural analysis of aging in Japan.* Durham, N.C.: Duke University Press.

Palmore, E. & Cleveland, W. (1976). Aging, terminal decline, and terminal drop. *Journal of Gerontology, 31*(1), 76–81.

Rachels, J. (1975). Active and passive euthanasia. *New England Journal of Medicine, 292*(2), 78–80.

Ramsey, P. (1978). *Ethics at the edges of life: Medical and legal intersections.* New Haven, Conn.: Yale University Press.

Reeves, R.B., Neale, R.E. & Kutscher, A.H. (1973). *Pastoral care of the dying and bereaved: Selected readings.* New York: Health Sciences Publishing Corp.

Reynolds, D.K. & Nelson, F.L. (1981). Personality, life situation and life expectancy. *Suicide and Life-Threatening Behavior, 11*(2), 99–110.

Richards, J.G. & McCallum, J. (1979). Bereavement in the elderly. *New Zealand Medical Journal, 89*(632), 201–204.

Riegel, K.F. & Riegel, R.M. (1972). Development, drop and death. *Developmental Psychology, 6*(2), 306–319.

Romaniuk, M. & Romaniuk, J.G. (1981). Looking back: An analysis of reminiscence functions and triggers. *Experimental Aging Research, 7*(4), 477–489.

Rosenbaum, M. (1983). Crime and punishment: The suicide pact. *Archives of General Psychiatry, 40*(9), 979–982.

Roth, N. (1978). Fear of death in the aging. *American Journal of Psychotherapy, 32*(4), 552–560.

Rowland, K.F. (1977). Environmental events predicting death for the elderly. *Psychological Bulletin, 84*(2), 349–372.

Sanders, J.F., Poole, T.E. & Rivero, W.T. (1980). Death anxiety among the elderly. *Psychological Reports, 46,* 53–54.

Saul, S. & Saul, S. (1977). Old people talk about "The right to die." *OMEGA: Journal of Death and Dying, 8*(2), 129–139.

Schoenfield, C.G. (1978). Mercy killing and the law: A psychoanalytically oriented analysis. *Journal of Psychology and Law, 6*(2), 215–244.

Scoggins, W.F. (1971). "Growing old": Death by installment plan. *Suicide and Life-Threatening Behavior, 1*(2), 143–147.

Shanas, E., Townsend, P., Wedderburn, H., Friis, H., Milhoj, P. & Stenhouwer, J. (1968). *Old people in three industrial societies.* New York: Atherton Press.

Shedletsky, R., Fisher, R. & Nadon, G. (1982). Assessment of palliative care for dying hospitalized elderly. *Canadian Journal on Aging, 1*(1–2), 11–15.

Sichor, D. & Bergman, S. (1979). Patterns of suicide among the elderly in Israel. *Gerontologist, 19*(5, Pt. 1), 487–495.

Siegler, I.C. (1975). The terminal drop hypothesis: Fact or artifact? *Experimental Aging Research, 1*(1), 169–185.

Sill, J.S. (1980). Disengagement reconsidered: Awareness of finitude. *Gerontologist, 20*(4), 457–462.

Slezak, M.E. (1981). Attitudes toward euthanasia as a function of death fears and demographic variables. *Dissertation Abstracts International, 41*(10–B), 3903.

Steuer, J., LaRue, A., Blum, J.E. *et al.* (1981). "Critical loss" in the eighth and ninth decades. *Journal of Gerontology, 36*(2), 211–213.

Storlie, F. J. (1980). Caring for a patient who wants to die: Should you let her? *Nursing, 10*(2), 50–53.

Strahan, C., Jr. (1980). The retired patient: Boredom, fears and suicide. *Delaware Medical Journal, 52*(9), 497–501.

Sullivan, C.A. (1982). Life review: A functional view of reminiscence. *Physical and Occupational Therapy in Geriatrics, 2*(1), 39–52.

Tait, D. (1983). Mortality and dementia among aging defectives. *Journal of Mental Deficiency Research, 27*(2), 133–142.

Tatro, S.E. & Marshall, J.M. (1982). Regression: A defense mechanism for the dying older adult. *Journal of Gerontological Nursing, 8*(1), 20–22.

Tideiksaar, R. (1979). Suicide in the elderly [letter]. *American Family Physician, 19*(3), 28–29.

Victor, H.R. (1981). Choice of the living will: Personality characteristics, death/dying attitudes, and locus of control orientation of signers and nonsigners; and the effects of the choice on death/dying attitudes. *Dissertation Abstracts International, 42*(2–B), 792.

Ward, R.A. (1980). Age and acceptance of euthanasia. *Journal of Gerontology, 35*(3), 421–431.

Weisman, A.D. (1972). *On dying and denying: A psychiatric study of terminality.* New York: Behavioral Publications.

Weisman, A.D. (1977). Does old age make sense? Decisions and destiny in growing older. *Humanitas, 13*(1), 111–120.

Weisman, A.D. (1980). Isolation in the aged: Individual dynamics, community and family involvement. Discussion: What do elderly, dying patients want, anyway? *Journal of Geriatric Psychiatry, 13*(1), 63–67.

Weisman, A.D. & Hackett, T.P. (1961). Predilection to death and dying as a psychiatric problem. *Psychosomatic Medicine, 23,* 232–257.

Westcott, N.A. (1983). Application of the structured life-review technique in counseling elders. *Personnel and Guidance Journal, 62*(3), 180–181.

Wilbanks, W. (1982). Trends in violent death among the elderly. *International Journal of Aging and Human Development, 14*(3), 167–175.

Woods, N. & Witte, K.L. (1981). Life satisfaction, fear of death and ego identity in elderly adults. *Bulletin of the Psychonomic Society, 18*(4), 165–168.

EPILOGUE: THE HEALTH CARE PROFESSIONAL, DEATH, AND DYING

Adams, R., Berant, N. & Sharon, R. (1978). Informing the individual of impending death—Yes or no? *New Zealand Nursing Journal, 71*(10), 12–15.

Baider, L. & Porath, S. (1981). Uncovering fear: Group experience of nurses in a cancer ward. *International Journal of Nursing Studies, 18*(1), 47–52.

Bailey, M.L. (1977). Attitudes toward death and dying in nursing students. *Dissertation Abstracts International, 38*(1–B), 139.

Bangert, S.E. (1976). An inservice education model, contextually designed, to promote attitude and behavior change of medical and health personnel. *Dissertation Abstracts International, 37*(3–A), 1396.

Bechervaise, M.D. (1979). Nursing Care Study: The riddle of communication—1. *Nursing Times, 75*(34), 1434–1436.

Bermensolo, P. & Groenwald, S. (1978). Are we death and dying our patients to death? *Oncology Nursing Forum, 5*(4), 8–10.

Bleeker, J.A. & Pomerantz, H.B. (1979). The influence of a lecture course in loss and grief on medical students: An empirical study of attitude formation. *Medical Education, 13*(2), 117–128.

Blumenfield, M., Levy, N.B. & Kaufman, D. (1978). The wish to be informed of a fatal illness. *OMEGA: Journal of Death and Dying, 9*(4), 323–326.

Bohart, J.B. & Bergland, B.W. (1979). The impact of death and dying counseling groups on death anxiety in college students. *Death Education, 2*(4), 381–391.

Bugen, L. (1979). State anxiety effects on counselor perceptions of dying stages. *Journal of Counseling Psychology, 26*(1), 89–91.

Butler, R.N. (1978). Toward a humanistic approach to dying patients. *American Pharmacy, 18*(4), 538.

Cassileth, B.R. (1979). Modification of medical student perceptions of the cancer experience. *Journal of Medical Education, 54*, 797–802.

Cassileth, B.R., et al. (1980). Academia and clinic: Information and participation preferences among cancer patients. *Annals of Internal Medicine, 92*(6), 832–836.

Clarke, P. J. (1981). Exploration of counter-transference toward the dying. *American Journal of Orthopsychiatry, 51*(1), 71–77.

Cooper, S., Bean, G., Alpert, R. & Baum, J.H. (1980). Medical students' attitudes toward cancer. *Journal of Medical Education, 55*(5), 434–439.

Crase, D. & Crase, D.R. (1979). Emerging dimensions of death education. *Health Education, 10*(1), 26–29.

Dickenson, G.E. & Pearson, A.A. (1980). Death education and physicians' attitudes toward dying patients. *OMEGA: Journal of Death and Dying, 11*(2), 167–174.

Doherty, G. (1976). Dying and the conspiracy of denial. *Essence, 1*(1), 34–37.

Dupont, M. (1980). Report of a patient care team with a cancer patient in the dying stage: Sensitivity of the team, information of and participation by the family. *SOINS, 25*(9), 51–53.

Earnshaw, S.E. (1979). Dealing with dying patients and their relatives. *British Medical Journal, 282*(6278), 1779.

Epley, R.J. & McCaghy, C.H. (1977). The stigma of dying: Attitudes toward the terminally ill. *OMEGA: Journal of Death and Dying, 8*(4), 379–393.

Feifel, H. (1977). Death and dying in modern America. *Death Education, 1*(1), 5–14.

Freud, S. (1957). Our attitude towards death. In *Standard edition of the complete psychological works of Sigmund Freud, 14*, 299–300. London: Hogarth Press.

Friedman, B.D. (1980). Coping with cancer: A guide for health care professionals. *Cancer Nursing, 3*(2), 105–110.

Gosselin, J.Y., Perez, E.L. & Gagnon, A. (1977). Attitude of psychiatrists toward terminally ill patients. *Psychiatric Journal of the University of Ottawa, 2*(3), 120–123.

Gosselin, J.Y., Perez, E.L. & Gagnon, A. (1981). The physician and the terminally ill patient. *Psychiatric Journal of the University of Ottawa, 6*(4), 252–256.

Hackett, T.P. (1976). Psychological assistance to the dying patient and his family. *Annual Review of Medicine, 5*, 371–378.

Hardt, D.V. (1976). A measure of the improvement of attitudes toward death. *Journal of School Health, 46*(5), 269–270.

Hardy, R.E., Green, D.R., Jordan, H.W. & Hardy, G. (1980). Communication between cancer patients and physicians. *Southern Medical Journal, 73*(6), 755–757.

Hardy, R.E. & Hardy, G. (1979). Patterns of communication to cancer patients: A descriptive analysis. *Journal of the Tennessee Medical Association, 72*(9), 656–658.

Harlow, J.L. (1976). The relationship between nurse behavior and attitudes toward terminal patients and nurse exposure to three desensitization experimental conditions. *Dissertation Abstracts International, 37*(6–A), 3518–3519.

Hartwich, P. (1979). The question of disclosing the diagnosis to terminally ill patients. *Archiv für Psychiatrie und Nervenkrankheiten, 227*(1), 23–32.

Hinton, J. (1980). Whom do dying patients tell? *British Medical Journal, 281*(6251), 1328–1330.

Hoggatt, L. & Spilka, B. (1979). The nurse and the terminally ill patient: Some perspectives and projected actions. *OMEGA: Journal of Death and Dying, 9*(3), 255–266.

Holden, C. (1979). Pain, dying and the health care system. *Science, 203*(4384), 984–985.

Howells, K. & Field, D. (1982). Fear of death and dying among medical students. *Social Science Medicine, 16*(15), 1421–1424.

Isaccs, B. (1979). Don't tell her—She'll worry. *Nursing Mirror, 149*(14), 27–29.

Jenkins, D.M. (1980). Case study (Terminal care). *New Zealand Nursing Journal, 73*(2), 16–17, 38.

Jensen, G.D. (1980). Expectation of death: Case reports with implications for medical and psychiatric care. *Psychotherapy and Psychosomatics, 33*(4), 198–204.

Jones, R.J. (1982). Doctors and dying [editorial]. *Journal of the American Medical Association, 247*(18), 2569–2570.

Kaye, J., Appel, M. & Joseph, R. (1981). Attitudes of medical students and residents toward cancer. *Journal of Psychology, 107*(First Half), 87–96.

Keeling, B. (1978). Giving and getting the courage to face death. *Nursing* (Horsham), *8*(11), 38–41.

Keeling, W. (1976). Live the pain, learn the hope: A beginner's guide to cancer counseling. *Personnel and Guidance Journal, 54*(10), 502–506.

Kincade, J. E. (1983). Attitudes of physicians, housestaff and nurses on care for the terminally ill. *OMEGA: Journal of Death and Dying, 13*(4), 333–344.

Kopel, K., O'Connell, W., Paris, J. & Girardin, P. (1975). A human relations laboratory approach to death and dying. *OMEGA: Journal of Death and Dying, 6*(3), 219–221.

Krumm, S., Vannatta, P. & Sanders, J. (1979). Group approaches for cancer patients: A group for teaching chemotherapy. *American Journal of Nursing, 79*(5), 916.

Kubler-Ross, E. (1969). *On death and dying.* New York: Macmillan.

Kubler-Ross, E. & Worden, J.W. (1977). Attitudes and experiences of death workshop and attendees. *OMEGA: Journal of Death and Dying, 8*(2), 91–106.

Levin, S., Berman, C., Bernstein, G. & Bonner, B. (1981). The dying patient: Attitudes and responses. *South African Medical Journal, 59*(1), 21–24.

Love, R.R., Hayward, J. & Stone, H.L. (1980). Attitudes about cancer medicine among primary care residents and their teachers. *Journal of Medical Education, 55*(3), 211–212.

Manganello, J.A. (1977). An investigation of counselor empathy with terminally ill patients on attitudes toward afterlife, fear of death, and denial. *Dissertation Abstracts International, 38*(4–B), 1891–1892.

Marie, H. (1978). Reorienting staff attitudes toward the dying. *Hospital Progress,*
59(8), 74–76.

McCorkle, R. (1982). Death education for advanced nursing practice. *Death Educa-*
tion, 5(4), 347–361.

McKitrick, D. (1981). Counseling dying clients. *OMEGA: Journal of Death and Dying,*
12(2), 165–187.

May, R. (1969). *Love and will.* New York: Dell.

Miles, M.S. (1977). The effects of a small group education/ counseling experience on
the attitudes of nurses toward death and toward dying patients. *Dissertation Ab-*
stracts International, 38(2–A), 636.

Mood, D.W. & Lick, C.F. (1979). Attitudes of nursing personnel toward death and
dying: II. Linguistic indicators of denial. *Research in Nursing and Health, 2*(3), 95–
99.

Moss, D.M., McGaghie, W.C. & Rubinstein, L.I. (1978). Medical resistance, crisis
ministry, and terminal illness. *Journal of Religion and Health, 17*(2), 99–116.

Mullins, L.C. (1981). A humanistic view of the nurse and the dying patient. *Journal of*
Gerontological Nursing, 7(3), 148–152.

Noll, G.A. & Sampsell, M. (1978). The community and the dying. *Journal of Com-*
munity Psychology, 6, 275–279.

Novack, D.H., Plumer, R., Smith, R.L. *et al.* (1979). Changes in physicians' attitudes
toward telling the cancer patient. *Journal of the American Medical Association,*
241(9), 897–900.

Novak, M.W. & Axelrod, C.D. (1979). Ancient and modern orientations to death:
The resurrection of myth in the treatment of the dying. *Journal of Phenomenologi-*
cal Psychology, 10(2), 151–164.

Posner, J. (1976). Death as a courtesy stigma. *Essence, 1*(2), 26–33.

Price, T. & Bergen, B.J. (1977). The relationship to death as a source of stress for
nurses on a coronary care unit. *OMEGA: Journal of Death and Dying, 8*(3), 229–
238.

Rando, T.A. (1984). *Grief, dying and death: Clinical interventions for caregivers.*
Champaign, Ill.: Research Press.

Ransohoff, J. (1978). Death, dying, and the neurosurgical patient. *Journal of Neuro-*
surgical Nursing, 10(4), 198–201.

Rea, M.P., Greenspoon, S. & Spilka, B. (1975). Physicians and the terminal patient:
Some selected attitudes and behavior. *OMEGA: Journal of Death and Dying, 6*(4),
291–302.

Redding, K. (1980). Coping strategies for the professional in working with oncology
patients. *Arizona Medicine, 37*(8), 565–568.

Ross, C.W. (1976). Death concerns and response to dying patient statements. *Disser-*
tation Abstracts International, 37(4–B), 1624–1625.

Salter, R. (1982). The art of dying. *Canadian Nurse, 78*(3), 20–21.

Schain, W.S. (1980). Patients' rights in decision making: The case for personalism
versus paternalism in health care. *Cancer, 46,* 1035–1041.

Schmale, A.H. (1980). The dying patient. *Advances in Psychosomatic Medicine, 10,*
99–110.

Schreibaum, D. (1975). Approaches and developments in the study of attitudes to
death: Descriptions of meetings with physicians and impressions of their attitude
on this subject. *Israel Annals of Psychiatry and Related Disciplines, 13*(3), 259–
269.

Schultz, R. & Aderman, D. (1976). How the medical staff copes with dying patients: A critical review. *OMEGA: Journal of Death and Dying, 7*(1), 11–21.

Shady, G.A. (1976). Death anxiety and care of the terminally ill: A review of the clinical literature. *Canadian Psychological Review, 17*(2), 137–142.

Souhami, R.L. (1978). Teaching what to say about cancer. *Lancet, 2*(8096), 935–936.

Spiegel, D. & Yalom, I.D. (1978). A support group for dying patients. *International Journal of Group Psychotherapy, 28*(2), 233–245.

Stanley, A.T. (1979). Is it ethical to give hope to a dying person? *Nursing Clinics of North America, 14*(1), 69–80.

Stedeford, A. (1979). Psychotherapy of the dying patient. *British Journal of Psychiatry, 135,* 7–14.

Stoller, E.P. (1980). The impact of death-related fears on attitudes of nurses in a hospital work setting. *OMEGA: Journal of Death and Dying, 11*(1), 85–96.

Taylor, P.B. & Gideon, M.D. (1982). Holding out hope to your dying patient: Paradoxical but possible. *Nursing (Horsham), 12*(2), 42–45.

Terrill, L.A. (1978). The clinical specialist in oncology and the dying patient. *Journal of Neurosurgical Nursing, 10*(4), 176–179.

Tousley, M.M. (1982). The use of family therapy in terminal illness and death. *Journal of Psychosocial Nursing and Mental Health Services, 20*(1), 17–22.

Trillin, A.S. (1981). Of dragons and garden peas: A cancer patient talks to doctors. *New England Journal of Medicine, 300*(12), 699–700.

Vachon, M.L., Lyall, W.A. & Freeman, S.J. (1978). Measurement and management of stress in health professionals working with advanced cancer patients. *Death Education, 1*(4), 365–375.

Valentine, A.S. (1979). A study of nursing intervention on the responses of patients receiving chemotherapy. *Oncology Nursing Forum, 6*(3), 6–7.

Wegmann, J.A. (1979). Avoidance behaviors of nurses as related to cancer diagnosis and/or terminality. *Oncology Nursing Forum, 6*(3), 8–14.

Wellisch, D.K., *et al.* (1978). Management of family emotional stress: Family group therapy in a private oncology practice. *International Journal of Group Psychotherapy, 28*(2), 225–231.

Zuehlke, T.E. & Watkins, J.T. (1975). The use of psychotherapy with dying patients: An exploratory study. *Journal of Clinical Psychology, 31*(4), 729–732.

Name Index

Abraham, K., 106, 169, 193
Achterberg, L. J., 242
Adams, M. A., 83, 86
Aiken, L. H., 245
Allen, A., 204, 209
Allport, G. W., 200, 225
Allyn, P., 144
Almquist, E., 273
Alpert, R., 211
Appels, A., 131
Arcand, R., 245
Arens, D. A., 187, 188
Arkin, A., 179
Azen, S. P., 130, 144

Bahnson, C. B., 202
Bailey, L. R., 244
Baines, M., 233, 234, 236, 238
Ball, J. F., 190
Barber, J., 233
Barchha, R. C., 184
Bartlett, R., 144
Bass, D. M., 234
Bateson, G., 209
Battin, D., 179
Bayer, R., 245, 252
Bean, G., 211
Beatty, L. F., 216, 217, 221
Bebbington, P., 51
Beck, A. T., 107, 108
Becker, D., 63, 64, 67
Beckwith, J. B., 27, 28, 46
Benjamin, B., 170, 185, 186
Bergman, A. B., 29, 30
Berman, A. L., 102, 108, 111, 117
Bernstein, N. R., 141, 145, 147, 148, 149,
         151, 152
Binik, Y. M., 135
Birtchnell, J., 51, 52, 60
Black, D., 40
Blades, B. C., 148
Bluebond-Langner, M., 55–56, 73
Bluglass, K., 36, 43
Blumenfield, M., 205–206
Bonica, J. J., 233

Borkani, N. O., 30
Bourne, S., 6, 9
Bowlby, J., 170, 171, 193
Brann, J., 243
Brehm, J. W., 213, 215
Breme, F. L., 36
Bromberg, S., 272
Brooks, J. G., 33
Brown, R. J., 142, 182
Brown, R. S., 233
Bruneau, J. P., 84
Brunnquell, D., 87, 91
Buckingham, R. W., 232, 245
Bunney, W. E., 104, 106
Burnet, M., 199
Burke, P., 35
Burns, W. J., 91
Butler, R. N., 258, 271, 280
Butterfield-Picard, H., 232, 245

Cahners, S. S., 149, 150
Cain, A., 17, 67
Cain, B., 17
Cameron, J., 254
Camfield, P., 33
Campbell, A. G., 21
Canter, R. C., 224
Caplan, G., 140–141
Carlson, G. A., 108
Cassel, C. K., 272, 278
Cassem, N. H., 130, 138
Catryn, L., 106
Cepeda, M. L., 40
Champlin, L., 263
Chang, Y. T., 130
Chappell, N. L., 267
Chase, T. M., 13
Cheater, F. M., 235, 236
Chernus, L. A., 19, 36
Ch'ien, L. T., 81, 82
Churchill, M. P., 93
Clarke, A. M., 150, 151
Clayton, P. J., 177, 179, 183, 184, 186
Cleveland, W., 264, 265
Cline, D. W., 105

Clyman, R. I., 13, 14
Cohen, K. P., 232
Cohen, L., 11
Cohen, M. M., 246
Cohen-Sandler, R., 102, 108, 111, 117
Cooper, S., 211
Cope, O., 150
Cornell, R. G., 144
Corr, C. A., 242, 245
Corr, D. M., 242, 245
Cotman, C. W., 105, 127
Cotter, J. M., 83
Cox, P. R., 185
Crawshaw, L., 36
Creek, L. V., 243, 245
Crout, T. K., 3–4, 9
Cullberg, J., 19

Dash, J., 89
David, C. J., 18
Davidson, F., 111
Davidson, G., 178
Davidson, T. N., 145, 147
Davis, J. M., 104
Davis, T. M., 144, 145
Deak, E. J., 261
DeFrain, J. D., 36, 37, 40, 42, 44
DenHouter, K. V., 108
Derogatis, L. R., 139
DeSilva, R. A., 136, 161
Devins, G. M., 278
Dienelt, M. N., 184
Dimsdale, J. E., 138
Dinsdale, F., 28
Doster, N. J., 273
Doyle, D., 233, 238
Drotar, D., 18
Dublin, L. I., 103
Durkheim, E., 185
Duszynski, D. R., 200

Edlich, R. F., 130, 145
Eiser, C., 82, 91, 93
Ekert, H., 83
Emery, J. L., 28, 36
Engel, G. L., 133, 134, 260, 263
Epperson, M. M., 155, 158
Erikson, E., 84, 269
Ernst, L., 36, 37, 40, 42, 44
Estok, P. J., 14

Farberow, N. L., 219
Fast, I., 67
Fawcett, J. A., 104

Fay, M., 218
Feller, I., 144
Fife, B. L., 83
Fiore, N., 210, 211–212
Fitzgerals, R. G., 170, 185
Flaherty, M., 84
Fleischman, T. B., 35
Floersch, J. E., 209
Flora, J. D., 144, 145
Fochtman, D., 88
Ford, J. R., 185
Forman, B. F., 218, 220, 221
Forrest, G. C., 14
Frederick, C. J., 102
Freeman, J. E., 81
Freud, S., 38, 58, 59, 61, 106, 126, 166–
    169, 175, 176, 177, 193, 197, 198,
    243, 283
Friedman, E. H., 139, 140
Friedman, M., 131
Froggatt, P., 30
Frost, N. R., 184
Fulton, R., 176, 177–178, 193, 194
Furman, E. P., 10, 60, 65, 71

Gaisford, J. C., 151, 152
Galen, 197
Gallagher, D. E., 187, 188, 189
Gardner, R. A., 64
Garfinkel, B. D., 102
Garland, S., 148
Garner, J., 232, 233
Garrow, I., 26
Garts, K., 148
Garusi, G. F., 215
Gazut, M., 208
Gentry, W. D., 131
George, S. L., 83, 93
Gerber, I., 178, 180, 181
Gianturco, D. T., 188
Gibbs, H. W., 242
Gifford, S., 104
Gitelson, J., 233
Glaser, B. G., 256, 257, 279
Glaser, K., 107, 108, 119, 127
Glass, D. C., 131
Glassman, S. M., 233
Gogan, J. L., 90
Golombek, H., 102
Gorer, G., 189
Gotay, C. C., 232, 245
Gottesman, D. J., 176, 177–178, 193, 194,
    215
Grave, G. D., 92

Greene, R. R., 271
Greene, W. A., 201
Greenough, W. T., 35
Greenstreet, R. L., 200
Greer, S., 198, 199, 200–201, 203, 226
Griffiths, W. J., 135
Grossarth-Maticek, R., 201
Guilleminault, C., 33
Gulledge, A. D., 139, 140
Gullo, S. V., 180–181
Guntheroth, W. G., 27, 30
Gutstein, S., 215
Gyllenskold, K., 97

Hackett, T. P., 130, 138, 258, 284
Hale, W. E., 132
Haley, J., 209
Halikas, H. A., 177
Hall, M. D., 87, 91
Hanefeld, F., 81
Hannon, N., 179
Hardy, R. E., 207
Harper, R. M., 33
Harrington, V., 13, 16
Hartmann, J. R., 83
Havighurst, R. J., 265
Hawkins, D. G., 42
Hayward, J., 206
Hellerstein, H. K., 139, 140
Helmrath, T. A., 15
Hendrin, H., 119
Herzog, D. B., 108, 117
Heyman, D. K., 188
Hiebert, J. H., 130, 145
Hildebrand, W. L., 13, 16
Hodges, D. M., 83
Holdsworth, C., 92
Hollinger, P. C., 102, 103
Holmes, T., 166
Hoppenbrouwers, T., 34
Hudgens, R. W., 184
Hufbauer, K., 26
Hughes, C. W., 135
Humphrey, G. B., 95
Hurry, J., 51

Iker, H., 201
Iles, J. P., 93
Imbus, S. H., 130, 143, 144
Irvin, N., 18
Ishii, K., 111

Jackson, D. D., 209
Jacobs, S. C., 186, 191, 195

Jenkins, C. D., 133
Jensen, G. D., 258, 259
Johnson, F. L., 83
Johnson, M. P., 26
Johnson, P. A., 68
Johnson, V., 140
Johnston, L., 234
Johnston, P. G. B., 81
Jolly, H., 13, 14
Jones, C., 148

Kagen-Goodheart, L., 91
Kahn, A. M., 143
Kaizuka, T., 111
Kalish, R., 265
Kalnins, I. V., 93
Kane, B., 54, 73
Karon, M., 85
Kassakian, M. G., 244
Katcher, A. H., 135
Katz, E. R., 84, 92
Kaufman, D., 206
Kavanagh, C., 148
Kellerman, J., 84, 86
Kelly, M. J., 220
Kennedy, B. J., 207–208
Kennedy, J. D., 140
Kennell, J. H., 11, 21
Kiely, W. F., 138
King, K. M., 139
King, R. A., 102, 111
Kipnis, D., 211
Klaus, M. H., 11, 21
Kleemeier, R. W., 263
Klein, D. F., 105
Klein, M., 169, 193
Klerman, G. L., 184
Knapp, R. J., 7
Koff, T. H., 232, 243
Kohut, H., 61, 74
Koocher, G. P., 86, 93
Kovacs, M., 107, 108
Krant, M. J., 234, 273
Kraus, J. F., 30
Krein, N., 18, 36, 37
Krueger, A., 97
Kubler-Ross, E., 267, 271, 283, 284
Kushner, L., 20

Ladd, J., 279
Lake, M., 8
Lamb, M. A., 222, 224, 225
Lamerton, R. C., 243
Landsdown, R., 93

Lattanzi, M. E., 251
Lauter, H., 276
Lebovici, S., 67
Lee, J., 40, 141, 162
Lehman, A., 14
Leonard, C. V., 219
Lesse, S., 106
Levy, N. B., 206
Lewak, N., 30
Lewis, E., 9, 13, 16, 19
Lewis, M. I., 258
Lewis, M. S., 215
Lickiss, J. N., 198
Lillehaugen, A., 207–208
Lindemann, E., 96, 170, 171, 176, 177, 193, 194
Lindenthal, J. J., 184
Lipman, A. G., 233, 236
Lipsitt, L. P., 30, 34–35
Long. R. T., 150
Longhofer, J., 209
Lopata, H. Z., 190, 191
Love, R. R., 206
Lowman, J., 39
Lown, B., 136, 137, 161
Lucas, R. H., 84
Lutkins, S. G., 185
Lynch, J. J., 135, 136, 161

MacDonald, R. N., 245
MacElveen-Hoehn, P., 245
MacKenzie, D., 192
MacKinnon, K. J., 233, 237
MacMahon, B., 168, 185
Maddison, D., 182, 187, 189
Magno, J. B., 232, 245
Mahan, C. K., 16
Maizler, J. S., 273
Maloney, L. J., 96
Mann, J. K., 154
Mansfield, L., 140
Marcelli, D., 111
Margolin, F., 63, 64, 67
Maris, R. W., 122
Marshall, J. M., 270
Marshall, V. W., 257, 266
Marvin, J. A., 150
Marx, M. M., 245
Masters, W., 140
Maurice, W. L., 177
Maxwell, M. B., 218
May, H. J., 36
May, R., 283
McCrady, V. L., 143

McGaugh, J. L., 105, 127
McIntire, M. S., 28
McIntosh, E. G., 245
McKenry, P. C., 119
McKnew, D. H., 106
McMahon, M., 273
McMordie, W. R., 265
McNaughton, M. W., 140
McPhee, M. S., 245
Mehr, M., 102
Meier, D. E., 278
Meislin, H. W., 154
Melzack, R., 233, 237
Mendelsohn, I. E., 150
Meyer, J. E., 276
Meyer, R., 16, 19
Miller, D., 110, 114
Miller, J. A., 89, 90
Miller, N. J., 148, 149, 150
Miller, P., 273
Mitchell, N. L., 56, 57, 74
Moonilal, J. M., 154
Morrison, J. R., 184
Moss, H. A., 81, 82
Mount, B. M., 233, 237
Mouren, M. C., 111
Mudd, P., 245, 246
Munster, A. M., 148
Murawski, B. J., 136
Murray, J. B., 200
Murray, K. H., 148
Myers, J. K., 184

Naeye, R. L., 29, 30, 31–32, 33
Nagy, M. H., 53–54, 73
Nannis, E. D., 81, 82
Nelson, F. L., 259
Nemec, E. D., 140
Neugarten, B., 265
Nielson, P. E., 6
Nikolaisen, S. M., 36, 40, 41
Nitschke, R., 95
Noonberg, A. R., 136
Nouvet, G., 28
Novack, D. H., 206
Noyes, R., Jr., 233

Oakes, A. R., 154
O'Donohue, N., 22
Offer, D., 102, 103
Oken, D., 206
Olton, D. S., 136
O'Malley, J. E., 83, 86
Orfirer, A. P., 18

Ostfeld, A., 186, 191, 195
Ostroff, R., 104
Oury, N., 83
Ouslander, J. G., 272

Paffenbarger, R. S., 132
Paget, J., 198
Palmore, E., 264, 265
Palombo, J., 59, 61, 62, 66, 69, 74
Parkes, C. M., 142, 167, 170–171, 172,
    181–182, 184, 185, 187, 192, 193,
    250, 254
Parrish, S., 12, 13
Pasquis, P., 28
Patel, A. R., 104
Paykel, E. S., 166, 184
Pehrsson, G., 97
Pendergrass, E. P., 212
Pepper, M. P., 184
Peppers, L. G., 7
Peterson, D. R., 30
Peterson, J. A., 187, 188, 189
Peterson, L. G., 216
Pettipas, M., 192
Petzel, S. V., 105
Pfeffer, C. R., 104, 106, 108, 111, 119, 124,
    126
Pfefferbaum, B., 84
Phipps, S., 18
Piaget, J., 52–53, 54, 73
Pierson, P. S., 30
Pincus, L., 169
Plank, E. N., 71
Plank, R., 71
Pless, I. B., 92
Ploof, S., 273
Polak, P. R., 40, 141, 142, 162
Pomeroy, M. A., 29
Poole, T. E., 268
Popkin, B. H., 233
Popkin, M. K., 216
Poznanski, E. O., 16
Preskorn, S. H., 135
Procci, W. R., 138
Prusoff, B. A., 166
Pugh, T. F., 168, 185
Puig-Antich, J., 120

Quirk, T. R., 4

Rabin, A. T., 16
Rachels, J., 276
Rahe, R., 166
Ramsey, P., 279

Rathbun, J. M., 108, 117
Ray, C. G., 29
Read, D. J., 31, 32
Rees, W. D., 185
Reich, P., 136, 220
Reynolds, D. K., 259
Rheingold, J., 56
Richards, W. S., 83
Richman, J., 111, 119
Richter, C. P., 134, 161
Riegel, K. F., 263
Riegel, R. M., 263
Riehm, H., 81
Rigler, D., 85
Rinker, M., 244
Rivero, W. T., 268
Rizzo, R. F., 245
Robertson, J., 170
Robins, E., 177
Roi, L. D., 139, 144, 145
Romaniuk, J. G., 271–272
Romaniuk, M., 271–272
Rosellini, R. A., 135
Rosenman, R. H., 131
Rosenthal, M. J., 106
Rosenthal, P. A., 72
Ross, J. W., 83
Rossman, P., 243
Roth, N., 268
Rowland, K. F., 260–261
Roy, M., 104
Royal, M. E., 71, 72
Rudolph, L. A., 83
Rusalem, R., 179
Ryndes, T., 233

Sacerdote, P., 90
Sachs, M. B., 92
Sachtleben, C. R., 212
Sahu, S., 16
Salladay, S. A., 71, 72
Sallan, S. E., 78, 80, 82, 93
Sanders, J. F., 268
Saraf, K. R., 105
Saul, L., 133
Saul, S., 278
Saunders, C. M., 230, 233, 234, 235, 236,
    238, 243, 246, 247, 254
Schain, W. S., 223
Schildkraut, J. J., 203
Schiller, P., 6
Schmale, A., 133, 201, 202
Shneidman, E. S., 219
Schreibaum, D., 288, 289

Schreiner, R. L., 13, 16
Schulman, K. R., 56, 57, 74
Schwartz, A. D., 83
Seiden, R. H., 102
Seitz, P. M., 18
Seligman, M. E. P., 134, 260
Sexauer, C. L., 95
Shaddy, R. E., 28
Shanas, E., 265
Shokeir, M., 12
Shustack, B., 135
Siegel, S. E., 84
Siegler, I. C., 264, 265
Sill, J. S., 266, 267
Silverman, P. R., 192
Sjolin, S., 97
Slade, C. I., 21
Slater, H., 151, 152
Slyter, H., 11
Smialek, Z., 36
Smith, W. J., 261
Snow, H., 198
Solomon, J. R., 150, 273
Soni, S. S., 81
Soulayrol, R., 111
Spence, D., 202
Spinetta, J. J., 85, 86, 94, 96
Steinitz, E. M., 15
Steinschneider, A., 31
Stern, M., 145
Steuer, J., 261
Stevenson, K. M., 38, 40
Stewart, C. A., 244
Stockard, J. L., 33
Stoddard, A., 231, 245
Stone, H. L., 206
Storlie, F. J., 260
Strahan, C., Jr., 261
Strauss, A. L., 256, 257, 279
Stroebe, M. S., 185, 187, 188
Stroebe, W., 187, 188
Struve, F. A., 105
Sturner, W. Q., 35
Sullivan, C. A., 271
Suter, B., 106
Swisher, S. N., 201

Tardif, C., 28
Tatro, S. E., 270
Taylor, J., 36, 37, 40, 42, 44
Tennant, C., 51
Terry, G. E., 93
Theriault, G., 135
Thomas, C. B., 200

Thomas, S. A., 136
Thompson, L. W., 187, 188, 189
Tiller, J. W., 83
Tishler, C. L., 119
Tobiason, J., 130, 145
Toolan, J. M., 106, 107, 117, 118, 119
Trillin, A. S., 210
Twycross, R. G., 233, 235, 236, 237, 242,
    245, 253

Uhlenhuth, E. H., 166

Valanis, B. G., 188
Valdes-Dapena, M. A., 27, 33
Vetafridda, V., 233
Viola, A., 182, 187, 189
Voke, J. M., 81

Waisbren, B. A., 145
Walker, B. A., 102
Walker, W. L., 189
Wallis, C., 185, 186
Walsh, T. D., 235, 236
Ward, B. J., 245
Ward, R. A., 277–278
Warrick, L. H., 18
Weakland, J., 209
Weinberg, N., 148, 149, 150
Weinstein, H. J., 78, 80, 82
Weisman, A. D., 258, 260, 269
Weisman, M. M., 103
Wellisch, D. K., 246
Werne, J., 26
Westcott, N. A., 272
Whitmore, K., 92
Wicklund, D., 213
Williams, M. L., 40
Williams, R. A., 36
Williams, R. B., 131
Williams, R. D., 134
Williams, W. V., 40, 141, 142, 162
Wilson, E., 192
Wilson, G. M., 104
Winnicott, D. W., 9
Witte, K. L., 267, 269
Wolfe, R. A., 145
Wolfenstein, M., 59, 74
Wolff, J. R., 6
Wolfgang, M. E., 103
Wolkmar, F. R., 35
Woods, N., 222, 224, 225, 267, 269
Wortman, C. B., 213, 215
Wright, L., 83
Wunder, S., 95

Yates, J. W., 244
Yeaworth, R., 188
Young, L. E., 201
Young, M., 185, 186

Zawacki, B. E., 130, 143, 144
Zilboorg, G., 56
Zschoche, D. A., 130
Zweig, A. R., 91

Subject Index

Abandonment, 62
Abbreviated Burn Severity Index, 145
Accidents, 130, 153–160
Adoption, loss of child by, 22
Age, conjugal bereavement and, 187–191
    death and, 256
Aiding Mothers Experiencing Neonatal Death
    (AMEND), 19
Alopecia, 91
American Cancer Society, 77
American Medical Association, policy on
    euthanasia, 276–277
Analgesics, terminally ill and, 234–238
Anger, bereavement and, 173
    generated by injury to loved one, 157–
    159
Anorexia, terminally ill and, 240
Anorexia nervosa, 115
Antileukemic chemotherapy, 80
Anxiety, family members and, 155
    separation, 62
Anxiolytic drugs, 155
Apnea, relationship between Sudden Infant
    Death Syndrome and, 31–33
Autopsy, psychological, 197
Awareness, of dying, 257–258
    of finitude, 266, 267

Baux rule, 144
Behavior, suicidal, 112–116
Bereavement, childhood, 50–75
    conjugal, 165–195
    guilt and, 173
    hospice services and, 248–251
    See also Grief
Beta-adrenergic blockers, 136, 137
Biofeedback, 136, 199
Biopsy, cone, 202
Body image, terminally ill and, 241
Bone marrow, 78
    aspiration, 80
Bradycardiac rhythms, 134
Bulimia, 115
Burn death, 152–153

Burn mortality, 130
    prediction of, 144–145
Burns, 130, 143–153
    See also Thermal injuries

Cancer, childhood and adolescent, 76–100
    communication and, 203–210
    coping behavior and, 212–225
    defense mechanisms and, 212–225
    depression and, 216–218
    diagnosis, 198
        crisis of, 213–216
    double bind concept and, 209–210
    etiology, psychological factors in, 198–
    203
    iatrogenic stresses and, 210–212
    personality and, 200
    psychological aspects of, 196–228
    psychophysiological mechanisms, 202–
    203
    psychosocial predictors of, 201–202
    self-esteem and, 222–224
    sexuality and, 221–225
    suicide and, 218–221
    treatment, 198
        crisis of, 216–221
    See also Leukemia
Care, curative, 232
    home, of terminally ill, 243–246
    hospice terminal, see Hospice terminal
        care
    palliative, 232–233
    of terminally ill, 229–254
Cardiac care, 138
Cardiac death, see Coronary heart disease
Catastrophic life-threatening events, 129–164
Catecholamines, cancer and, 203
Central nervous system, irradiation of, in
    treatment of leukemia, 82
Chemotherapy, leukemia treatment, 80–81
    neurological complications of, 81
Child abuse, 27
Childhood bereavement, see Bereavement,
    childhood

Children, adjustment to parental death, 61–66
bereavement and, *see* Bereavement, childhood
conceptual awareness of death, 53–56
efforts to protect, from reality of death, 62–64
experience of death and, 51–52
fear of death, 56–58
guilt reactions to parental death, 64–66
thermal injuries and, 149–151
traumatic aspects of parental death, 66–71
understanding of death, 52–56
Chlordiazepoxide, 155
Communication, cancer patients and, 203–210
Concrete operations (development phase), 53
Cone biopsy, 202
Congenital malformations, newborns with, 21–22
Conjugal bereavement, 165–195
age as factor, 187–191
clinical management of, 187–192
epidemiological conclusions, 186–187
health care management and, 191–192
mortality patterns among the bereaved, 185–187
physical and psychological morbidity during, 181–183
psychiatric morbidity during, 183–185
sequelae of, 181–187
suicide and, 185
Coping, psychological dynamics of, 156–160
Coronary heart disease, 130, 131–142
coital coronary, 139–140
complex interplay of factors in, 132–134
intervention with family survivors, 140–142
physical activity and, 132
psychological problems of hospitalization and convalescence, 138–139
symptoms, 131
Corticosteroids, cancer and, 203
Craniospinal irradiation, 82
Crisis service, 140–142
Critical care center, 153–155

Death, age and, 256
anticipatory grief and, 96–98
attitude toward, 283
burn, 152–153
cardiac, *see* Coronary heart disease
children and experience of, 51–52
children's awareness of, 53–56
children's fear of, 56–58
children's understanding of, 52–56
elderly and, 255–281
environmental events predicting, 260–263
expectation of, 258–260
fear of, 243, 256, 257, 268
health care professionals and, 282–292
parents, *see* Parental death
predilection to, 258
preparation for, defense mechanisms and, 268
"social," 147–148
sudden, *see* Coronary heart disease; Sudden death
suicidal, *see* Suicide
viewing of body after, 248–249
Defense mechanisms, preparation for death and, 268
Denial, family members and, 156–157
thermal injury deformities and, 148
Depression, cancer and, 216–218
death and, 272–273
reactive, 168, 174, 213
suicide and, 106–108, 114, 121
Detachment, 10
Developmental phases, Piagetian, 52–53
Diazepam, 155
Dignity, dying person's, 244
Diplegia, 81
Diplopia, 81
Disengagement theory, 256, 265–267
Disfigurement, thermal injuries, and, 147–148
Doctor-patient relationship, fetal death and, 5–9
perinatal death and, 5–9
stillbirths and, 5–9
Double blind concept, cancer patients and, 209–210
Dying, awareness of, 257–258
Dying person, psychosocial needs of, 243–245
Dying process, 257–258
ethical considerations, 274–279
role of regression in, 269–271
Dying trajectory, 256, 257

Eating disorders, suicide and, 115–116
Education, *see* Prenatal education
Elderly, the, death and, 255–281
euthanasia and, 277–279
preoccupations with death, 268–269

psychology of the dying older person, 267–274
thermal injuries and, 151–152
Emotional disorders, suicide and, 105–110
Erythrocytes, 79
Euthanasia, 275–279
active, 276, 277, 278
American Medical Association's policy on, 276–277
direct, 276, 277
elderly and, 277–279
indirect, 276, 277
involuntary, 275–276
passive, 276, 277, 278
religion and, 278
voluntary, 275–277
Expectation of death, 258–260

Family, with life-threatening injury to member of, 155–160
Fear of death, 243, 256, 257, 268
Fetal death(s), decline in number of, 2
doctor-patient relationship and, 5–9
Finitude, awareness of, 266, 267
Formal operations (development phase), 53

Grief, anticipatory, 96–98, 175–181
Freudian thought on, 175
neoanalytic formulations of, 176–177
preventive value of, assessment of, 178–181
sociopsychological and sociocultural aspects of, 177–178
childhood, 58–61
defined, 58, 166
family members of multiple-trauma victims and, 159–160
normal, 168–169, 170–175
parental, 9–14, 15–16
pathognomonic of, 171
pathological, 167–170
psychodynamics of, 166–170
See also Bereavement
Guilt, bereavement and, 173

Health care professionals, death and, 282–292
perinatal deaths and, 5, 6
stillbirths and, 5, 6
"Heart attack," see Myocardial infarction
Heart block, 135
Heart disease, coronary, see Coronary heart disease
Helplessness, learned, 213

Home care of terminally ill, 243–246
Homicides, among adolescents, 103, 104
Hopelessness, sudden death and, 134–135
Hospice terminal care, 229–254
bereavement services, 248–251
closure to, 251
contacts with surviving family members, 250–251
polypharmacology of, 233–238
Hostility, generated by injury to loved ones, 157–159
Hyperplasia, 32
Hypnotherapy, 89–90
Hypotonia, 81
Hypoxemia, 27, 28

Iatrogenic stresses, cancer patients and, 210–212
Identification, 10
Impulsive character disorders, suicide and, 109–110
Indirect self-destructive behavior, 259
Intellectual functioning, decline in, death process and, 263–264
Irradiation, craniospinal, 82
leukemia treatment, 82
palliative, 238

Learned helplessness, 213
Leukemia, acute lymphocytic, 77–83
children's adjustment to realities of, 90
defined, 78, 79
description, 78–79
diagnosis, 79–81
terminal, problem of, 92–96
loss of control and, 83–85
maintenance modalities, 82–83
normalization of hospital life, 88
nursing care, primary, 89
relaxation techniques and, 89–90
psychological issues in care and management of patients, 83–92
reentry to home and school, 91–92
relapse, 92–96
separation from family, 85–86
therapeutic aspects of play activities, 86–88
Librium, 155
Life review, 269, 271–272
Life-sustaining treatments, 131
Life-threatening events, 129–164
Living will, 275
Lymphoblasts, 78
Lymphocytes, 78

Malformations, congenital, *see* Congenital malformations
Marital relationship, perinatal death and, 18–19
   stillbirth and, 18–19
   Sudden Infant Death and, 41–43
Melancholia, 168, 169
Mercy killing, 276, 277
Miscarriage, 2, 17
Mitochondria, 32
Monocytes, 78
Mortality, burn, 144–145
Motor vehicle accidents, *see* Accidents; Multiple-trauma injuries
Mourning, childhood and, 58–62
   defined, 58, 167
   psychodynamics of, 166–170
   thermal injuries and, 149–150
Multiple-trauma injuries, 130, 153–160
   replaying the events, 159
Myelination, 34
Myocardial infarction, 130
   defined, 131
   sexual activity and, 139–140
   See also Sudden death

Narcissism, primary, 61
Narcissistic injury, 61
Neonatal intensive care units, 2, 5
Nerve blocks, 238
Neuropathy, 81
Neutrophils, 78

Oral hygiene, terminally ill and, 240
Pain control, 233
Pain killers, *see* Analgesics
Palliative care, 232–233
Palliative irradiation, 238
Parental death, children's adjustment to, 61–66
   traumatic aspects of, 66–71
Parents, grieving, effective management of, 9–14
   single, Sudden Infant Death Syndrome and, 45
Perinatal death(s), 1–24
   decline in number of, 2
   doctor-patient relationship and, 5–9
   establishing personal identity of infant, 9–10
   experiencing, 2–9
   funeral arrangements, 13–14
   grieving parents, effective management of, 9–14
   inadequate recognition of actual loss, 5–6
   naming the child, 10–11
   photographing deceased infant, 13
   prenatal preparation for, 20–21
   psychiatric sequelae to, 14–19
   reactions of other children, 17–18
   stress in marital relationship and, 18–19
Personality, cancer and, 200
   precancerous, 200–201
   Type A, 131
Petechiae, leukemia and, 79
   Sudden Infant Death Syndrome and, 27, 28
Physical activity, coronary heart mortality and, 132
Physician-patient relationship, *see* Doctor-patient relationship
Physiology, human, sudden death and, 135–138
Piagetian developmental phases, 52–53
Play, therapeutic, aspects of, 86–88
Pregnancy, 2, 4
   replacement, 16–17
Premature vetricular contractions, 136
Prenatal education, perinatal death and, 20–21
   stillbirth and, 20–21
Preoperational stage, 53
Preventive psychiatry, 141
Primary narcissism, 61
Prodromes, 122
Professionals, health care, see Health care professionals
Psychiatry, preventive, 141
Psychological autopsy, 197
Psychology of dying older person, 267–274
Psychopharmacological treatment, suicidal adolescents and, 120
Psychotherapy, suicidal adolescents and, 119–120

Regression, role of, in dying process, 269–271
Religion, conjugal bereavement and, 189
   euthanasia and, 278
   terminally ill and, 242–243
Relocation, as factor in death of elderly, 261–263
Retirement, as factor in death of elderly, 263
"Right to die," 274–275

Schizophrenia, suicide and, 106, 108–109
Self-esteem, cancer and, 222–224
   terminally ill and, 241

Self-hypnosis, 90
Selfobjects, 61, 62
Sensorimotor stage, 52
Separation anxiety, 62
Sexuality, cancer and, 221—225
    coronary heart disease and, 139—140
SIDS, *see* Sudden Infant Death Syndrome
Significant other, death of, as factor in death
    of elderly, 261
Single parents, *see* Parents, single
"Social death," 147—148
Spiritual pain, terminally ill and, 242—243
Stillbirth, 1—24
    antepartum, 8
    defined, 5
    doctor-patient relationship and, 5—9
    establishing personal identity of infant, 9—
        10
    experiencing, 2—9
    funeral arrangements, 13—14
    grieving parents, management of, 9—14
    inadequate recognition of actual loss, 5—6
    intrapartum, 8
    naming the child, 10—11
    photographing the infant, 13
    prenatal preparation for, 20—21
    psychiatric sequelae to, 14—19
    reactions of other children, 17—18
    seeing the baby, 11—13
    stress in marital relationship and, 18—19
Sudden death, 130
    family crisis service and, 140—142
    hopelessness and, 134—135
    human physiology and, 135—138
    See also Myocardial infarction
Sudden Infant Death Syndrome (SIDS), 25—
        49
    age distribution, 29
    apnea theory, 31—33
    autopsies and, 27—29
    clinical description of, 27—29
    concern for other children in the family,
        40—41
    diagnosis, 27—28
    epidemiology, 29—31
    etiology, 29—31
    gross examination, 28
    impact on martial relationship, 41—43
    incidence of, 29—31
    initial impact of discovery, 36—39
    microscopic examination, 28—29
    operational definition, 26—27
    psychological issues for the family of
        victims, 35—49

psychophysiological theories, 33—35
    replacement child, 43—45
    single parent and, 45
    theoretical approaches to, 31—35
Suicide, accidents raising suspicion of, 116,
        117
    attempted, 103
    behavior and, 112—116
    biochemical factors, 104—105
    burn patients and, 151
    cancer patients and, 218—221
    conjugal bereavement and, 185
    depression and, 106—108, 114, 121
    diagnostic issues, 116—117
    emotional disorders and, 105—110
    etiology of, 104—112
    familial determinants, 110—112
    genetic predispositions, 104
    impulsive character disorders and, 109—
        110
    incidence of, 102, 103
    prevention of, 121—124
    psychotherapy and, 119—120
    race and, 102
    research and, 102, 103
    schizophrenia and, 106, 108—109
    sociocultural determinants, 110—112
    statistics on, 102—103
    symptoms, recognition and identification
        of, 117
    treatment, 117—120
    young people and, 101—128

Tachycardia, 135, 136
Terminal care, hospice, *see* Hospice terminal
        care
Terminal decline, 256, 265
Terminal disease, management of, 232—243
Terminal drop theory, 256, 263—265
Terminally ill, anorexia and, 240
    body image and, 241
    breathing difficulties, 238—239
    home care of, 243—246
    hospice care of, 229—254
    insomnia and, 239—240
    oral hygiene and, 240
    related physical, psychological and
        spiritual concerns of, 238—243
    religion and, 242—243
    self-esteem and, 241
    spiritual pain and, 242—243
Thermal injuries, 143—153
    coping strategies, 148—149
    disfigurement and, 147—148

geriatric, 151–152
life-death choices and, 143–144
postburn adjustment and adaptation, 145–148
special needs and, 149–151
See also Burns
Titration, 234
Trauma, childhood, psychological outcome of, 69–70
parental, death and, 66–71
Type A personality, 131

Valium, 155
Ventricular fibrillation, 130
Viewing of body after death, 248–249

"Waiting vulture syndrome," 178
White blood cells, 78
Will, living, 275
Work-related accidents, *see* Accidents;
Multiple-trauma injuries

Youth, suicide and, *see* Suicide